MW00884874

The Castor Oil Complete Collection

Over 500 Pages of Castor Oil-Based
Solutions for Body, Health, and Beauty.
Your Natural Elixir to
Lasting Holistic Wellness

By

Vincent Vega

Disclaimer notice

Please be aware that the information provided in this document is intended solely for educational and entertainment purposes. Every effort has been made to ensure the content is accurate, reliable, current, and complete.

However, no guarantees, either explicit or implicit, are made. Readers acknowledge that the author is not providing legal, financial, medical, or professional advice.

The content has been sourced from various references. It is strongly recommended that you consult a licensed professional before attempting any of the of the methods described in this document.

By reading this document, you agree that the author is not liable for any direct or indirect losses resulting from the use of the information within, including but not limited to errors, omissions, or inaccuracies.

Table of Contents

Introduction

Welcome to an extraordinary journey into castor oil, a timeless natural remedy that has captured the hearts and minds of healers and health enthusiasts for centuries. This 10-book-in-1 collection is a testament to castor oil's remarkable versatility and profound benefits, an unassuming yet powerful elixir. As the author, my inspiration for this extensive project stemmed from a personal quest for holistic health solutions that transcend conventional medicine. What began as a curiosity transformed into a passionate mission to share the transformative potential of castor oil with the world, inspiring hope and a healthier future.

My journey with castor oil started years ago when I found myself constantly searching for natural alternatives to traditional treatments. Frustrated with conventional medicine's side effects and limitations, I turned to the wisdom of ancient practices and natural remedies. In castor oil, I discovered a hidden gem—an oil that not only provided relief and healing but also enriched my overall well-being. The more I learned about its history, properties, and uses, the more I felt compelled to delve deeper and share my findings. Along the way, I encountered numerous individuals who had experienced the transformative power of castor oil, from skincare to pain relief, and their stories serve as a testament to its efficacy.

This collection is designed to be your ultimate guide to unlocking the full potential of castor oil. Each volume meticulously explores different facets of castor oil's applications, offering a blend of historical insights, scientific validation, and practical advice. The journey begins with a deep dive into castor oil's historical and cultural significance, tracing its roots from ancient civilizations to modern-day uses. This comprehensive approach ensures that you have all the information you need to trust in the power of castor oil for your holistic health.

From there, the series transitions into specific domains, starting with skincare. Imagine discovering an oil that moisturizes and rejuvenates your skin and combats acne, eczema, and other skin conditions. The skincare volume is a treasure trove of recipes and techniques to harness castor oil's remarkable properties for a radiant complexion. Next, we venture into hair care, revealing how castor oil can transform your hair—promoting growth, reducing dandruff, and restoring shine and vitality.

Digestive health is another critical area where castor oil shines. The dedicated volume on this topic provides insights into how this oil can support your digestive system, relieve constipation, and detoxify your liver. For those interested in the soothing power of scents, the aromatherapy volume explores how castor oil can enhance the benefits of essential oils, offering blending techniques and therapeutic applications to elevate your aromatherapy practice.

Pain relief is another domain where castor oil proves invaluable. Whether dealing with joint pain, muscle aches, or chronic discomfort, the pain relief volume offers natural, topical solutions that harness the anti-inflammatory properties of castor oil. For practical everyday use, the home remedies volume empowers you with simple yet effective solutions for common ailments, making castor oil a go-to remedy for your entire family.

Detoxification is crucial for maintaining optimal health, and castor oil also plays a significant role here. Learn how to use castor oil to support your body's natural detox processes, enhancing overall well-being. For those looking to customize their aromatherapy treatments, another volume offers advanced insights into blending castor oil with essential oils, creating personalized therapeutic experiences.

Finally, the collection addresses the unique needs of children and pets, offering safe and gentle remedies to support their health and well-being. This holistic approach ensures that every household member can benefit from the wonders of castor oil.

This collection is not just a series of books but a gateway to a healthier, more natural way of living. Embrace this journey with me, and let the wisdom of castor oil enrich your life, bringing you closer to nature's healing touch. Each page invites discovery, learning, and transformation, paving the way for a more empowered and healthier you.

BOOK 1: Castor Oil Unveiled

Castor Oil Unveiled

A Complete Guide to Its Uses and Benefits

By

Vincent Vega

Disclaimer notice

Please be aware that the information provided in this document is intended solely for educational and entertainment purposes. Every effort has been made to ensure the content is accurate, reliable, current, and complete.

However, no guarantees, either explicit or implicit, are made. Readers acknowledge that the author is not providing legal, financial, medical, or professional advice.

The content has been sourced from various references. It is strongly recommended that you consult a licensed professional before attempting any of the of the methods described in this document.

By reading this document, you agree that the author is not liable for any direct or indirect losses resulting from the use of the information within, including but not limited to errors, omissions, or inaccuracies.

Chapter 1: What is castor oil?

1.1 Definition and origins

Castor oil, derived from the seeds of the castor plant (*Ricinus communis*), has a rich history and diverse applications dating back thousands of years. This paragraph explores its definition, origins, historical uses, and modern-day significance in various industries and applications.

Castor oil is a vegetable oil extracted from the seeds of the castor plant (*Ricinus communis*). The plant is native to tropical regions of Africa and Asia but is now widely cultivated around the world for its seeds. The plant is an annual flowering shrub that can grow up to 10 meters tall and produces large, spiny seed pods containing seeds about the size of a coffee bean.

1.1.1 Historical Significance

Castor oil, with its roots in ancient Egypt, holds a significant place in history. The Egyptians, recognizing its potential, extracted the oil from the seeds and used it as a versatile remedy for a range of ailments. From treating eye irritations and skin infections to digestive disorders, castor oil was a multipurpose solution. Its purgative properties made it a popular choice for alleviating constipation and other gastrointestinal issues in ancient civilizations.

In ancient Greece, castor oil was highly regarded for its medicinal properties. Physicians such as Hippocrates and Dioscorides used it to treat various conditions, including joint pain, inflammation, and skin disorders. The oil's anti-inflammatory and analgesic properties were particularly valued in treating arthritis and rheumatism.

1.1.2 Modern Uses and Applications

Castor oil continues to be valued for its versatility and therapeutic properties. It is widely used in various industries, including pharmaceuticals, cosmetics, food, and manufacturing. Here are some of the vital modern applications of castor oil:

Pharmaceutical Industry: Castor oil is used as a laxative to relieve constipation due to its ability to stimulate intestinal motility. It is also used in the formulation of medications and ointments for skin disorders and infections.

Cosmetic and Personal Care Products: Castor oil is a common ingredient in skincare products such as moisturizers, creams, and lip balms due to its emollient and hydrating properties. It is also used in hair care products to promote hair growth and strengthen hair follicles.

Industrial Applications: Castor oil is used in the manufacturing of various products, including lubricants, paints, dyes, and plastics. Its viscosity and lubricating properties make it suitable for use in hydraulic fluids and as a biodegradable lubricant.

Health and Wellness: Castor oil is gaining popularity in alternative and holistic medicine practices beyond its traditional medicinal uses. It is used in detoxification therapies, such as castor oil packs applied to the abdomen to promote liver detoxification and lymphatic circulation.

1.1.3 Production and Extraction

The production of castor oil is a meticulous process that ensures its purity and quality. The seeds, carefully harvested from the castor plant, undergo a drying process before the oil is extracted. The extraction methods, which may vary, typically involve mechanical pressing or solvent extraction. Mechanical pressing, particularly for producing cold-pressed castor oil, is preferred as it retains more of the oil's natural nutrients and beneficial compounds compared to solvent-extracted oils.

1.1.4 Chemical Composition and Properties

Castor oil mainly comprises ricinoleic acid, a monounsaturated fatty acid that constitutes about 90% of its total fatty acid content. Ricinoleic acid is known for its unique chemical structure, giving castor oil distinctive properties, including its viscosity, hydrophobic nature, and oxidative stability. Other fatty acids in castor oil include oleic acid, linoleic acid, stearic acid, and palmitic acid, each contributing to its overall composition and characteristics.

Castor oil has a long and storied history as a versatile and valuable natural resource. Its uses have evolved from ancient civilizations to modern industries, ,but its fundamental properties and benefits remain highly regarded. As research continues to uncover new applications and benefits of castor oil, its role in health, industry, and everyday products will likely expand further, continuing a legacy that spans millennia.

1.2 Historic uses in various civilizations

Historical uses of castor oil across civilizations reveal its enduring significance and diverse applications throughout human history. From the castor plant (*Ricinus communis*), native to tropical regions of Africa and Asia, castor oil has played a pivotal role in various cultures and societies worldwide.

1.2.1 Ancient Egypt and Mesopotamia

Castor oil's historical roots can be traced back to ancient civilizations such as Egypt and Mesopotamia. In ancient Egypt, the oil extracted from castor seeds was highly prized for its medicinal and therapeutic properties. Egyptians used it to treat various ailments, including eye irritations, skin conditions, and digestive disorders. The oil's purgative effects made it a popular remedy for constipation and other gastrointestinal issues. Castor oil was applied topically to soothe skin irritations and promote wound healing.

In Mesopotamia, castor oil was similarly revered for its medicinal uses. Ancient texts from this region document its application as a treatment for various diseases and ailments. Physicians and healers recognized its potential to alleviate pain, reduce inflammation, and promote overall health. The oil's versatility and efficacy made it a valuable commodity in early medical practices.

1.2.2 Ancient Greece and Rome

During the classical era, castor oil continued to be valued for its medicinal properties in ancient Greece and Rome. Greek physician Hippocrates, often referred to as the "father of medicine," advocated for using castor oil to treat joint pain, inflammation, and skin disorders. Dioscorides, a renowned Greek pharmacologist, also documented its therapeutic benefits in his seminal work *De Materia Medica*.

In Rome, castor oil gained popularity as a versatile remedy. It was used both internally and externally to address a range of health issues, from digestive complaints to skin ailments. The Roman naturalist Pliny the Elder praised its effectiveness in treating wounds and promoting healing. The widespread use of castor oil across the Roman Empire underscored its status as a valuable medicinal resource.

1.2.3 Traditional Chinese Medicine and Ayurveda

In traditional Chinese medicine (TCM), castor oil has been utilized for its detoxifying and purgative properties. It was incorporated into herbal formulations to promote gastrointestinal health, cleanse the body of toxins, and alleviate digestive discomfort. TCM practitioners also valued castor oil for its ability to stimulate circulation and reduce inflammation.

In Ayurvedic medicine, an ancient healing system practiced in India, castor oil is known as "Erand Tel." It is revered for its therapeutic benefits in treating joint pain, arthritis, and skin disorders. Ayurvedic texts highlight its use in detoxification therapies, such as *Panchakarma*, where castor oil is ingested or applied externally to support the body's natural cleansing processes.

1.2.4 Medieval and Renaissance Europe

During the medieval and Renaissance periods in Europe, castor oil continued to be a staple in medical treatments. It was used by physicians and herbalists to treat various ailments, ranging from fevers and infections to skin conditions and menstrual disorders. Its purgative properties were particularly valued for promoting bowel movements and relieving constipation.

1.2.5 Modern Era and Contemporary Uses

In the modern era, castor oil remains a prominent ingredient in pharmaceuticals, cosmetics, and industrial products. Due to its unique chemical composition and properties, its applications extend to lubricants, paints, dyes, and plastics. Castor oil's versatility has also led to its inclusion in natural and alternative health therapies, which are used in detoxification protocols, massage therapies, and skincare products.

Throughout history, castor oil has transcended geographical and cultural boundaries, earning a reputation as a valuable therapeutic agent. From ancient Egypt to modern-day applications, its enduring legacy underscores its efficacy and versatility in promoting health and well-being. As scientific research continues to uncover new uses and benefits, castor oil's role in medicine and industry is poised to evolve, ensuring its relevance in future generations.

1.3 Modern applications and relevance

Castor oil continues to find diverse and innovative applications in the modern world. Its unique chemical composition and beneficial properties make it a valuable ingredient across various industries, including pharmaceuticals, cosmetics, food, and manufacturing. From traditional medicinal uses to contemporary innovations, castor oil's versatility underscores its enduring relevance in today's global market.

Pharmaceutical Industry

Castor oil remains a crucial component in various medications and treatments in the pharmaceutical sector. Its potent anti-inflammatory and analgesic properties make it a preferred ingredient in topical ointments, creams, and salves for relieving joint pain, muscle soreness, and arthritis. Castor oil's ability to penetrate deeply into the skin layers enhances its efficacy in delivering active ingredients and soothing irritated tissues. Moreover, its mild laxative effect continues to be utilized in specific laxative formulations for alleviating constipation.

Research into castor oil's potential extends to broader therapeutic applications. Studies have explored its antimicrobial properties, suggesting its use in wound healing preparations and antimicrobial agents. Furthermore, ongoing investigations into its anti-cancer properties highlight its potential role in cancer therapy and prevention, although further research is needed to validate these claims.

Cosmetics and Personal Care Products

Castor oil's emollient and moisturizing properties make it a popular ingredient in cosmetics and personal care products. It is widely used in skincare formulations such as cleansers, moisturizers, and lip balms because it hydrates the skin and prevents moisture loss. Castor oil's humectant properties help draw moisture from the air into the skin, making it particularly beneficial for dry and sensitive skin types.

Additionally, castor oil is used in hair care products to nourish and strengthen hair follicles, promoting healthy hair growth and reducing breakage. It is often incorporated into hair serums, conditioners, and scalp treatments to improve hair texture and manage frizz. Its high concentration of ricinoleic acid contributes to its ability to stimulate circulation in the scalp, potentially aiding in preventing hair loss.

Industrial Applications

Beyond personal care, castor oil plays a significant role in industrial applications. Its viscosity and lubricating properties make it an ideal ingredient in lubricants and hydraulic fluids used in machinery and automotive applications. Castor oil's ability to withstand high temperatures and pressures enhances its durability and effectiveness in these industrial settings.

Moreover, castor oil is utilized to manufacture bio-based products such as biodegradable plastics, paints, coatings, and adhesives. Its renewable and eco-friendly nature makes it a sustainable alternative to petroleum-based chemicals, contributing to environmental conservation efforts.

Agricultural and Veterinary Uses

In agriculture, castor oil and its derivatives are employed as natural pesticides and insecticides due to their toxic properties against pests and insects. They are applied to crops and plants to protect them from infestations while minimizing environmental impact compared to synthetic pesticides. Additionally, castor oil has been explored in veterinary medicine for its potential therapeutic benefits in treating skin conditions, wounds, and infections in animals.

Emerging Research and Future Directions

As scientific research advances, new applications for castor oil continue to emerge. Recent studies have explored its potential in regenerative medicine, including tissue engineering and wound healing therapies. Castor oil's anti-inflammatory and immunomodulatory properties hold promise for treating chronic inflammatory conditions and autoimmune diseases.

Moreover, advancements in nanotechnology have enabled the development of nanoemulsions and nanoparticles containing castor oil, which enhance its delivery and bioavailability in targeted therapies. These innovations pave the way for personalized medicine approaches and novel drug delivery systems using castor oil as a carrier.

Castor oil's journey from ancient medicinal practices to modern scientific exploration underscores its enduring significance and relevance in multiple industries. Its therapeutic properties and sustainable and eco-friendly attributes position castor oil as a valuable resource for addressing global health challenges and advancing technological innovations. As research unveils its potential benefits and applications, castor oil is poised to remain a cornerstone in medicine, industry, and beyond.

Chapter 2: Castor oil chemistry

2.1 Composition and key components

1) Fatty Acid Profile

The composition of castor oil predominantly consists of triglycerides, with ricinoleic acid being the primary fatty acid present. Ricinoleic acid constitutes about 85-95% of the fatty acids in castor oil, distinguishing it from other vegetable oils. This hydroxylated fatty acid is responsible for many of castor oil's therapeutic properties, including its anti-inflammatory, analgesic, and antimicrobial effects. Besides ricinoleic acid, castor oil also contains other fatty acids such as oleic acid (approximately 2-6%), linoleic acid (1-5%), stearic acid (0.5-1.5%), and palmitic acid (0.5-1%). These fatty acids contribute to the oil's overall texture, viscosity, and stability.

2) Hydroxy Fatty Acids

Ricinoleic acid, unique to castor oil, is a monounsaturated omega-9 fatty acid with a hydroxyl group (-OH) attached to the 12th carbon atom. This structural feature gives ricinoleic acid its distinctive chemical and biological properties. The hydroxyl group enhances ricinoleic acid's solubility in water and its ability to penetrate deeply into the skin, making it an effective emollient and moisturizer.

3) Other Components

In addition to fatty acids, castor oil contains several other bioactive compounds that contribute to its therapeutic and industrial applications. These include:

- Phytosterols: These plant-derived sterols help improve skin barrier function and reduce inflammation.

- Tocopherols: Also known as vitamin E, tocopherols are antioxidants that protect the skin from oxidative stress and promote skin health.

- Squalene: A natural hydrocarbon that provides moisture and protection to the skin, enhancing its softness and suppleness.

- Minerals: Castor oil contains trace amounts of minerals such as zinc, copper, iron, and magnesium, which play roles in various biological processes.

2.1.1 Properties and Benefits

The chemical composition of castor oil contributes to its wide-ranging benefits across different applications:

- Moisturizing and Emollient: The high content of ricinoleic acid and other fatty acids makes castor oil an excellent moisturizer and emollient. It helps soften and hydrate the skin, making it beneficial for dry, rough, or chapped skin conditions.

- Anti-inflammatory: Ricinoleic acid exhibits potent anti-inflammatory properties by inhibiting the synthesis of inflammatory mediators such as prostaglandins. This property makes castor oil effective in reducing inflammation and relieving pain associated with various skin and joint conditions.

- Antimicrobial: Castor oil has shown antimicrobial activity against bacteria, fungi, and viruses. It can be used topically to prevent infections and promote wound healing.

- Laxative: When taken orally, castor oil acts as a stimulant laxative due to its ricinoleic acid content. It stimulates intestinal motility and increases water and electrolyte secretion, thereby promoting bowel movements.

2.1.2 Industrial Applications

Beyond its therapeutic benefits, castor oil finds extensive use in various industrial sectors:

- Lubricants: The high viscosity and lubricating properties of castor oil make it suitable for use in lubricants, greases, and hydraulic fluids.

- Plastics and Polymers: Castor oil derivatives are used as plasticizers and additives in the manufacturing of biodegradable plastics, resins, and coatings.

- Cosmetics: Castor oil is a key ingredient in cosmetics and personal care products such as lipsticks, soaps, and hair care formulations due to its emollient and moisturizing properties.

- Pharmaceuticals: It is used in the formulation of pharmaceuticals, including topical creams, ointments, and drug delivery systems.

2.1.3 Environmental Sustainability

Castor oil is derived from the castor bean plant, which is fast-growing and resilient to drought conditions. It requires minimal water and pesticide inputs compared to other oilseed crops, making it environmentally sustainable. Moreover, castor oil and its derivatives are biodegradable, offering eco-friendly alternatives to petroleum-based products in various industries. The composition of castor oil, characterized by its high ricinoleic acid content and diverse array of bioactive compounds, underpins its multifaceted applications in health, industry, and sustainability. As scientific research continues to uncover new therapeutic uses and industrial innovations, castor oil remains a versatile and valuable resource with promising potential for future developments.

2.2 Unique properties

Castor oil possesses several unique properties that distinguish it from other vegetable oils, making it valuable in various industries and applications. Understanding these properties is crucial for appreciating their versatility and benefits in different contexts.

Viscosity

One of the most distinctive characteristics of castor oil is its high viscosity. Viscosity refers to the oil's resistance to flow, and castor oil is notably thicker and more dense than many other vegetable oils. This property is primarily attributed to its high ricinoleic acid content, a hydroxylated fatty acid with a bulky hydroxyl group (-OH) at the 12th carbon position. The presence of this hydroxyl group increases the oil's polarity and intermolecular forces, leading to its thick consistency.

Density

The density contributes to its ability to penetrate deeply into tissues when applied topically, making skin moisturization and treatments practical. The density also influences its use in industrial applications requiring specific densities for lubricants and other formulations.

High Boiling Point

Castor oil's relatively high boiling point, typically around 313°C (595°F), provides a stable foundation for its use in high-temperature environments. This stability is a key factor in its suitability for use in lubricants, hydraulic fluids, and other industrial applications where thermal stability is essential. Understanding this stability can provide a sense of reassurance to professionals in these industries.

Solubility

Despite its high viscosity, castor oil's excellent solubility in non-polar solvents like alcohol and ether enhances its versatility in formulations. This solubility allows castor oil to be used as a dispersing agent, emulsifier, or carrier oil in pharmaceuticals, cosmetics, and industrial products. Understanding this versatility can spark interest in the potential applications of castor oil among professionals in these fields.

Hygroscopicity

Castor oil has hygroscopic properties, meaning it can absorb moisture from the air. This attribute makes it beneficial in formulations where moisture retention or prevention of moisture loss is desired, such as cosmetic creams, lotions, and hair care products. The hygroscopic nature of castor oil contributes to its emollient and humectant properties, helping to soften and hydrate the skin.

Biodegradability

One of castor oil's environmentally favorable properties is its biodegradability. Derived from the seeds of the castor bean plant (*Ricinus communis*), castor oil and its derivatives break down naturally in the environment over time. This biodegradability reduces its environmental impact compared to petroleum-based oils and synthetic chemicals, making it a sustainable choice for various applications.

Non-Toxicity

Castor oil is generally considered safe (GRAS) by the U.S. Food and Drug Administration (FDA) when used in appropriate concentrations. It is non-toxic and does not cause skin sensitization or allergic reactions in most people, making it suitable for topical applications in cosmetics, personal care products, and pharmaceuticals. However, as with any substance, individuals with specific allergies or sensitivities should exercise caution and consult a healthcare professional if needed. The unique properties of castor oil, including its high viscosity, density, thermal stability, solubility, hygroscopicity, biodegradability, and non-toxicity, contribute to its wide-ranging applications in health, industry, and sustainability. These properties make castor oil versatile in cosmetics, pharmaceuticals, lubricants, and other specialized formulations.

Chapter 3: Production and extraction

3.1 Methods of extraction

Extracting castor oil is critical to maintaining its purity, quality, and suitability for various applications. Two primary methods are commonly used: cold-pressing and solvent extraction. Each method has distinct advantages and considerations, impacting the final product's characteristics and applications.

3.1.1 Cold-Pressed Extraction

Process Overview

Cold-pressed extraction, also known as mechanical pressing or expeller pressing, is a traditional method for extracting oils from seeds without applying heat or chemical solvents. This method preserves the oil's natural properties and is preferred for producing high-quality castor oil suitable for medicinal, cosmetic, and pharmaceutical applications.

Seed Preparation: The first step involves cleaning and drying the castor seeds to remove impurities and moisture, ensuring optimal oil yield and quality.

Pressing: The dried seeds are then fed into a continuous screw press or expeller. The expeller applies mechanical pressure to crush the seeds and extract the oil. As the seeds are crushed, the oil is released and collected.

Filtration: The extracted oil undergoes filtration to remove any remaining solids or impurities, producing clear and pure oil.

Storage: Cold-pressed castor oil is typically stored in dark, airtight containers to protect it from light and oxidation, preserving its freshness and efficacy.

Advantages

Quality Retention: Cold-pressed extraction retains the oil's natural flavor, aroma, and nutritional value, as it does not involve heat or chemical treatments that could degrade these properties.

Health Benefits: The resulting oil is rich in essential fatty acids, including ricinoleic acid, which has potent anti-inflammatory and antimicrobial properties that are beneficial for skin and hair care.

Environmental Sustainability: This method is environmentally friendly since it does not use chemical solvents or generate harmful by-products, aligning with sustainable practices.

3.1.2 Solvent Extraction

<u>Process Overview</u>

Solvent extraction is an alternative method used primarily for industrial applications where high oil yield is essential. It involves using chemical solvents to dissolve the oil from the castor seeds, then separating the solvent from the oil through evaporation.

Seed Preparation: Similar to cold-pressed extraction, the seeds undergo cleaning and drying to prepare them for extraction.

Extraction: The seeds are then crushed or ground into a fine powder and mixed with a hexane solvent. The solvent dissolves the oil, creating a mixture called miscella.

Separation: The collection is then subjected to a series of evaporators to remove the solvent. The remaining crude oil is purified through distillation and filtration to remove impurities and residual solvents.

Refinement: The refined oil undergoes additional processing steps to adjust its color, odor, and other properties, making it suitable for specific industrial applications.

<u>Advantages</u>

High Oil Yield: Solvent extraction achieves higher oil yields compared to cold-pressed methods, making it economically advantageous for large-scale production.

Industrial Applications: The refined oil is used in various industries, including lubricants, coatings, and biofuels, due to its purity and specific characteristics.

Consistency: The controlled extraction process ensures consistent quality and composition of the oil, meeting stringent industry standards.

<u>Considerations</u>

Purity and Safety: Cold-pressed castor oil is often preferred for cosmetic and pharmaceutical uses due to its purity and absence of residual solvents. Solvent extraction, while efficient, requires stringent purification to ensure safety and quality.

Environmental Impact: Solvent extraction may pose ecological concerns due to the use and disposal of chemical solvents. Proper handling and disposal practices are essential to minimize environmental impact.

Application Specificity: The choice between extraction methods depends on the intended application of the castor oil. Cold-pressed oil is suitable for direct skin and hair care applications, while solvent-extracted oil is preferred for industrial and commercial uses.

Both cold-pressed and solvent extraction methods play crucial roles in producing castor oil for diverse applications. Cold-pressed extraction preserves the oil's natural properties and is favored for high-quality consumer products, while solvent extraction ensures high yields and purity required for industrial applications. Understanding these extraction methods allows manufacturers and consumers to choose the most appropriate castor oil based on their specific needs and preferences.

3.2 The production hubs and cultivation at the global level

Global production of castor oil is primarily concentrated in several critical regions known for their conducive climates and agricultural practices. Understanding these production hubs and cultivation methods provides insights into the global supply chain of castor oil.

India

India is the world's largest producer of castor oil, accounting for over 80% of global production. The country's tropical climate, particularly in states like Gujarat, Rajasthan, and Andhra Pradesh, provides ideal conditions for castor plant cultivation. Castor plants thrive in semi-arid regions with well-drained soil and sufficient sunlight.

Cultivation Practices

Sowing: Castor seeds are typically sown during the monsoon season (June-July) with adequate soil moisture. The seeds are planted at about 5-7 centimeters deep and require spacing to facilitate growth and proper development.

Growth and Maintenance: Castor plants are hardy and drought-resistant once established. Farmers often practice intercropping with other crops like pulses or cereals to optimize land use and yield. Weeding and pest management are essential during the growth stages to ensure healthy plant growth.

Harvesting: The castor plant matures within 120 to 150 days after sowing. Harvesting usually begins in October or December, depending on the region and climatic conditions. Farmers manually cut the mature plants and collect the seed pods.

Processing: Post-harvest, the seeds undergo drying to reduce moisture content and prevent mold formation. The dried seeds are then either stored or processed for oil extraction.

China

China is another significant producer of castor oil, particularly in regions like Guangxi, Guangdong, and Yunnan provinces. The country benefits from favorable climatic conditions, including warm temperatures and sufficient rainfall during the growing season.

Cultivation Practices

Climate Adaptation: Castor plants in China are cultivated in subtropical and tropical regions. These areas experience warm summers and mild winters, which support the castor plant's growth and development throughout the year.

Farming Techniques: Chinese farmers often use mechanized farming techniques for planting and harvesting castor plants. This approach helps streamline the agricultural process and improve overall efficiency.

Market Dynamics: China's production of castor oil is driven not only by domestic demand but also by export markets. The country is crucial in the global supply chain, catering to diverse industrial and consumer applications.

Brazil

Brazil is a significant producer of castor oil, particularly in the northeastern states such as Bahia and Ceará. The country's tropical climate and fertile soils support the cultivation of castor plants, making it a key player in the global castor oil market.

Cultivation Practices

Regional Focus: Castor cultivation in Brazil is concentrated in semi-arid regions where rainfall is limited but sufficient for crop growth. The northeastern states benefit from irrigation systems that supplement natural rainfall during dry periods.

Government Support: The Brazilian government supports castor cultivation through agricultural policies and incentives aimed at promoting sustainable farming practices and enhancing crop yields.

Export Market: Brazil exports a significant portion of its castor oil production to international markets, including Europe, North America, and Asia. The country's robust production capacity and export infrastructure contribute to its competitiveness in the global market.

Other Global Regions

Emerging Markets

Africa: Countries like Ethiopia, Mozambique, and South Africa are on the brink of becoming significant castor oil producers. These regions, with their favorable agro-climatic conditions, are venturing into castor cultivation, a move that promises to diversify agricultural activities and boost economic growth.

Southeast Asia: Countries like Thailand and Indonesia have also started cultivating castor plants to meet domestic and regional demand for castor oil. These regions benefit from tropical climates and are exploring sustainable farming practices to boost castor production.

Global production hubs for castor oil are strategically located in regions with favorable climatic conditions and supportive agricultural practices. Understanding these cultivation methods and regional dynamics is key to comprehending the intricate global supply chain of castor oil, catering to diverse industrial, pharmaceutical, and consumer markets worldwide.

3.3 Sustainability and environmental impact

Sustainability and environmental impact are critical considerations in castor oil production, influencing agricultural practices, processing methods, and overall industry practices worldwide. Understanding these aspects is crucial as global demand for castor oil rises, driven by its versatile applications across various sectors.

3.3.1 Agricultural Practices

1) Crop Rotation and Intercropping

Sustainable castor oil production often involves crop rotation and intercropping with other crops. This practice helps improve soil fertility, reduce pest and disease incidence, and optimize land use efficiency. Farmers rotate castor plants with crops like pulses, cereals, or legumes, enhancing soil health and mitigating the risk of monoculture.

2) Water Management

Efficient water management is essential in regions where water resources are scarce or prone to variability. Farmers adopt drip irrigation or rainwater harvesting techniques to minimize water consumption and ensure adequate moisture for castor plant growth. Sustainable water practices support crop yield and conserve precious water resources for other agricultural and community needs.

3) Soil Health and Conservation

Healthy soils are fundamental to sustainable agriculture. Practices like minimal tillage, organic fertilization, and cover cropping help maintain soil structure, increase organic matter content, and reduce erosion. These practices enhance the productivity of castor plants and contribute to long-term soil health and sustainability.

3.3.2 Environmental Impact

Biodiversity Conservation

Castor cultivation can impact local biodiversity depending on agricultural practices and land management. Sustainable farming practices that preserve natural habitats conserve native species and minimize chemical inputs help mitigate adverse impacts on biodiversity. Maintaining biodiversity supports ecosystem resilience and contributes to overall environmental health.

Pesticide and Chemical Use

Responsible pesticide and chemical management is crucial in sustainable castor oil production. Integrated pest management (IPM) strategies prioritize biological controls, cultural practices, and resistant varieties to reduce reliance on synthetic pesticides. This approach minimizes environmental contamination, protects beneficial organisms, and promotes ecosystem balance.

Carbon Footprint

The carbon footprint of castor oil production includes greenhouse gas emissions from agricultural activities, processing, transportation, and energy consumption. Sustainable practices such as carbon sequestration through agroforestry, renewable energy adoption, and efficient logistics help reduce the overall carbon footprint of castor oil production. Life cycle assessments (LCAs) provide insights into carbon emissions and guide strategies for emission reduction across the supply chain.

3.3.3 Industry Initiatives

Certifications and Standards

Certification schemes such as organic certification, Fair Trade, and sustainability standards are crucial in promoting sustainable practices in the castor oil industry. These certifications ensure compliance with environmental regulations, fair labor practices, and ethical sourcing principles, enhancing market competitiveness and consumer trust.

Research and Innovation

Ongoing research and innovation in agricultural techniques, processing technologies, and product development contribute to sustainable castor oil production. Biotechnology, precision agriculture, and waste utilization innovations help optimize resource efficiency, reduce environmental impact, and improve overall sustainability metrics.

3.3.4 Challenges and Opportunities

Climate Change Resilience

Climate variability challenges sustainable castor oil production, impacting crop yield, water availability, and pest dynamics. Adaptation strategies such as drought-resistant varieties, climate-smart agriculture, and ecosystem-based approaches are essential for building resilience and maintaining productivity in a changing climate.

Market Demand and Consumer Awareness

Growing consumer awareness and demand for sustainably produced goods drive industry efforts toward sustainability. Transparent supply chains, eco-labeling, and corporate social responsibility (CSR) initiatives enable consumers to make informed choices and support sustainable practices in castor oil production.

Sustainability in castor oil production involves balancing economic viability with environmental stewardship and social responsibility. Adopting holistic approaches that integrate sustainable agricultural practices, environmental conservation, and industry collaboration is essential for advancing the sustainability agenda. By prioritizing sustainability, the castor oil industry can mitigate environmental impact, promote biodiversity conservation, and meet global demand for responsibly sourced products in an increasingly interconnected world.

Chapter 4: Castor oil in traditional medicine

4.1 Traditional uses

Traditional medicine systems like Ayurveda and Traditional Chinese Medicine (TCM) have long recognized the therapeutic properties of castor oil, integrating it into their holistic healing practices for centuries. Here's a detailed exploration of its traditional uses in these esteemed medical systems:

4.1.1 Ayurveda

Overview: Ayurveda, the ancient Indian system of medicine, considers castor oil (known as "Erand Taila" in Sanskrit) a valuable therapeutic agent. It is classified as a "Vata" pacifying oil, primarily used to balance the Vata dosha, which is one of the three fundamental principles (doshas) that govern physiological and psychological functions in the body. The Vata dosha is responsible for movement and nervous system functions in the body.

Digestive Health: In Ayurveda, castor oil is commonly used to alleviate digestive disorders such as constipation, bloating, and abdominal discomfort. It is administered orally to promote bowel movement and cleanse the intestines. The oil's laxative properties are believed to stimulate peristalsis and help eliminate ama (toxins) from the digestive tract.

Joint and Muscle Pain: External application of castor oil is employed in Ayurvedic therapies like Abhyanga (oil massage) and Pinda Sweda (hot herbal bolus massage) to relieve joint stiffness, muscle pain, and inflammation. The oil's deep-penetrating and warming qualities are believed to nourish tissues, improve circulation, and reduce pain associated with conditions like arthritis.

Skin Conditions: Castor oil is valued in Ayurveda for its emollient and moisturizing properties. It is used topically to soothe dry, irritated skin and treat minor cuts, wounds, and skin infections. The oil's anti-inflammatory effects are thought to alleviate itching, reduce redness, and promote skin healing.

Hair and Scalp Care: Ayurvedic texts recommend castor oil for hair and scalp treatments to strengthen hair follicles, promote hair growth, and prevent premature graying. Regular scalp massage with castor oil is believed to nourish the roots, improve hair texture, and enhance overall hair health.

4.1.2 Traditional Chinese Medicine (TCM)

Concepts of TCM: In Traditional Chinese Medicine, castor oil (referred to as "Bi Ma Zi" or "Ma Zi Ren You") is associated with the concept of "Yang" and is used to invigorate blood circulation, dispel cold and dampness, and promote detoxification.

Digestive Health: TCM utilizes castor oil to address stagnant Qi (energy) and relieve constipation. It is believed to lubricate the intestines, soften stools, and facilitate smoother bowel movements. Castor oil is administered in small quantities and often combined with other herbs to enhance its therapeutic effects on the digestive system.

External Applications: Topical use of castor oil in TCM includes treating joint pain, muscle sprains, and rheumatic conditions. Castor oil packs or poultices are applied to affected areas to alleviate pain, reduce inflammation, and improve mobility. The oil's warming nature is thought to enhance circulation and promote healing.

Skin Disorders: Castor oil is applied externally in TCM to treat skin ailments such as boils, eczema, and fungal infections. Its antimicrobial properties are valued for clearing heat and toxins from the skin, reducing inflammation, and supporting skin regeneration.

Hair Care: Like Ayurveda, TCM employs castor oil for hair and scalp health. It is believed to nourish the scalp, promote blood circulation to the hair follicles, and strengthen hair roots. Regular application of castor oil is recommended to maintain lustrous hair and prevent hair loss.

Castor oil's integration into Ayurvedic and Traditional Chinese Medicine reflects its versatile therapeutic applications across diverse health conditions. These traditional medicine systems highlight its efficacy in promoting digestive health, alleviating pain and inflammation, enhancing skin and hair care, and supporting overall well-being. As modern research continues to validate these traditional uses, castor oil maintains its significance as a natural remedy cherished for its holistic healing properties in global healthcare practices.

4.2 Folk remedies and cultural significance

Folk remedies using castor oil have deep cultural significance across various regions and societies, reflecting its enduring popularity as a versatile natural remedy. Here's an exploration of its folkloric uses and cultural importance:

Latin American Traditions: in Latin America, castor oil, known as "aceite de ricino," holds a prominent place in folk medicine. It is widely used to relieve constipation, often administered orally in small doses. This practice is passed down through generations, with families relying on castor oil as a gentle yet effective remedy for digestive discomforts.

Caribbean Islands: throughout the Caribbean islands, castor oil is celebrated for its therapeutic properties. It is used externally to soothe muscle aches, joint pains, and inflammation. A popular remedy involves massaging warm castor oil onto the affected area, believed to improve circulation and alleviate pain due to its anti-inflammatory effects.

Asian Traditions: in parts of Asia such as India and China, castor oil has been integrated into traditional medicine practices for centuries. In India, Ayurvedic texts recommend castor oil for various health conditions, including digestive disorders, joint pain, skin ailments, and hair care. It is also used in rituals and ceremonies for its purifying and cleansing properties.

European Folklore: in European folklore, castor oil was historically used as a laxative to cleanse the digestive system. It was believed to expel toxins and promote overall health. It was also applied topically in some cultures to treat skin conditions like rashes, cuts, and bruises, owing to its soothing and healing properties.

African Traditions: across many regions of Africa, castor oil is valued for its medicinal benefits. It is utilized to alleviate constipation and promote regular bowel movements. Additionally, it is applied topically to treat minor skin irritations, insect bites, and to nourish hair and scalp.

Modern Folk Practices: in contemporary times, folk remedies involving castor oil have evolved to include its use in natural skincare and hair care routines. DIY treatments such as castor oil masks for hair growth, castor oil packs for detoxification, and facial serums for moisturizing and anti-aging purposes are gaining popularity.

Beyond its medicinal uses, castor oil holds a deep cultural significance in rituals, ceremonies, and traditional practices worldwide. It is often associated with purification, healing, and spiritual cleansing in various cultural contexts, symbolizing renewal and vitality. This cultural significance underscores the global heritage of traditional medicine and the enduring appeal of castor oil as a natural healing agent.

Castor oil's folk remedies and cultural significance underscore its enduring appeal as a natural healing agent across diverse societies. From its roots in ancient medicine to its adaptation to modern folk practices, castor oil continues to be cherished for its therapeutic benefits in promoting digestive health, relieving pain, nurturing skin and hair, and preserving cultural heritage through generations.

Chapter 5: Modern Medical Applications

5.1 Pharmaceutical and industrial uses

Castor oil's versatility extends beyond its traditional and folk uses into pharmaceutical and industrial applications, where its unique properties find diverse utilization. Here's an exploration of its pharmaceutical and industrial uses:

5.1.1 Pharmaceutical Applications

Castor oil is a vital ingredient in various pharmaceutical products due to its medicinal properties and ability to act as an effective carrier for active ingredients. Some critical pharmaceutical uses include:

Laxative: Castor oil is widely used as a laxative to relieve constipation. It works by stimulating bowel movements and promoting the expulsion of stool. Its effectiveness is attributed to its high concentration of ricinoleic acid, which activates receptors in the intestines, leading to increased fluid secretion and peristalsis.

Skin Care: Pharmaceutical-grade castor oil is incorporated into skincare products such as creams, ointments, and lotions. It is valued for its emollient properties, providing moisturization and forming a protective barrier on the skin to prevent moisture loss. Additionally, it is used in treatments for conditions like dermatitis, eczema, and psoriasis due to its anti-inflammatory and soothing effects.

Wound Healing: Due to its antimicrobial and anti-inflammatory properties, castor oil is used in wound care formulations. It promotes faster healing by reducing inflammation, preventing infection, and supporting tissue regeneration.

Drug Delivery: Castor oil is employed in pharmaceutical formulations as a vehicle or carrier oil for delivering active ingredients. It enhances the solubility and bioavailability of poorly soluble drugs, thereby improving their efficacy.

5.1.2 Industrial Applications

Castor oil finds extensive use in various industrial sectors owing to its unique chemical composition and functional properties:

Cosmetics: In the cosmetics industry, castor oil is utilized in the formulation of lipsticks, mascaras, and other makeup products. It acts as a binding agent, imparting gloss and sheen to cosmetic formulations while providing moisturizing benefits to the skin and lips.

Lubricants and Greases: Castor oil's high viscosity and lubricating properties make it suitable for use in lubricants, greases, and hydraulic fluids. It enhances the lubricity and durability of these products, particularly in applications where high temperature and pressure conditions are present.

Plastics and Polymers: Ricinoleic acid derived from castor oil is used in the production of biodegradable plastics and polymers. These materials offer a sustainable alternative to conventional petroleum-based plastics, contributing to environmental conservation efforts.

Textiles: Castor oil is employed in the textile industry as a sizing agent and softener for fabrics. It improves the flexibility and tensile strength of textile fibers, enhancing the quality and durability of finished textile products.

Paints and Coatings: Due to its excellent wetting and dispersing properties, castor oil is used in the formulation of paints, varnishes, and coatings. It helps to achieve uniform coverage, improve adhesion to surfaces, and enhance the durability of painted surfaces.

As research continues to uncover new applications and benefits of castor oil, particularly in areas such as pharmaceuticals, biotechnology, and renewable energy, its role is expected to expand further. Innovations in extraction techniques, sustainability practices, and biorefinery processes are paving the way for enhanced utilization of castor oil derivatives in diverse industrial and pharmaceutical applications.

Castor oil's pharmaceutical and industrial uses underscore its significance as a versatile natural resource. From its traditional role as a potent laxative and skincare remedy to its modern applications in pharmaceutical formulations, cosmetics, lubricants, and biodegradable materials, castor oil continues to play a pivotal role in enhancing human health and industrial efficiency.

5.2 Clinical trials and medical research

Clinical trials and medical research involving castor oil have explored its potential therapeutic benefits across various health conditions. Here's an overview of the findings and ongoing investigations in this field:

Laxative Effectiveness. Castor oil is well-known for its laxative properties, primarily attributed to its high concentration of ricinoleic acid. Clinical trials have validated its efficacy in relieving constipation. Research has shown that ricinoleic acid stimulates the smooth muscle contractions in the intestines, leading to increased bowel movements and evacuation of stool. Clinical studies have compared castor oil with other laxatives and placebo treatments, demonstrating its superior effectiveness in promoting bowel regularity.

Skin Conditions. Studies have investigated the use of castor oil in dermatological applications, particularly for treating various skin conditions. Its emollient properties help moisturize the skin and form a protective barrier. Clinical trials have evaluated its efficacy in managing dry skin, eczema, psoriasis, and other inflammatory dermatoses. Research suggests that castor oil's anti-inflammatory and antimicrobial properties may reduce skin irritation and improve skin barrier function.

Wound Healing. Castor oil has been studied for its potential role in wound healing. Clinical trials have explored its application in promoting wound closure, reducing inflammation, and preventing infections. Research indicates that castor oil may accelerate the healing process by stimulating tissue regeneration and enhancing the formation of granulation tissue. Studies have also investigated its use in chronic wounds and diabetic ulcers, highlighting its promising therapeutic benefits.

Anti-inflammatory Effects. Ricinoleic acid, the primary component of castor oil, exhibits anti-inflammatory properties. Clinical research has examined its potential in alleviating inflammatory conditions such as arthritis, joint pain, and muscle soreness. Studies have explored the mechanism by which ricinoleic acid modulates inflammatory pathways, suggesting its potential as a natural anti-inflammatory agent.

Antimicrobial Properties. Castor oil possesses antimicrobial properties that have been investigated in clinical studies. Research has evaluated its effectiveness against various bacteria, fungi, and viruses. Clinical trials have explored its use in topical formulations for treating infections, including fungal infections and microbial skin conditions. The antimicrobial activity of castor oil is attributed to compounds like ricinoleic acid, which disrupt microbial cell membranes and inhibit their growth.

Gastrointestinal Disorders. Clinical trials have examined the therapeutic potential of castor oil in gastrointestinal disorders beyond its laxative effects. Research has explored its use in managing irritable bowel syndrome (IBS), inflammatory bowel disease (IBD), and other functional gastrointestinal disorders. Studies have investigated the impact of castor oil on gut microbiota, intestinal inflammation, and symptom management in these conditions.

Cancer Research. Preliminary studies have explored the anticancer properties of castor oil and its derivatives. Research has investigated its potential to inhibit cancer cell proliferation, induce apoptosis (programmed cell death), and modulate cancer cell signaling pathways. Clinical trials are underway to evaluate castor oil's safety, efficacy, and potential synergistic effects in combination with conventional cancer treatments.

Future Directions. Ongoing research continues to explore new therapeutic applications of castor oil and its derivatives. Advances in biotechnology, nanomedicine, and drug delivery systems are expanding the scope of clinical trials and medical research involving castor oil. Collaborative efforts between researchers, healthcare professionals, and pharmaceutical companies aim to uncover novel uses and formulations that harness the therapeutic potential of this natural remedy.

Clinical trials and medical research have provided valuable insights into the therapeutic benefits of castor oil across various health conditions. From its established role as a potent laxative to its potential applications in dermatology, wound healing, inflammation, and beyond, castor oil remains a subject of scientific interest and exploration in clinical settings. Future studies hold promise to further elucidate its mechanisms of action and expand its clinical applications in healthcare and pharmaceutical industries.

5.3 FDA regulations and safety considerations

Due to its diverse applications and health claims, castor oil is subject to regulatory oversight by the U.S. Food and Drug Administration (FDA). Here's an overview of FDA regulations and safety considerations regarding the use of castor oil:

1) GRAS Status

Castor oil is Generally Recognized as Safe (GRAS) for use in food and cosmetic products when used by FDA regulations. This means that it is considered safe for its intended use without the need for pre-market approval from the FDA. It is commonly used as an ingredient in food additives and flavorings and as a laxative in over-the-counter drugs.

2) Labeling Requirements

FDA regulations require that castor oil products adhere to specific labeling requirements. Manufacturers must accurately label the product's ingredients, intended uses, and any potential associated risks. This ensures that consumers are informed about castor oil-based products' contents and proper usage.

3) Cosmetic Uses

Castor oil is widely used in cosmetic products such as creams, lotions, and hair care products. The FDA regulates these products under the Federal Food, Drug, and Cosmetic Act (FD&C Act), ensuring they are safe for consumer use. Cosmetic products containing castor oil must comply with FDA regulations regarding labeling, safety, and manufacturing practices.

4) Drug Applications

Castor oil is also used in pharmaceutical products, primarily as a stimulant laxative for relieving occasional constipation. Over-the-counter laxatives containing castor oil must meet FDA safety, efficacy, and labeling requirements. Manufacturers must provide sufficient evidence through clinical studies to support the product's effectiveness and safety profile.

5) Adverse Effects

While generally safe for topical and oral use, excessive consumption of castor oil can cause adverse effects such as abdominal cramping, diarrhea, and electrolyte imbalance. FDA regulations mandate that products containing castor oil must include warnings about potential side effects and advise consumers to consult healthcare professionals before use, especially for prolonged or excessive use.

6) Quality and Purity Standards

The FDA monitors the quality and purity of castor oil used in food, cosmetic, and pharmaceutical products. Manufacturers must adhere to Good Manufacturing Practices (GMP) to ensure product consistency, purity, and safety. This includes proper handling, storage, and testing of raw materials and finished products to prevent contamination and ensure product quality.

7) Regulatory Compliance

Companies marketing products containing castor oil must comply with FDA regulations to obtain and maintain market authorization. This includes submitting product formulations, safety data, and labeling information to the FDA for review and approval. Non-compliance with FDA regulations can result in regulatory actions such as product recalls, warnings, or legal penalties.

8) International Standards

In addition to FDA regulations, international standards and regulations may apply to importing, exporting, and marketing products containing castor oil. Companies involved in global trade must comply with relevant laws in each country or region where their products are marketed.

Continuous monitoring and compliance with FDA requirements are not just regulatory obligations, but also a commitment to maintaining consumer trust and promoting the responsible use of castor oil in various applications. By adhering to these regulations, manufacturers and marketers of castor oil-based products can provide consumers with assurance of product quality, safety, and appropriate usage guidelines.

Chapter 6: Benefits of castor oil

6.1 Health benefits for skin, hair and general well-being

Castor oil offers a plethora of health benefits for skin, hair, and overall wellness, making it a popular choice in natural health and beauty routines:

Skin Benefits

Castor oil is renowned for its moisturizing properties, making it an excellent emollient for dry and rough skin. Rich in fatty acids, particularly ricinoleic acid, it penetrates deeply into the skin, hydrating and nourishing it from within. Regular application can soften skin texture, reduce dry patches, and enhance overall health.

Anti-inflammatory Properties

Castor oil's anti-inflammatory properties make it effective in soothing irritated skin conditions such as acne, dermatitis, and eczema. It helps alleviate itching, redness, and swelling, relieving sensitive skin areas.

Anti-aging Benefits

Castor oil contains antioxidants that combat free radicals, contributing to premature aging. Regular use can help reduce the appearance of fine lines, wrinkles, and age spots, promoting a more youthful and radiant complexion.

Hair Growth and Scalp Health

When applied to the scalp, castor oil stimulates blood circulation and nourishes hair follicles, promoting healthy growth. It is rich in nutrients like vitamin E, omega-6 fatty acids, and proteins, strengthening the hair shaft, reducing hair breakage, and improving overall hair texture and shine.

Thickening and Conditioning

Due to its viscosity, castor oil coats the hair shaft, adding volume and thickness to fine or thinning hair. It also acts as a natural conditioner, moisturizing the hair strands and preventing moisture loss, resulting in softer, more manageable hair.

Wound Healing

Castor oil's antimicrobial and anti-inflammatory properties contribute to its effectiveness in wound healing. It promotes tissue repair and accelerates the healing process of minor cuts, scrapes, and bruises.

Boosts Immunity

Consuming castor oil orally is believed to support overall wellness by boosting the immune system. Its antibacterial properties may help fight off infections and support gastrointestinal health.

Laxative and Digestive Aid

Traditionally used as a natural laxative, castor oil aids in relieving constipation by stimulating intestinal motility. It acts as a lubricant, facilitating the movement of stool through the digestive tract.

Detoxification

Castor oil packs applied to the abdomen are believed to support detoxification by improving lymphatic circulation and promoting the elimination of toxins from the body.

Joint and Muscle Pain Relief

Massaging sore joints and muscles with castor oil can provide relief from pain and inflammation. Its anti-inflammatory properties help reduce swelling and improve mobility.

Incorporating castor oil into skincare, haircare, and wellness routines can yield significant benefits due to its natural healing and nourishing properties. Whether used topically or consumed orally, castor oil offers a holistic approach to enhancing skin health, promoting hair growth, supporting overall wellness, and addressing various health concerns. As with any natural remedy, it's essential to consult with a healthcare professional before starting new treatments, especially for internal use or sensitive skin conditions.

6.2 Therapeutic uses and anecdotal evidence

Therapeutic uses of castor oil span centuries and cultures, supported by anecdotal evidence that highlights its diverse applications in health and wellness:

Skin Conditions

Castor oil is celebrated for its ability to soothe and heal various skin ailments. Its high concentration of ricinoleic acid, a monounsaturated fatty acid, possesses anti-inflammatory, antimicrobial, and moisturizing properties. These qualities make it effective in treating acne, eczema, dermatitis, and dry skin. Many users apply castor oil topically to alleviate itching, reduce inflammation, and promote skin healing.

Hair Care

For centuries, castor oil has been a go-to remedy for enhancing hair growth and maintaining healthy locks. Its nourishing properties penetrate the scalp, stimulating circulation and follicle health. Regular application of castor oil can strengthen hair shafts, prevent breakage, and improve overall hair texture and shine. It is often used in hair masks, conditioners, and scalp treatments to address dandruff and hair thinning.

Laxative and Digestive Aid

One of castor oil's oldest and most well-known uses is as a natural laxative. When ingested, castor oil stimulates the intestines, promoting bowel movements and relieving constipation. This effect is attributed to ricinoleic acid, which binds to receptors in the intestinal lining, triggering contractions that facilitate the passage of stool. Due to potential side effects, oral use should be done cautiously and under medical guidance.

Pain Relief

Castor oil is also valued for its analgesic properties, particularly in easing joint pain, muscle soreness, and inflammation. Massaging castor oil onto affected areas can help alleviate pain and improve mobility. The oil's anti-inflammatory actions can reduce swelling and enhance circulation, providing relief from conditions like arthritis, sprains, and strains.

Wound Healing

The antimicrobial and anti-inflammatory properties of castor oil contribute to its effectiveness in wound care. It accelerates healing by protecting wounds from infection and promoting tissue regeneration. Applying castor oil topically to cuts, scrapes, and minor burns can help soothe pain, reduce redness, and facilitate faster recovery.

Menstrual Cramps

Some women use castor oil packs on the abdomen to alleviate menstrual cramps and discomfort. The packs are believed to improve blood flow to the pelvic area, reduce inflammation, and relieve pain associated with menstrual cycles. However, more scientific research is needed to fully understand its efficacy.

Detoxification

Castor oil packs are also utilized in detoxification practices to promote liver and lymphatic system health. By applying a cloth soaked in castor oil to the abdomen and covering it with heat, toxins are believed to be drawn out through the skin, aiding in detoxification. This method is often recommended as part of holistic health routines to support overall well-being.

Immune Support

Some individuals use castor oil to boost immune function and support overall health. Its antimicrobial properties may help fight off infections, while its anti-inflammatory effects contribute to reducing inflammation throughout the body.

Eye Care

In traditional medicine, castor oil has been used to alleviate dry eyes and discomfort. A drop or two of castor oil is sometimes applied to the eyes to lubricate and soothe dryness. However, caution must be exercised when using castor oil near sensitive areas like the eyes, and consulting with an eye care professional is advisable.

General Wellness

Beyond specific therapeutic uses, many people incorporate castor oil into their daily routines for its overall health benefits. Whether used topically or ingested, it's valued for its potential to support skin health, hair growth, digestive function, and more.

While anecdotal evidence and historical uses highlight the versatility of castor oil in various health applications, scientific research supporting its efficacy in many of these areas is still evolving. To ensure safety and effectiveness, it's essential to consult healthcare professionals before using castor oil, especially internally or for treating medical conditions.

6.3 Comparative analysis with other oils and treatments

Comparing castor oil with other oils and treatments reveals distinct characteristics and applications, showcasing its unique benefits and versatility in various health and wellness contexts:

6.3.1 Castor Oil vs. Coconut Oil

Composition: Castor oil, rich in ricinoleic acid, offers unique properties such as anti-inflammatory and antimicrobial effects. In contrast, coconut oil, abundant in lauric acid, provides antibacterial and moisturizing benefits. This comparison enlightens the audience about the distinct properties of these oils.

Skin and Hair Care: Both oils are popular in skincare and hair care. Castor oil is thicker and more dense, making it suitable for deep moisturization and scalp treatments, whereas coconut oil is lighter and absorbs quickly, which is ideal for overall skin hydration and conditioning hair without leaving a greasy residue.

Digestive Health: Castor oil is known for its laxative properties, aiding in relieving constipation, while coconut oil is often used to promote gut health due to its potential antimicrobial and anti-inflammatory effects on the digestive tract.

6.3.2 Castor Oil vs. Olive Oil

Composition: Olive oil is primarily composed of oleic acid, a monounsaturated fatty acid, which contributes to its moisturizing and antioxidant properties. Castor oil's ricinoleic acid content provides it with unique anti-inflammatory and healing benefits.

Skin Care: Olive oil is lighter than castor oil and is often used as a facial moisturizer and massage oil. Castor oil's thicker consistency makes it suitable for addressing dry, cracked skin and promoting wound healing.

Hair Care: Castor oil is favored for its potential to stimulate hair growth and enhance hair thickness, while olive oil is used to condition and soften hair.

6.3.3 Castor Oil vs. Jojoba Oil

Composition: Jojoba oil resembles human sebum, quickly absorbing and well-tolerated by all skin types. Castor oil's composition is thicker and contains ricinoleic acid, offering unique healing and moisturizing properties.

Skin Care: Jojoba oil is often used as a facial cleanser, moisturizer, and makeup remover due to its similarity to natural oils produced by the skin. Castor oil's antimicrobial properties make it beneficial for treating acne and skin infections.

Hair Care: Both oils are used for hair conditioning, but castor oil's ability to penetrate deeply into the scalp and strengthen hair follicles sets it apart for promoting hair growth and addressing scalp conditions like dandruff.

6.3.4 Castor Oil vs. Tea Tree Oil

Composition: Tea tree oil is renowned for its antimicrobial and antifungal properties due to its high concentration of terpenes. Castor oil's ricinoleic acid content provides anti-inflammatory and moisturizing benefits.

Skin Care: Tea tree oil is effective against acne, fungal infections, and insect bites. Castor oil's thicker consistency makes it suitable for soothing dry, irritated skin and reducing inflammation.

Hair Care: Tea tree oil treats dandruff and scalp infections. Castor oil promotes hair growth and strengthens hair strands.

6.3.5 Castor Oil vs. Essential Oils

Composition: Essential oils are highly concentrated plant extracts with distinct therapeutic properties. Castor oil is a carrier oil that enhances the absorption and efficacy of essential oils when combined.

Application: Essential oils are typically used in aromatherapy, massage, and topical treatments for specific health concerns like stress relief, pain management, and skin conditions. Castor oil serves as a base for diluting essential oils and delivering them to the skin or scalp.

6.3.6 Castor Oil vs. Pharmaceutical Treatments

Safety and Side Effects

Castor oil is generally considered safe for topical and oral use in recommended doses but may cause gastrointestinal discomfort if ingested in large quantities. Pharmaceutical treatments often target specific medical conditions with potent effects but may carry side effects and require medical supervision.

Holistic Approach

Castor oil is embraced for its holistic benefits in promoting overall wellness, digestive health, and skincare without the synthetic compounds often found in pharmaceuticals.

In conclusion, while castor oil stands out for its unique composition and therapeutic properties, such as anti-inflammatory, antimicrobial, and moisturizing effects, each oil and treatment have distinct applications and benefits. Choosing the right oil depends on individual needs, preferences, and desired outcomes, with castor oil proving to be a versatile addition to natural health and beauty regimens. Always consult healthcare professionals for personalized advice, especially when integrating oils into medical treatments or addressing specific health concerns.

Chapter 7: Side effects and cautions

7.1 Potential risks and contraindications

Castor oil, derived from the seeds of the Ricinus communis plant, has been used for centuries for its medicinal properties and wide range of applications. While it is generally considered safe for use in various forms, there are potential risks and contraindications that users need to be aware of to ensure safe and effective use.

7.1.1 Allergic Reactions

One of the primary concerns with castor oil is the potential for allergic reactions. Some individuals may be sensitive or allergic to ricinoleic acid, the main component of castor oil. Symptoms of an allergic reaction can include:

- Skin Irritation: Redness, itching, and rash may occur when castor oil is applied topically.

- Respiratory Issues: In rare cases, inhaling castor oil vapors or fumes can cause respiratory discomfort, such as difficulty breathing, wheezing, or coughing.

- Anaphylaxis: Though extremely rare, a severe allergic reaction called anaphylaxis can occur, characterized by swelling of the face and throat, difficulty breathing, and a rapid drop in blood pressure, which requires immediate medical attention.

7.1.2 Gastrointestinal Issues

When taken orally, castor oil acts as a powerful laxative, stimulating bowel movements by increasing the movement of the intestines. While this can be beneficial for relieving constipation, it can also lead to several gastrointestinal issues if not used correctly:

- Diarrhea: Overconsumption of castor oil can cause severe diarrhea, leading to dehydration and electrolyte imbalances.

- Nausea and Vomiting: Some individuals may experience nausea or vomiting after ingesting castor oil, particularly if taken on an empty stomach or in large doses.

- Abdominal Cramps: The strong laxative effect of castor oil can cause painful abdominal cramps and discomfort.

7.1.3 Pregnancy and Lactation

Pregnant women should exercise caution when using castor oil. While it has been traditionally used to induce labor, this practice should only be done under the supervision of a healthcare professional due to the potential risks:

- Premature Labor: Unsupervised use of castor oil to induce labor can lead to premature labor, which can be dangerous for both the mother and the baby.

- Miscarriage: In early pregnancy, the use of castor oil can potentially induce miscarriage due to its strong stimulant effects on the uterus.

7.1.4 Chronic Health Conditions

Individuals with certain chronic health conditions should consult with their healthcare provider before using castor oil:

- Gastrointestinal Disorders: Those with inflammatory bowel disease (IBD), irritable bowel syndrome (IBS), or other gastrointestinal disorders should avoid using castor oil as a laxative, as it may exacerbate their condition.

- Kidney Disease: People with kidney disease should use castor oil cautiously, especially when taken orally, due to the potential risk of dehydration and electrolyte imbalances.

7.1.5 Drug Interactions

Castor oil may interact with certain medications, affecting their efficacy or increasing the risk of adverse effects:

- Diuretics: When used in combination with diuretics, the laxative effect of castor oil can increase the risk of dehydration and electrolyte imbalances.

- Anticoagulants: Castor oil may enhance the effects of anticoagulant medications, increasing the risk of bleeding.

- Medications for High Blood Pressure: The dehydrating effect of castor oil can potentially interfere with medications used to manage high blood pressure.

7.1.6 Pediatric Use

Caution is also advised when using castor oil in children:

- Dosage: Children are more susceptible to the potent effects of castor oil, so proper dosage and administration are crucial to avoid adverse reactions.

- Hydration: Ensuring adequate hydration is important to prevent dehydration, especially when using castor oil as a laxative.

7.1.7 Topical Use Concerns

For topical applications, castor oil should be used with care:

- Open Wounds: Applying castor oil to open wounds or irritated skin can cause further irritation and delay healing.

- Sensitive Skin: Individuals with sensitive skin should perform a patch test before widespread use to avoid adverse reactions.

While castor oil offers numerous benefits, it is important to be aware of potential risks and contraindications. Consulting with a healthcare professional, particularly for individuals with existing health conditions or those who are pregnant or breastfeeding, is essential to ensure safe and effective use. Proper dosage, administration, and monitoring can help mitigate risks and maximize the therapeutic benefits of castor oil.

7.2 Allergic reactions and sensitivity

Castor oil, derived from the seeds of the Ricinus communis plant, is widely recognized for its therapeutic properties and applications in health and beauty. However, like any natural product, it carries the potential for allergic reactions and sensitivities in some individuals. Understanding these risks and how to manage them is crucial for safe usage.

Allergic reactions occur when the immune system mistakenly identifies a harmless substance as a threat and responds accordingly. In the case of castor oil, certain compounds, particularly ricinoleic acid, can trigger these reactions. Symptoms of an allergic reaction to castor oil can range from mild to severe and include:

- *Skin Irritation*: this is the most common allergic response to topical application of castor oil. Symptoms may include redness, itching, and rash at the site of application. These reactions are typically localized but can be uncomfortable and persistent.

- *Contact Dermatitis*: a more severe form of skin irritation, contact dermatitis can result in blisters, hives, and swelling. This reaction occurs when the skin becomes inflamed due to direct contact with an allergen.

- *Respiratory Symptoms*: inhaling castor oil vapors or fumes can lead to respiratory issues such as sneezing, coughing, and difficulty breathing. This is less common but can occur in individuals with heightened sensitivities.

- *Anaphylaxis*: though extremely rare, anaphylaxis is a severe, potentially life-threatening allergic reaction that requires immediate medical attention. Symptoms include swelling of the face and throat, difficulty breathing, rapid heartbeat, and a dramatic drop in blood pressure.

7.2.1 Sensitivities and Intolerances

Beyond allergic reactions, some individuals may experience sensitivities or intolerances to castor oil. These are non-allergic responses that can still cause discomfort and should be monitored:

Gastrointestinal Sensitivities

When ingested, castor oil can cause stomach cramps, nausea, and diarrhea due to its strong laxative effect. Individuals with sensitive digestive systems should use caution and consult a healthcare professional before using castor oil internally.

Skin Sensitivities

Even in the absence of an allergy, some people may find castor oil too harsh for their skin, leading to dryness, flaking, or a burning sensation. This is often due to the oil's thick consistency and potent nature.

Preventive Measures and Management

To minimize the risk of allergic reactions and sensitivities, several precautionary steps can be taken.

Patch Testing: before applying castor oil extensively, perform a patch test. Apply a small amount of oil to a discrete area of skin, such as the inner forearm, and wait 24-48 hours. If no irritation or reaction occurs, it is likely safe to use.

Dilution: diluting castor oil with a carrier oil, such as coconut or almond oil, can reduce its potency and lessen the likelihood of skin irritation. This is especially important for individuals with sensitive skin.

Consultation with Healthcare Providers: those with known allergies or sensitivities should consult with a healthcare provider before using castor oil. This is particularly important for individuals with pre-existing skin conditions, respiratory issues, or gastrointestinal sensitivities.

Avoiding Ingestion for Sensitive Individuals: given its strong laxative effect, castor oil should be used with caution or avoided altogether by individuals with sensitive digestive systems or certain medical conditions.

Awareness of Cross-Reactivity: individuals allergic to certain plants or seeds may be at higher risk for an allergic reaction to castor oil due to cross-reactivity. Awareness and caution are advised.

While castor oil offers numerous benefits for health and beauty, it is important to be aware of the potential for allergic reactions and sensitivities. By understanding these risks and taking appropriate preventive measures, individuals can safely incorporate castor oil into their routines and enjoy its therapeutic properties without adverse effects. Always prioritize safety and consult with healthcare professionals when in doubt to ensure the best outcomes.

7.3 Safe use guidelines for different applications

Castor oil is renowned for its versatility and myriad health benefits, but safe usage is crucial to maximize its efficacy while minimizing potential risks. This guide outlines safe application practices for different uses of castor oil, ensuring that you can harness its benefits effectively and safely.

7.3.1 Topical Applications

Skin Care

Patch Test: Always perform a patch test before using castor oil extensively on your skin. Apply a small amount to a discrete area and wait 24-48 hours to check for any adverse reactions.

Dilution: Due to its thick consistency, dilute castor oil with a carrier oil like coconut or almond oil. A 1:1 ratio is typically effective, but you can adjust according to your skin's tolerance.

Application: Use castor oil sparingly on the face to avoid clogging pores. It's particularly beneficial for dry, rough patches and can be applied directly to problem areas.

Hair Care

Scalp Treatments: Mix castor oil with lighter oils (e.g., jojoba or olive oil) to facilitate easier application and rinsing. Massage the blend into your scalp to promote hair growth and reduce dandruff.

Hair Conditioning: For deep conditioning, apply castor oil to your hair, focusing on the ends. Leave it in for at least 30 minutes, or overnight for intense hydration, then wash thoroughly with shampoo.

7.3.2 Internal Use

Digestive Health

Laxative: Castor oil can be used as a potent laxative. The recommended dose for adults is typically 15-60 mL, but it's crucial to consult a healthcare professional before internal use to determine the appropriate dosage and frequency.

Precautions: Pregnant women, nursing mothers, and individuals with gastrointestinal disorders should avoid internal use without medical advice due to the oil's strong laxative effect.

Oral Health

Oil Pulling: Use castor oil for oil pulling to promote oral hygiene. Swish 1-2 tablespoons of castor oil in your mouth for 10-20 minutes, then spit it out and rinse your mouth with water. This practice can help reduce bacteria and improve gum health.

7.3.3 Therapeutic Uses

Pain Relief

Castor Oil Packs: Soak a piece of flannel or cotton cloth in castor oil, place it on the affected area, cover with plastic wrap, and apply heat using a heating pad or hot water bottle. This method is effective for alleviating muscle and joint pain. Leave the pack on for 45-60 minutes, then clean the area with a mild soap and water.

Anti-Inflammatory

Arthritis and Joint Pain: Regularly massaging castor oil into inflamed joints can help reduce pain and inflammation. For enhanced effects, combine it with essential oils like eucalyptus or peppermint, which also have anti-inflammatory properties.

7.3.4 Cosmetic Uses

Eyelashes and Eyebrows

Application: Use a clean mascara wand or a cotton swab to apply a small amount of castor oil to your eyelashes and eyebrows before bed. This can promote thicker, healthier growth over time.

Lip Care

Lip Balm: Mix castor oil with beeswax and a few drops of your favorite essential oil to create a nourishing lip balm. Apply as needed to keep your lips moisturized and prevent chapping.

7.3.5 Precautions and Considerations

1. Allergies and Sensitivities: Individuals with known sensitivities to castor oil should avoid its use. Always conduct a patch test before extensive application.

2. Storage: Store castor oil in a cool, dark place to maintain its stability and prevent rancidity.

3. Consultation with Professionals: Always seek advice from healthcare professionals, especially when considering internal use or if you have pre-existing health conditions.

Chapter 8: Purchase and storage of castor oil

8.1 Choose quality products

Selecting high-quality castor oil is not just a choice, but a necessity for your safety and well-being. Especially when used for health and beauty applications, the safety of the product is paramount. Among the various types available, organic, cold-pressed castor oil stands out for its purity and superior properties. Here's a detailed guide on why choosing such products matters and how to identify the best options on the market.

8.1.1 Importance of Quality

Purity: high-quality castor oil, especially when labeled organic and cold-pressed, is free from harmful chemicals and additives. This purity is crucial for applications involving sensitive skin, internal consumption, or therapeutic uses, as it minimizes the risk of adverse reactions.

Nutrient Retention: cold-pressing is a method that extracts oil without using heat, preserving the oil's natural nutrients, enzymes, and beneficial compounds. Heat can degrade these elements, reducing the oil's efficacy. Cold-pressed castor oil retains its natural composition, making it more potent and useful.

Environmental and Ethical Considerations: Your choice of organic castor oil, produced without synthetic pesticides or fertilizers, promotes environmental sustainability and reduces the ecological footprint. Additionally, choosing products from ethical sources ensures fair trade practices and supports communities involved in production. Your choice makes a difference and connects you with these communities, fostering a sense of compassion and understanding.

8.1.2 Characteristics of High-Quality Castor Oil

Color and Consistency: pure, cold-pressed castor oil is typically pale yellow with a thick, dense consistency. Any significant deviations, such as a very dark color or watery texture, may indicate impurities or processing issues.

Odor: quality castor oil has a mild, slightly earthy smell. A strong, unpleasant odor can be a sign of rancidity or contamination.

Packaging: high-quality castor oil is usually packaged in dark glass bottles to protect it from light, which can degrade the oil and reduce its shelf life. Avoid plastic containers, as they can leach harmful chemicals into the oil.

8.1.3 Labels and Certifications

1) Organic Certification

Look for certification labels such as USDA Organic or equivalent international standards. This certification guarantees that the oil is produced according to strict organic farming practices, freeing it from synthetic chemicals and GMOs.

2) Cold-Pressed Label

Ensure the product explicitly states it is cold-pressed. This information is often highlighted on the front label, but you may need to check the product description or packaging details.

3) Third-Party Testing

Some brands offer third-party lab testing to verify the purity and quality of their castor oil. These tests can confirm the absence of contaminants and the presence of beneficial compounds. Look for products that provide access to these test results.

8.1.4 Brands and Sourcing

Reputable Brands

Opt for brands with a good reputation and positive reviews. Established brands are more likely to adhere to high production standards and offer quality products.

Sourcing Information

Transparency about sourcing practices is a good indicator of quality. Brands that disclose where their castor beans are grown and how the oil is processed are generally more trustworthy.

8.1.5 Price Considerations

Cost vs. Quality: While high-quality, organic, cold-pressed castor oil may be more expensive, the benefits outweigh the costs. Cheaper options often compromise on purity and effectiveness, potentially introducing harmful substances.

Value for Money: Consider the concentration and effectiveness of the oil. A higher upfront cost for a pure, potent product can be more cost-effective compared to frequent purchases of lower-quality oil in the long run.

Choosing organic, cold-pressed castor oil is crucial for ensuring the highest quality and effectiveness of the product. By paying attention to certifications, brand reputation, and product characteristics, you can make an informed decision and fully benefit from castor oil's numerous health and beauty applications. Investing in high-quality castor oil promotes better health outcomes and supports sustainable and ethical production practices.

8.2 Storage recommendations and shelf-life considerations

Proper storage of castor oil is essential to maintaining its quality, potency, and shelf life. Like many other natural oils, castor oil can degrade over time if not stored correctly, losing its beneficial properties and becoming less effective. Understanding the best practices for storing castor oil can help you maximize its lifespan and ensure it remains a valuable part of your health and beauty regimen.

8.2.1 Why Proper Storage Matters

1) Preserving Potency

The beneficial compounds in castor oil, such as ricinoleic acid, can degrade when exposed to unfavorable conditions. Proper storage helps maintain the oil's potency and effectiveness.

2) Preventing Contamination

Improper storage can lead to contamination from environmental factors, such as air and moisture, which can spoil the oil and make it unsafe for use.

3) Extending Shelf Life

By following the correct storage methods, you can extend the shelf life of castor oil and ensure it remains usable for a longer period.

8.2.2 Ideal Storage Conditions

Temperature. Store castor oil at a consistent, cool temperature. Avoid exposing it to heat sources, such as direct sunlight or appliance proximity. A temperature range of 50°F to 70°F (10°C to 21°C) is generally ideal.

Light. Light, incredibly UV light, can break down the beneficial compounds in castor oil. Store the oil in a dark, cool place, such as a pantry or cupboard, away from windows and other light sources. Using dark-colored glass bottles can also help protect the oil from light exposure.

Air Exposure. Oxygen can oxidize the oil, leading to rancidity. Always ensure the bottle is tightly sealed after each use to minimize air exposure. Using smaller bottles can help reduce the amount of air in contact with the oil as it is used.

Humidity. Moisture can lead to contamination and spoilage. Store castor oil in a dry environment to prevent moisture from getting into the bottle.

8.2.3 Packaging Considerations

Choose dark glass bottles for storing castor oil. Glass is non-reactive and doesn't leach chemicals into the oil, unlike some plastics. The dark color helps protect the oil from light exposure.

Smaller bottles are preferable as they reduce the amount of air exposure over time. If you purchase castor oil in bulk, consider transferring it to smaller bottles for daily use, keeping the bulk container sealed and stored correctly.

8.2.4 Shelf Life

Castor oil generally has a shelf life of 1 to 2 years when stored properly. However, this can vary depending on the quality of the oil and how well it is stored.

Castor oil can become rancid over time. Signs of spoilage include a sour or off smell, changes in color, and a change in consistency. If you notice any of these signs, it's best to discard the oil.

Expiration Date: Check the expiration date provided by the manufacturer. Even if the oil appears fine, following these guidelines is good practice to ensure the oil's effectiveness and safety.

8.2.5 Extending Shelf Life

While not always necessary, refrigeration can help extend the shelf life of castor oil, particularly in warmer climates. If you refrigerate the oil, allow it to come to room temperature before use, as it can become thick and difficult to pour when cold.

Adding natural antioxidants like vitamin E oil can help extend the shelf life of castor oil by preventing oxidation. However, this should be done with caution and knowledge of proper dosages to avoid significantly altering the oil's properties.

8.2.6 Usage Tips

Always use clean hands or tools when dispensing castor oil to avoid introducing contaminants into the bottle.

If you transfer castor oil into smaller bottles, label them with the date of transfer and the expiration date. This helps you keep track of the oil's age and ensures you use it within its optimal time frame.

Proper storage of castor oil is crucial to maintaining its quality and extending its shelf life. By following the guidelines on temperature, light, air exposure, and humidity, and using appropriate packaging materials, you can ensure that your castor oil remains potent and effective for its intended uses. Paying attention to signs of spoilage and adhering to the manufacturer's expiration dates further helps make the most out of this versatile oil.

8.3 Consumer advice and common misconceptions

Castor oil is renowned for its numerous health and beauty benefits, but consumers often encounter various tips and misconceptions regarding its use. To make informed decisions and maximize the benefits of castor oil, it's important to distinguish between fact and fiction. This paragraph provides essential consumer tips and addresses some common misconceptions surrounding castor oil.

8.3.1 Consumer Tips

When purchasing castor oil, look for cold-pressed, organic options. Cold-pressed castor oil retains more nutrients and beneficial compounds than oil extracted using heat or chemicals. Organic certification ensures the oil is free from pesticides and synthetic additives.

Before using castor oil extensively on your skin or hair, perform a patch test. Apply a small amount of oil to a small area of your skin and wait 24 hours to check for any adverse reactions. This helps prevent potential allergic reactions or sensitivities.

Castor oil should be stored in a cool, dark place, preferably in a dark glass bottle, to protect it from light and air exposure. Proper storage extends the oil's shelf life and preserves its efficacy.

If you're new to using castor oil, start with small amounts to see how your body reacts. Gradually increase usage as you become more comfortable and familiar with its effects.

If you plan to use castor oil for therapeutic purposes, such as treating a specific medical condition, it's advisable to consult a healthcare professional or a dermatologist. They can provide guidance tailored to your individual needs.

8.3.2 Common Misconceptions

While castor oil has numerous benefits, it is not a miracle cure for all ailments. Some people believe it can cure severe medical conditions overnight, but such claims are often exaggerated. Castor oil should be seen as a supportive remedy rather than a standalone treatment for serious health issues.

There is a misconception that castor oil is always safe for internal use. While it has been used as a laxative, ingesting castor oil can lead to side effects like stomach cramps, diarrhea, and dehydration. It should be used internally only under the guidance of a healthcare professional.

Another common misconception is that using more castor oil will yield better results. In reality, using too much can lead to skin irritation or buildup in the hair, making it greasy and difficult to manage. Moderation is vital to achieving the desired benefits.

Some users expect immediate results from castor oil, especially for hair growth and skin improvement. However, the benefits of castor oil often manifest over time with consistent use. Patience and regular application are necessary for optimal results.

It's a common belief that castor oil is suitable for everyone. However, individual reactions to castor oil can vary. Some people may experience allergic reactions or sensitivities. It's important to recognize that what works for one person may not work for another.

Not all castor oils are created equal. The extraction method, source of the castor beans, and additional ingredients can significantly affect the quality and effectiveness of the oil. Consumers should educate themselves about different types of castor oil and choose products that best suit their needs.

Understanding castor oil's correct usage and potential limitations can help consumers make informed decisions and avoid common pitfalls. Users can safely incorporate castor oil into their health and beauty routines by focusing on quality, conducting patch tests, and starting with small amounts. Dispelling misconceptions ensures a realistic expectation of the benefits castor oil can offer. With proper knowledge and application, castor oil can be a valuable addition to your self-care arsenal.

BOOK 2: Castor Oil for Skincare

Castor Oil for Skincare

Unlocking the Secret of Naturally Radiant and Rejuvenated Skin

By

Vincent Vega

Disclaimer notice

Please be aware that the information provided in this document is intended solely for educational and entertainment purposes. Every effort has been made to ensure the content is accurate, reliable, current, and complete.

However, no guarantees, either explicit or implicit, are made. Readers acknowledge that the author is not providing legal, financial, medical, or professional advice.

The content has been sourced from various references. It is strongly recommended that you consult a licensed professional before attempting any of the of the methods described in this document.

By reading this document, you agree that the author is not liable for any direct or indirect losses resulting from the use of the information within, including but not limited to errors, omissions, or inaccuracies.

Chapter 1: Benefits of Castor Oil for Skin

Castor oil has long been celebrated for its multifaceted benefits in skincare. From deep hydration to anti-aging properties, this natural oil offers a wide array of advantages that cater to various skin concerns. In this chapter, we explore the scientifically-backed benefits of using castor oil as a staple in your skincare regimen.

1.1 Moisturizing Properties

Deep Hydration:

- Emollient Power: Castor oil's thick consistency allows it to deeply penetrate the skin, providing lasting hydration that helps restore moisture balance.

- Barrier Function: It forms a protective barrier on the skin, preventing water loss and keeping it soft and supple throughout the day.

- Suitable for Dry Skin: Ideal for dry and dehydrated skin types, castor oil effectively alleviates rough patches and flakiness, promoting a smoother texture.

1.2 Anti-Aging Benefits

Reduction of Fine Lines and Wrinkles:

- Stimulates Collagen Production: Rich in ricinoleic acid and essential fatty acids, castor oil stimulates collagen and elastin production, which helps reduce the appearance of fine lines and wrinkles.

- Improves Elasticity: By maintaining skin elasticity, castor oil helps to keep the skin firm and youthful.

- Antioxidant Protection: The presence of antioxidants like vitamin E in castor oil protects the skin from oxidative stress, preventing premature aging caused by free radicals.

1.3 Anti-inflammatory and Healing Properties

Soothes Irritation and Inflammation:

- Ricinoleic Acid: Known for its anti-inflammatory properties, ricinoleic acid in castor oil helps reduce redness, swelling, and itching associated with skin irritations such as acne, eczema, and dermatitis.

- Calms Sensitive Skin: It provides relief to sensitive skin conditions, promoting comfort and minimizing discomfort.

1.4 Antimicrobial and Acne-Fighting Abilities

Antibacterial Action:

- Natural Cleansing: Castor oil's antimicrobial properties help cleanse the skin, eliminating bacteria and impurities that contribute to acne breakouts.

- Prevents Clogged Pores: By reducing excess sebum production and preventing pore blockages, castor oil aids in maintaining clear and healthy skin.

- Gentle Yet Effective: It offers a gentle approach to treating acne without harsh chemicals, making it suitable for sensitive and acne-prone skin.

1.5 How to Incorporate Castor Oil into Your Skincare Routine

Facial Moisturization:

- Daily Application: Use castor oil as a facial moisturizer by applying a small amount to clean, damp skin. Massage gently until fully absorbed for maximum hydration.

- Blending with Other Oils: Customize your skincare routine by blending castor oil with other beneficial oils like jojoba or argan oil to address specific skin concerns such as dryness or aging.

Targeted Treatments:

- Spot Treatments: Apply a dab of castor oil directly onto blemishes or areas of concern as a spot treatment to reduce inflammation and promote healing.

- Overnight Treatments: For intensive hydration and rejuvenation, apply castor oil as an overnight treatment, allowing its nourishing properties to work overnight for refreshed skin in the morning.

Castor oil stands as a versatile and effective natural remedy for achieving healthy, radiant skin. From its powerful moisturizing abilities to its anti-aging and healing properties, incorporating castor oil into your skincare routine can transform your skin's texture and appearance. Understanding these benefits empowers you to harness the full potential of castor oil for a radiant and youthful complexion.

Chapter 2: Castor Oil for Facial Skincare

Facial skincare is essential for maintaining healthy, glowing skin. With its rich composition and beneficial properties, castor oil offers a natural and effective solution for various facial skincare needs. In this chapter, we explore how castor oil can be incorporated into your daily facial skincare routine to cleanse, moisturize, and enhance your skin's overall health and appearance.

2.1 Cleansing with Castor Oil

Oil Cleansing Method:

Gentle Makeup Removal: Castor oil effectively dissolves makeup, sunscreen, and impurities without stripping the skin of its natural oils.

Deep Pore Cleansing: It penetrates deep into pores to remove dirt, excess sebum, and pollutants, preventing clogged pores and breakouts.

Balancing Sebum Production: Regular use of castor oil in the oil cleansing method can help balance sebum production, reducing the occurrence of oily skin.

DIY Castor Oil Cleansers:

Simple Recipes: You can easily create your castor oil cleanser by blending it with other oils, like olive oil or grapeseed oil, tailored to your skin type. This simplicity empowers you to take control of your skincare routine.

Addition of Essential Oils: Enhance the cleansing experience by adding a few drops of essential oils like lavender or tea tree oil for added benefits.

2.2 Facial Moisturization with Castor Oil

Hydrating and Nourishing:

Deep Moisture: Castor oil's emollient properties make it an excellent facial moisturizer, providing deep hydration and locking in moisture.

Improves Skin Texture: Regular application softens and smoothens the skin, improving overall texture and radiance.

Blending with Other Oils:

Customizable Formulations: Blend castor oil with lighter oils such as almond or rosehip seed oil to create a customized facial serum or moisturizer.

Anti-Aging Benefits: Incorporating oils rich in antioxidants like vitamin E enhances the anti-aging benefits, protecting against free radical damage and promoting youthful skin.

2.3 Anti-Acne Treatments

Reducing Inflammation:

Anti-inflammatory Properties: The ricinoleic acid in castor oil soothes inflammation, redness, and irritation associated with acne. This reassures you that castor oil is a reliable solution for acne-related issues.

Prevents Breakouts: Its antibacterial properties help combat acne-causing bacteria, preventing new breakouts and promoting clearer skin.

Spot Treatments:

Direct Application: Apply a small amount of castor oil directly onto acne spots or blemishes as a targeted treatment overnight.

Healing Properties: It aids in healing acne scars and marks, promoting faster skin regeneration and smoother skin texture.

2.4 Incorporating Castor Oil into Facial Masks

Hydrating Masks:

DIY Recipes: Combine castor oil with natural ingredients like honey, yogurt, or oatmeal to create hydrating and nourishing facial masks.

Soothing and Refreshing: Masks enriched with castor oil rejuvenate tired skin, leaving it refreshed and revitalized.

2.5 Facial Massage and Castor Oil Packs

Massage Benefits:

Stimulates Circulation: Facial massage with castor oil improves blood circulation, promoting a healthy glow and even skin tone.

Relaxation and Tension Relief: It relaxes facial muscles, reducing tension and promoting a relaxed, youthful appearance.

Castor Oil Packs:

Detoxification: How to make and use castor oil packs for detoxifying the skin and improving overall skin health.

Enhanced Absorption: Packs enhance the absorption of nutrients into the skin, maximizing the benefits of castor oil.

Incorporating castor oil into your facial skincare routine can significantly enhance the health and appearance of your skin. From cleansing and moisturizing to treating acne and rejuvenating with facial masks and massages, the versatile properties of castor oil make it a valuable asset for achieving radiant and healthy facial skin. By understanding its benefits and applications, you can tailor your skincare regimen to harness the full potential of castor oil for beautiful, glowing skin.

Chapter 3: Castor oil for body care

While facial skincare often receives the most attention, caring for the skin on your body is equally important. Castor oil, known for its moisturizing and healing properties, can significantly improve the health and appearance of your body's skin. In this chapter, we explore how to use castor oil to nourish and rejuvenate the skin all over your body.

3.1 Body Moisturization

Hydrating Dry Skin:

- Deep Penetration: Castor oil's thick, rich consistency allows it to penetrate deeply into the skin, providing long-lasting hydration.

- Preventing Moisture Loss: It forms a protective barrier on the skin, preventing moisture loss and keeping the skin soft and supple.

- Ideal for Dry Areas: It is particularly effective on notoriously dry areas like elbows, knees, and heels, transforming rough patches into smooth skin.

Full-Body Moisturizers:

- DIY Body Lotion: Create a homemade body lotion by blending castor oil with lighter oils such as coconut or jojoba oil for easy application.

- Post-Bath Routine: Apply castor oil to damp skin after a bath or shower to lock in moisture and enhance absorption.

3.2 Stretch Marks and Scars

Reducing the Appearance of Stretch Marks:

- Improves Elasticity: The fatty acids in castor oil help improve skin elasticity, reducing the appearance of stretch marks over time.

- Prevents New Stretch Marks: Regular application during periods of rapid growth or weight changes can help prevent the formation of new stretch marks.

Healing Scars:

- Promotes Skin Regeneration: Castor oil encourages the growth of new skin cells, helping to fade scars and even out skin tone.

- Application Techniques: Massage castor oil onto scars daily to promote healing and reduce their visibility.

3.3 Soothing Irritated Skin

Calming Eczema and Psoriasis:

- Anti-inflammatory Effects: Ricinoleic acid in castor oil has anti-inflammatory properties that soothe irritated and inflamed skin conditions like eczema and psoriasis.

- Moisturizing Benefits: Its deep moisturizing effect helps relieve dryness and scaling associated with these conditions.

Relieving Itchiness:

- Soothing Irritation: Applying castor oil to itchy areas provides relief and reduces the urge to scratch, which can further irritate the skin.

3.4 Body Scrubs and Exfoliants

Exfoliating Dry Skin:

- DIY Scrubs: Create exfoliating body scrubs by mixing castor oil with natural exfoliants like sugar, salt, or ground coffee.

- Removes Dead Skin Cells: Regular exfoliation with castor oil scrubs helps remove dead skin cells, revealing smoother, more radiant skin underneath.

Softening and Smoothing:

- Improves Texture: The combined action of exfoliation and moisturizing from castor oil results in softer and smoother skin.

- Usage Tips: Use body scrubs once or twice a week for best results, focusing on rough areas like elbows and knees.

3.5 Castor Oil Baths

Relaxing and Hydrating:

- Castor Oil Baths: Add a few tablespoons of castor oil to your bathwater for a deeply hydrating and relaxing soak.

- Skin Benefits: This method allows your entire body to absorb the moisturizing and healing properties of castor oil.

Detoxifying Effects:

- Detox Baths: Combine castor oil with Epsom salts for a detoxifying bath that helps draw out impurities and relax sore muscles.

- Enhanced Absorption: Warm bathwater helps open pores, enhancing the absorption of castor oil into the skin.

3.6 Special Treatments with Castor Oil

Targeted Treatments:

- Foot Care: Use castor oil to treat dry, cracked heels by applying it generously and covering with socks overnight for softer feet.

- Hand Care: Moisturize and repair dry hands by massaging castor oil into the skin and cuticles, particularly before bedtime.

Massage Oil:

- Therapeutic Massages: Castor oil makes an excellent massage oil, providing a smooth glide and deep hydration while also helping to relieve muscle tension.

- Blending with Essential Oils: Enhance the experience by blending castor oil with essential oils like lavender or eucalyptus for added therapeutic benefits.

Incorporating castor oil into your body skincare routine can transform the health and appearance of your skin. From intense hydration and scar healing to soothing irritations and providing luxurious body treatments, castor oil offers a multitude of benefits. By understanding and utilizing its properties, you can achieve soft, smooth, and radiant skin all over your body.

Chapter 4: Castor oil for specific skin conditions

Castor oil is a versatile skincare ingredient and a potent remedy for various skin conditions. Its anti-inflammatory, antimicrobial, and deeply moisturizing properties make it practical for managing chronic skin issues such as eczema, dermatitis, and psoriasis. This chapter delves into how castor oil can be used to alleviate the symptoms and improve the appearance of these specific skin conditions.

4.1 Eczema and Dermatitis

Eczema and dermatitis are common inflammatory skin conditions characterized by red, itchy, and inflamed patches of skin. Castor oil's unique composition provides a natural and gentle approach to managing these conditions.

4.1.1 Soothing Irritated and Inflamed Skin

Anti-inflammatory Properties

Ricinoleic Acid: The high concentration of ricinoleic acid in castor oil gives it powerful anti-inflammatory properties that help reduce swelling and redness associated with eczema and dermatitis.

Calming Effect: Applying castor oil to affected areas can soothe irritation and provide immediate relief from itching and discomfort.

Deep Moisturization

Hydration: Castor oil's ability to deeply penetrate the skin ensures long-lasting hydration, which is crucial for preventing flare-ups and maintaining skin health.

Barrier Protection: By forming a protective barrier on the skin's surface, castor oil helps lock in moisture and shield the skin from external irritants.

4.1.2 Managing Symptoms with Castor Oil

Regular Application:

Daily Use: Consistent application of castor oil on eczema-prone areas can help manage and reduce the frequency of flare-ups.

Massage and Absorption: Massaging castor oil into the skin enhances absorption and boosts blood circulation, promoting faster healing.

Combined Treatments:

Blending with Essential Oils: For enhanced benefits, blend castor oil with essential oils such as lavender or chamomile, which have soothing and anti-inflammatory properties.

Overnight Treatment: Apply a generous layer of castor oil to affected areas before bedtime and cover them with cotton gloves or socks to maximize hydration and healing overnight.

4.2 Psoriasis

Psoriasis is a chronic autoimmune condition that results in the rapid buildup of skin cells, leading to scaling, redness, and inflammation. Castor oil's hydrating and soothing properties make it an effective natural treatment for managing psoriasis symptoms.

4.2.1 Hydration and Calming of Psoriatic Skin

Deep Hydration

Moisture Retention: Castor oil's thick consistency helps retain moisture in the skin, preventing dryness and reducing the appearance of scales.

Nourishment: Its rich nutrient content nourishes the skin, promoting a healthier appearance and texture.

Calming Effect

Reduces Inflammation: The anti-inflammatory properties of ricinoleic acid help calm psoriatic skin, reducing redness and irritation.

Soothes Discomfort: Applying castor oil to psoriatic plaques can alleviate itching and discomfort, providing much-needed relief.

4.2.2 Reduce Scaling and Itching

Softening Scales

Exfoliating Action: Regular application of castor oil softens the thick scales associated with psoriasis, making them easier to remove and improving the skin's appearance.

Gentle Exfoliation: Combine castor oil with a mild exfoliant like oatmeal or sugar to gently slough off dead skin cells without causing further irritation.

Itch Relief

Anti-itch Properties: The moisturizing and anti-inflammatory properties of castor oil provide effective itch relief, reducing the urge to scratch and minimizing skin damage.

Cooling Sensation: For additional relief, mix castor oil with a few drops of peppermint oil to create a cooling sensation that soothes itchy skin.

Castor oil offers a natural and effective way to manage specific skin conditions like eczema, dermatitis, and psoriasis. Its anti-inflammatory, deeply moisturizing, and soothing properties help alleviate symptoms, promote healing, and improve the overall health and appearance of the skin. By incorporating castor oil into your skincare routine, you can achieve significant relief and better control over these chronic skin issues.

Chapter 5: DIY skin care recipes with castor oil

Creating your own skincare products at home allows you to tailor ingredients to meet your specific skin needs. Castor oil, with its rich, emollient properties, is a versatile base for a variety of DIY skincare recipes. This chapter explores how to make hydrating and nourishing facial masks, anti-aging and brightening face masks, and exfoliating body scrubs using castor oil. These simple, yet effective, recipes will help you achieve radiant, healthy skin.

5.1 Facial Masks

Facial masks are a great way to deliver concentrated nutrients to your skin. Castor oil's deep moisturizing properties make it an excellent base for creating masks that address different skin concerns.

Hydrating and Nourishing Masks for Different Skin Concerns

1) Hydrating Avocado and Castor Oil Mask

- Ingredients:
    - 1 ripe avocado
    - 1 tablespoon castor oil
    - 1 teaspoon honey
- Instructions:
1. Mash the avocado in a bowl until smooth.
2. Add the castor oil and honey, and mix well.
3. Apply the mask to your face, avoiding the eye area.
4. Leave on for 15-20 minutes, then rinse off with warm water.
    - Benefits: This mask is perfect for dry and dehydrated skin. Avocado is rich in healthy fats and vitamins, while honey is a natural humectant that attracts moisture to the skin.

2) Soothing Oatmeal and Castor Oil Mask

- Ingredients:
    - 2 tablespoons oatmeal

- o 1 tablespoon castor oil

- o 2 tablespoons yogurt

- Instructions:

1. Cook the oatmeal according to the package instructions and let it cool.

2. Mix the cooled oatmeal with castor oil and yogurt.

3. Apply the mixture to your face and let it sit for 15-20 minutes.

4. Rinse off with lukewarm water.

- Benefits: This mask is ideal for sensitive or irritated skin. Oatmeal has anti-inflammatory properties, and yogurt contains lactic acid, which gently exfoliates while soothing the skin.

Anti-aging and Brightening Face Masks

1) Anti-aging Banana and Castor Oil Mask

- Ingredients:

- o 1 ripe banana

- o 1 tablespoon castor oil

- o 1 teaspoon rosehip oil

- Instructions:

1. Mash the banana in a bowl until smooth.

2. Add the castor oil and rosehip oil, and mix thoroughly.

3. Apply the mask evenly to your face.

4. Leave it on for 15-20 minutes, then rinse off with warm water.

- Benefits: Bananas are rich in vitamins A and E, which help to reduce the appearance of fine lines and wrinkles. Rosehip oil is known for its ability to promote skin regeneration and improve skin tone.

2) Brightening Turmeric and Castor Oil Mask

- Ingredients:

- o 1 tablespoon turmeric powder

- o 1 tablespoon castor oil

- o 2 tablespoons plain yogurt

- Instructions:

1. Mix the turmeric powder, castor oil, and yogurt in a bowl until you have a smooth paste.

2. Apply the mask to your face, avoiding the eye area.

3. Leave it on for 10-15 minutes, then rinse off with lukewarm water.

- Benefits: Turmeric is known for its brightening and anti-inflammatory properties. Combined with the moisturizing effects of castor oil and the gentle exfoliation from yogurt, this mask can help improve skin tone and texture.

5.2 Body Scrubs and Exfoliants

Exfoliating is an essential part of any skincare routine as it helps to remove dead skin cells, revealing smoother, more radiant skin underneath. Castor oil can be used to create effective body scrubs that not only exfoliate but also moisturize the skin.

Exfoliating Dry Skin with Castor Oil Scrubs

1) Sugar and Castor Oil Body Scrub

- Ingredients:
    - 1 cup granulated sugar
    - 1/2 cup castor oil
    - 10 drops of your favorite essential oil (optional)
- Instructions:

1. Combine the sugar and castor oil in a bowl and mix well.

2. Add the essential oil if desired and stir to combine.

3. In the shower, apply the scrub to wet skin and massage in circular motions.

4. Rinse off with warm water and pat dry.

- Benefits: Sugar is a natural exfoliant that gently removes dead skin cells. The castor oil provides deep hydration, leaving the skin feeling soft and smooth. Essential oils can be added for a pleasant fragrance and additional skin benefits.

2) Coffee and Castor Oil Body Scrub

- Ingredients:
    - 1 cup coffee grounds
    - 1/2 cup castor oil
    - 1/4 cup brown sugar
- Instructions:

1.   Mix the coffee grounds, castor oil, and brown sugar in a bowl.

2.   Apply the scrub to wet skin in the shower, massaging in circular motions.

3.   Focus on rough areas like elbows, knees, and feet.

4.   Rinse thoroughly with warm water and pat dry.

- Benefits: Coffee grounds help to improve blood circulation and reduce the appearance of cellulite. Brown sugar acts as a gentle exfoliant, while castor oil moisturizes the skin, leaving it soft and nourished.

Softening and Smoothing Body Exfoliants

1) Sea Salt and Castor Oil Scrub

- Ingredients:

    o   1 cup sea salt

    o   1/2 cup castor oil

    o   Zest of one lemon

- Instructions:

1.   Combine the sea salt and castor oil in a bowl.

2.   Add the lemon zest and mix thoroughly.

3.   In the shower, apply the scrub to wet skin and massage gently.

4.   Rinse off with warm water and pat dry.

- Benefits: Sea salt is a natural exfoliant that helps to detoxify and cleanse the skin. The lemon zest adds a refreshing scent and brightening effect, while castor oil hydrates and softens the skin.

2) Almond and Castor Oil Scrub

- Ingredients:

    o   1 cup finely ground almonds

    o   1/2 cup castor oil

    o   1 tablespoon honey

- Instructions:

1.   Mix the ground almonds, castor oil, and honey in a bowl until well combined.

2.   Apply the scrub to wet skin, massaging in gentle, circular motions.

3.   Rinse thoroughly with warm water and pat dry.

- Benefits: Ground almonds provide gentle exfoliation, honey acts as a natural humectant and antibacterial agent, and castor oil deeply moisturizes, leaving the skin feeling soft and smooth.

Creating your own skincare products with castor oil allows you to customize treatments to meet your skin's unique needs. Whether you're looking to hydrate and nourish your face, reduce the signs of aging, brighten your complexion, or exfoliate and soften your body, castor oil is a versatile and effective ingredient. By incorporating these DIY recipes into your skincare routine, you can achieve healthy, glowing skin in a natural and cost-effective way.

Chapter 6: Advanced Skincare Techniques

As you delve deeper into skincare, incorporating advanced techniques can significantly enhance the effectiveness of your regimen. With its multifaceted benefits, castor oil can be a valuable addition to these advanced practices. This chapter explores integrating castor oil into advanced skin care techniques, including facial steaming, oil cleansing methods, lymphatic drainage massage, and overnight treatments. These methods will help you maximize the benefits of castor oil for your skin, ensuring a healthier, more radiant complexion.

6.1 Facial Steaming with Castor Oil

1. Benefits of Facial Steaming

Facial steaming with castor oil is a powerful technique that opens up pores, allowing for deeper cleansing and better absorption of skincare products. This method, with its unique benefits, is a key part of advanced skincare techniques.

Improves Circulation: The heat from the steam increases blood circulation, which can lead to a brighter complexion.

Promotes Relaxation: Steaming can be a soothing experience, helping to reduce stress and promote relaxation.

2. How to Incorporate Castor Oil

Pre-steam Preparation: Cleanse your face thoroughly to remove any makeup or surface impurities. Apply a thin layer of castor oil to your face, focusing on areas prone to congestion.

Steaming Process: Fill a bowl with hot water and add a few drops of essential oils like eucalyptus or lavender for additional benefits. Lean over the bowl, covering your head with a towel to trap the steam. Steam your face for 5-10 minutes.

Post-steam Care: After steaming, gently wipe your face with a soft towel to remove excess oil and impurities. Follow up with your regular skincare routine, including toner and moisturizer.

6.2 Oil Cleansing Method

1. Understanding the Oil Cleansing Method (OCM)

Principle: The oil cleansing method uses oils to dissolve and remove impurities, makeup, and excess sebum from the skin.

Benefits: OCM helps maintain the skin's natural moisture balance, reduces the occurrence of blackheads and breakouts, and leaves the skin feeling soft and hydrated.

2. Using Castor Oil for OCM

Choosing the Right Oil Mix: Castor oil is often blended with other carrier oils like jojoba, olive, or grapeseed oil to suit different skin types. For oily skin, use a higher ratio of castor oil (30%); for dry skin, use a lower ratio (10-20%).

Application Process: Pour a small amount of the oil blend into your hands and massage it onto your dry face for 1-2 minutes. Focus on areas with makeup, congestion, or dryness.

Removal: Soak a washcloth in warm water, wring it out, and place it over your face for 30 seconds to a minute. Gently wipe away the oil and impurities. Repeat, if necessary, then rinse your face with cool water.

6.3 Lymphatic Drainage Massage

1. Benefits of Lymphatic Drainage

Lymphatic drainage massage is a gentle technique that offers multiple benefits. It helps reduce facial puffiness by encouraging the drainage of lymphatic fluids, improves skin tone and texture, and aids in detoxifying the skin, removing waste products, and reducing inflammation.

Improves Skin Tone: Regular lymphatic drainage can improve skin tone and texture, promoting a youthful appearance.

Detoxifies: It aids in detoxifying the skin, removing waste products, and reducing inflammation.

2. Incorporating Castor Oil

Preparation: Start with a clean face and apply a small amount of castor oil to your skin to provide a smooth surface for the massage.

Technique: Using gentle pressure, use your fingertips to massage in upward and outward motions along your jawline, cheeks, and forehead. Focus on areas where lymph nodes are located, such as under the jaw and around the neck.

Duration: Perform the massage for 5-10 minutes, then follow up with your regular skincare routine.

6.4 Overnight Treatments with Castor Oil

1. Benefits of Overnight Treatments

Extended Hydration: Leaving castor oil on your skin overnight allows for extended hydration and nourishment.

Enhanced Repair: Overnight treatments can enhance the skin's natural repair processes, leading to improved texture and appearance.

Deep Penetration: The extended contact time allows castor oil to penetrate deeply into the skin, delivering its beneficial properties more effectively.

2. Overnight Treatment Techniques

Pure Castor Oil Application: For intense hydration, apply a thin layer of castor oil to your face and neck before bed. Massage gently until absorbed. Ensure you use a pillowcase that can withstand oil stains.

Customized Oil Blends: Blend castor oil with other nourishing oils like argan or rosehip oil to create a customized overnight treatment. This can enhance specific benefits such as anti-aging or brightening.

Targeted Treatments: Apply castor oil to specific problem areas, such as dry patches, fine lines, or acne spots. Cover these areas with a thin layer of oil and leave it on overnight.

6.5 Advanced Exfoliation Techniques

1. Chemical Exfoliation

- AHAs and BHAs: Alpha-hydroxy acids (AHAs) and beta-hydroxy acids (BHAs) are effective for chemical exfoliation, removing dead skin cells and promoting cell turnover.

- Combining with Castor Oil: After using a chemical exfoliant, apply castor oil to soothe and hydrate the skin. This helps to mitigate any potential irritation and enhances the exfoliation results.

2. Physical Exfoliation

- Microdermabrasion: This technique uses a device to gently exfoliate the outer layer of the skin, improving texture and appearance.

- Post-treatment Care: After a microdermabrasion session, apply castor oil to help calm the skin and provide intense moisture, aiding in the skin's recovery process.

6.6 Castor Oil Packs

1. Benefits of Castor Oil Packs

- Detoxification: Castor oil packs are used to detoxify the skin and improve overall skin health.

- Reduces Inflammation: They help reduce inflammation and can be used on areas with chronic pain or swelling.

2. How to Use Castor Oil Packs

- Preparation: Soak a piece of flannel or cotton cloth in castor oil. Apply it to the area you wish to treat.

- Application: Cover the cloth with plastic wrap and place a heating pad or hot water bottle on top. Leave it on for 30-60 minutes.

- Post-treatment: After removing the pack, cleanse the area with a mild soap and water. Follow up with a moisturizer if needed.

Incorporating advanced skincare techniques with castor oil can significantly enhance your skincare routine. From facial steaming and oil cleansing to lymphatic drainage massage and overnight treatments, castor oil offers numerous benefits that can transform your skin's health and appearance.

By understanding and applying these advanced methods, you can achieve a radiant, youthful complexion while addressing specific skin concerns more effectively. Embrace the power of castor oil in your advanced skincare regimen for optimal results.

Chapter 7: Incorporating castor oil into your daily skin care routine

Consistency is critical to achieving and maintaining healthy skin. Incorporating castor oil into your daily skincare routine can offer numerous benefits, from deep hydration to anti-inflammatory effects. This chapter will guide you through the steps to seamlessly integrate castor oil into your daily regimen, ensuring you maximize its properties for radiant and healthy skin.

7.1 Morning Skincare Routine

1. Cleansing

Step-by-step Guide:

Gentle Cleanser: Start your day with a gentle, non-stripping cleanser to remove nighttime oils and impurities. Look for a product that balances the skin's pH.

Optional: Oil Cleansing: If you prefer, use a small amount of castor oil as a cleanser. Massage it onto dry skin, then remove it with a warm, damp cloth. This method is particularly beneficial for dry or sensitive skin types.

Benefits:

Hydration: Castor oil helps maintain skin moisture, preventing dryness throughout the day.

Cleansing: Its natural antimicrobial properties help to keep the skin clear and healthy.

2. Toning

Step-by-step Guide:

Choose the Right Toner: After cleansing, apply a hydrating toner. Look for ingredients like hyaluronic acid or rose water.

Application: Apply the toner with a cotton pad or your hands, gently pressing it into your skin.

Benefits:

Balance: Toners help to restore the skin's natural pH balance.

Preparation: Prepares your skin for the next steps in your skincare routine, enhancing absorption.

3. Moisturizing

Step-by-step Guide:

Blend with Moisturizer: Mix a few drops of castor oil with your regular moisturizer. This helps to enhance the moisturizing effect.

Application: Apply the blend evenly over your face and neck, massaging gently.

Benefits:

Hydration: Provides deep, lasting moisture.

Barrier Protection: Helps to lock in hydration and protect against environmental damage.

4. Sunscreen

Step-by-step Guide:

Choose a Broad-spectrum Sunscreen: Select a sunscreen with at least SPF 30.

Application: Apply generously over your face and neck, ensuring even coverage.

Benefits:

Protection: Shields your skin from harmful UV rays, preventing premature aging and skin damage.

Enhances Overall Skincare: Sunscreen is a crucial final step to protect the benefits of your skincare routine.

7.2 Evening Skincare Routine

1. Makeup Removal

Step-by-step Guide:

Castor Oil for Removal: Use castor oil to remove makeup, especially waterproof products. Apply a small amount to a cotton pad and gently wipe away makeup.

Follow with Cleanser: After removing makeup, cleanse your skin with a gentle cleanser to ensure all residues are gone.

Benefits:

Effective Removal: Castor oil efficiently breaks down makeup without harsh chemicals.

Nourishing: Leaves the skin feeling soft and moisturized after makeup removal.

2. Deep Cleansing

Step-by-step Guide:

Double Cleansing: Start with an oil cleanser (like castor oil) followed by a water-based cleanser. This ensures thorough cleansing without stripping the skin.

Application: Massage the oil cleanser onto dry skin, then use a foaming or gel cleanser on wet skin.

Benefits:

Thorough Cleansing: Removes all traces of makeup, sunscreen, and impurities.

Maintains Balance: Helps to keep the skin's natural oils intact.

3. Toning

Step-by-step Guide:

Hydrating Toner: Use the same hydrating toner as in the morning routine.

Application: Apply with a cotton pad or your hands, pressing it gently into the skin.

Benefits:

Prep for Treatment: Prepare your skin to absorb treatments more effectively.

Soothing: Castor oil is a gentle soother, calming and refreshing the skin after cleansing, providing a comforting experience.

4. Treatments and Serums

Step-by-step Guide:

Targeted Treatments: Apply any targeted treatments, such as serums for acne, hyperpigmentation, or anti-aging.

Layering: Apply lighter serums first, followed by thicker ones.

Benefits:

Customized Care: Addresses specific skin concerns with targeted ingredients.

Enhanced Results: By incorporating castor oil into your skincare routine, you can significantly improve the efficacy of your skincare routine, boosting your confidence and motivation.

5. Moisturizing and Overnight Care

Step-by-step Guide:

Night Cream: Use a nourishing night cream or facial oil. Add a few drops of castor oil for extra hydration.

Application: Apply evenly over your face and neck, massaging gently.

Benefits:

Repair and Renew: Supports the skin's natural repair processes overnight.

Deep Hydration: Ensures the skin stays hydrated and nourished.

7.3 Weekly Skincare Enhancements

1. Exfoliation

Step-by-step Guide:

Exfoliating Scrub: Use a gentle scrub 1-2 times a week. Mix castor oil with a natural exfoliant like sugar or coffee grounds.

Application: Apply to damp skin and massage gently in circular motions. Rinse with warm water.

Benefits:

Removes Dead Skin Cells: Promotes cell turnover and smooths the skin.

Enhances Glow: Reveals a brighter, more radiant complexion.

2. Masks

Step-by-step Guide:

Hydrating Mask: Use a hydrating mask once a week. Apply a castor oil-based mask for deep moisture.

Application: Apply the mask to clean skin and leave it on for 15-20 minutes. Rinse with warm water and follow with your regular routine.

Benefits:

Intense Hydration: Provides an extra boost of moisture.

Rejuvenation: Helps to rejuvenate and refresh the skin.

3. Specialized Treatments

Step-by-step Guide:

Spot Treatments: Use castor oil as a spot treatment for acne or dry patches. Apply a small amount directly to the affected area.

Overnight Treatments: For deeper hydration, apply a thin layer of castor oil to your face before bed once a week.

Benefits:

Targeted Care: Addresses specific skin issues effectively.

Enhanced Hydration: Provides intense moisture to combat dryness.

7.4 Tips for Integrating Castor Oil

1. Patch Test

Importance: Always perform a patch test before integrating castor oil into your routine to ensure you don't have an adverse reaction.

2. Customize to Your Skin Type

Dry Skin: Use castor oil more frequently and combine it with other hydrating ingredients.

Oily/Combination Skin: Use castor oil sparingly and focus on areas prone to dryness.

Sensitive Skin: Mix castor oil with a gentle carrier oil like jojoba to reduce potential irritation.

3. Consistency is Key

Daily Use: For best results, incorporate castor oil into your daily routine. Consistent use will maximize its benefits.

Monitor Results: Keep track of how your skin responds to ensure that castor oil is benefiting your routine. Adjust usage as needed based on your skin's needs.

Integrating castor oil into your daily skincare routine can provide a myriad of benefits, from deep hydration and nourishment to enhanced skin texture and appearance. Following the outlined steps and tips, you can seamlessly incorporate this versatile oil into your morning and evening routines. Consistency and customization are essential to unlocking the full potential of castor oil, ensuring your skin remains healthy, radiant, and resilient. Embrace castor oil as a staple in your skincare regimen and experience the transformative effects it can offer.

BOOK 3: Castor Oil for Hair Care

Castor Oil for Hair Care

Get Luxuriant Locks with Nature's Secret Remedy

By

Vincent Vega

Disclaimer notice

Please be aware that the information provided in this document is intended solely for educational and entertainment purposes. Every effort has been made to ensure the content is accurate, reliable, current, and complete.

However, no guarantees, either explicit or implicit, are made. Readers acknowledge that the author is not providing legal, financial, medical, or professional advice.

The content has been sourced from various references. It is strongly recommended that you consult a licensed professional before attempting any of the of the methods described in this document.

By reading this document, you agree that the author is not liable for any direct or indirect losses resulting from the use of the information within, including but not limited to errors, omissions, or inaccuracies.

Chapter 1: Understanding hair structure and growth

Understanding hair's structure and growth cycle is fundamental to appreciating how castor oil can benefit hair health. This chapter provides a comprehensive overview of hair anatomy, the phases of the hair growth cycle, and the factors that influence hair health. With this foundational knowledge, you will be better equipped to make informed decisions about your hair care routine.

1.1 Anatomy of Hair

Hair is a complex structure composed of several layers, each with a specific function. Knowing these layers helps us understand how different treatments, including those with castor oil, can impact hair health.

Hair Shaft

Cuticle: The outermost layer, composed of overlapping cells that protect the inner layers. A healthy cuticle ensures smooth, shiny hair.

Cortex: The middle layer, rich in keratin and pigments. It provides strength, color, and elasticity to the hair.

Medulla: The innermost layer, often absent in finer hair. Its function is not fully understood but may contribute to the overall strength of the hair shaft.

Hair Follicle

Follicle Structure: The hair follicle is a tunnel-like segment of the epidermis that extends into the dermis. It is the root of the hair, where growth begins.

Dermal Papilla: Located at the follicle's base, it supplies nutrients and oxygen to the hair through a network of blood vessels.

Sebaceous Glands: These glands produce sebum, an oily substance that conditions the hair and scalp.

Hair Bulb

Hair Matrix: The growth zone within the hair bulb where cells divide rapidly to form new hair.

Melanocytes: Cells that produce melanin, giving hair its color.

1.2 Hair Growth Cycle

Hair growth follows a cycle composed of three main phases. Each phase plays a crucial role in your hair's length, strength, and health.

Anagen Phase

Active Growth: This is the active growth phase, lasting between 2 to 7 years. During this period, cells in the hair bulb rapidly divide, adding length to the hair shaft.

Duration: The length of the anagen phase determines how long your hair can grow. Factors such as genetics, health, and age influence this duration.

Catagen Phase

Transitional Phase: Lasting about 2 to 3 weeks, the catagen phase is a short transitional stage where hair growth slows down, and the hair follicle begins to shrink.

End of Active Growth: The hair detaches from the blood supply but remains in place within the follicle.

Telogen Phase

Resting Phase: Lasting around 3 months, this phase is when the hair follicle remains dormant. Old hair is eventually shed, and new hair begins to grow, starting a new cycle.

Shedding: It is normal to lose about 50-100 hairs daily as part of this phase.

1.3 Factors Affecting Hair Health

Several factors influence hair health, from genetic predispositions to external conditions. Understanding these can help you take better care of your hair and optimize your use of castor oil.

1) Genetics

Hereditary Traits: Genetics play a significant role in determining hair characteristics such as texture, density, and growth rate.

Pattern Baldness: Conditions like male and female pattern baldness are largely influenced by genetic factors.

2) Nutrition

Dietary Impact: A balanced diet rich in vitamins, minerals, and proteins is essential for healthy hair growth. Nutrients like biotin, vitamin E, and omega-3 fatty acids are particularly beneficial.

Deficiencies: Lack of essential nutrients can lead to hair thinning, dullness, and increased hair loss.

3) Hormonal Changes

Life Stages: Hormonal fluctuations during puberty, pregnancy, menopause, and andropause can significantly impact hair growth and health.

Conditions: Hormonal disorders like thyroid imbalances can lead to hair issues.

4) Lifestyle Factors

Stress: Chronic stress can disrupt the hair growth cycle, leading to increased hair shedding and thinning.

Sleep: Adequate sleep is crucial for the body's repair and regeneration processes, including hair growth.

Exercise: Regular physical activity improves blood circulation, which helps deliver essential nutrients to the hair follicles.

5) Environmental Influences

Pollution: Exposure to pollutants can damage the hair and scalp, leading to dryness, breakage, and scalp irritation.

Weather: Extreme weather conditions, such as intense sun exposure, cold, and humidity, can affect hair health.

Chemical Treatments: Frequent chemical treatments like coloring, perming, and relaxing can weaken hair structure.

6) Hair Care Practices

Gentle Handling: Avoiding harsh brushing, tight hairstyles, and rough towel drying can prevent breakage and hair loss.

Product Choice: Using the right hair care products, including those containing castor oil, can improve hair health. Opt for products free from sulfates, parabens, and silicones.

Understanding the structure and growth cycle of hair and the factors that affect its health provides a solid foundation for effective hair care. With this knowledge, you can better appreciate the benefits of incorporating castor oil into your hair care routine.

Castor oil's moisturizing, strengthening, and nourishing properties make it an excellent choice for promoting healthy hair growth and overall health. By considering the unique needs of your hair and the various factors that influence its health, you can develop a comprehensive hair care regimen that ensures your hair remains strong, vibrant, and resilient.

Chapter 2: Properties and composition of castor oil for hair

Castor oil, derived from the seeds of the castor plant (Ricinus communis), has been used for centuries for its remarkable therapeutic and cosmetic properties. In hair care, castor oil is celebrated for its ability to moisturize, strengthen, and promote hair growth. This chapter delves into the unique properties and composition of castor oil that make it an essential component in hair care routines.

2.1 Chemical Composition of Castor Oil

Understanding the chemical makeup of castor oil is key to appreciating its benefits for hair. The oil is rich in fatty acids, vitamins, and other nutrients that contribute to its effectiveness.

Fatty Acids

- Ricinoleic Acid: This is the most prominent fatty acid in castor oil, comprising about 90% of its content. Ricinoleic acid is known for its anti-inflammatory and antimicrobial properties, which help maintain a healthy scalp environment.

- Oleic Acid: This monounsaturated fatty acid is known for its moisturizing properties. It helps to seal in moisture, making hair softer and more manageable.

- Linoleic Acid: An essential polyunsaturated fatty acid, linoleic acid helps to balance scalp oils and maintain the health of hair follicles.

- Stearic Acid: This saturated fatty acid has cleansing properties and helps to protect the hair by forming a protective barrier on the hair shaft.

Vitamins and Minerals

- Vitamin E: An antioxidant that helps to repair and build tissue, vitamin E is essential for healthy hair growth. It helps to prevent oxidative stress and promotes blood circulation to the scalp.

- Omega-6 Fatty Acids: These are crucial for hair growth and overall scalp health. They help to stimulate hair follicles and promote hair regeneration.

Other Nutrients

- Proteins: Castor oil contains small amounts of proteins that help to strengthen hair and repair damage.

- Sterols: Plant-based sterols in castor oil help to reduce inflammation and support a healthy scalp.

2.2 Unique Properties of Castor Oil

The chemical composition of castor oil gives it several unique properties that are beneficial for hair care. These properties help to address common hair concerns and improve overall hair health.

1) Moisturizing Properties

Deep Hydration: Castor oil is an excellent humectant, meaning it helps to retain moisture. When applied to hair, it penetrates deeply into the hair shaft, providing intense hydration and preventing dryness.

Scalp Moisturization: The oil's ability to moisturize extends to the scalp as well, helping to alleviate dryness and flakiness. This is particularly beneficial for individuals with dry or irritated scalps.

2) Anti-inflammatory and Antimicrobial Properties

Scalp Health: Ricinoleic acid's anti-inflammatory properties help to soothe irritated and inflamed scalps. This can be particularly beneficial for conditions like dandruff and seborrheic dermatitis.

Preventing Infections: The antimicrobial properties of castor oil help to keep the scalp free from infections that can impede hair growth. This includes bacterial and fungal infections that can cause scalp issues and hair loss.

3) Strengthening Properties

Protein-Rich: The proteins in castor oil help to strengthen the hair shaft, reducing the likelihood of breakage and split ends. This is especially important for damaged or chemically treated hair.

Elasticity and Flexibility: Regular use of castor oil can improve the elasticity and flexibility of hair, making it less prone to breakage during styling and brushing.

4) Promoting Hair Growth

Stimulating Hair Follicles: Castor oil's high concentration of ricinoleic acid helps to increase blood circulation to the scalp. Improved circulation ensures that hair follicles receive the necessary nutrients and oxygen to grow healthy hair.

Reducing Hair Loss: By keeping the scalp healthy and free from infections, and by providing essential nutrients, castor oil can help to reduce hair loss and promote thicker, fuller hair.

2.3 Why Castor Oil Works for Hair

The unique properties and chemical composition of castor oil make it a powerful tool in hair care. Let's explore how these elements come together to benefit different aspects of hair health.

Moisturizing and Conditioning

Hydration: Castor oil's ability to retain moisture makes it an excellent conditioner for dry and frizzy hair. By sealing in moisture, it keeps hair hydrated, smooth, and manageable.

Softening: The fatty acids in castor oil soften the hair, making it easier to detangle and style. This can help to prevent breakage and improve the overall appearance of the hair.

Enhancing Scalp Health

Reducing Inflammation: The anti-inflammatory properties of ricinoleic acid help to reduce scalp inflammation, which can be caused by conditions such as dandruff, eczema, and psoriasis.

Preventing Infections: The antimicrobial properties of castor oil protect the scalp from infections that can lead to hair loss and scalp discomfort. This includes preventing fungal infections that cause dandruff and other scalp issues.

Strengthening Hair

Repairing Damage: The proteins and fatty acids in castor oil help to repair damaged hair by filling in gaps in the hair shaft. This strengthens the hair from within, making it less prone to breakage.

Improving Elasticity: Regular use of castor oil can improve the elasticity of hair, making it more resilient to stretching and styling. This is particularly beneficial for individuals with brittle or damaged hair.

Stimulating Hair Growth

Nutrient Delivery: By increasing blood circulation to the scalp, castor oil ensures that hair follicles receive the necessary nutrients to promote healthy hair growth. This can lead to thicker, fuller hair over time.

Reducing Hair Loss: Castor oil's ability to strengthen hair and maintain a healthy scalp environment helps to reduce hair loss. This makes it an excellent choice for individuals experiencing thinning hair or hair loss.

The properties and composition of castor oil make it a highly effective solution for a wide range of hair care needs. Its unique blend of fatty acids, vitamins, and proteins work together to moisturize, strengthen, and promote the growth of healthy hair. By understanding these properties, you can better appreciate how castor oil can be integrated into your hair care routine to achieve optimal results.

Whether you are looking to hydrate dry hair, reduce scalp inflammation, or stimulate hair growth, castor oil offers a natural and effective solution. Embrace the benefits of castor oil and experience the transformative effects it can have on your hair.

Chapter 3: Types of castor oil for hair

Castor oil is renowned for its numerous benefits for hair health, but not all castor oil is created equal. There are several types of castor oil available, each with distinct properties and uses. This chapter explores the various types of castor oil, their unique characteristics, and how they can be best utilized for different hair care needs.

3.1 Types of Castor Oil

1. Cold-Pressed Castor Oil

2. Jamaican Black Castor Oil

3. Hydrogenated Castor Oil

4. Comparing Types

3.1.1 Cold-Pressed Castor Oil

Cold-pressed castor oil is extracted by pressing the castor seeds without applying heat. This method preserves the oil's natural nutrients, making it a pure and potent product.

Characteristics

Color and Consistency: Cold-pressed castor oil is usually pale yellow in color and has a thick, viscous consistency.

Nutrient Content: This type of castor oil retains most of its natural nutrients, including fatty acids, vitamins, and minerals, due to the lack of heat during extraction.

Benefits for Hair

Moisturizing: Cold-pressed castor oil is an excellent moisturizer. It penetrates deep into the hair shaft, providing long-lasting hydration.

Strengthening: The high ricinoleic acid content strengthens hair, reducing breakage and split ends.

Scalp Health: Its antimicrobial and anti-inflammatory properties help maintain a healthy scalp, preventing dandruff and scalp infections.

Best Uses

Deep Conditioning: Ideal for deep conditioning treatments to restore moisture and strength to dry, damaged hair.

Scalp Massages: This is effective for scalp massages to improve blood circulation and promote hair growth.

Leave-In Treatments: Can be used as a leave-in conditioner to maintain moisture throughout the day.

3.1.2 Jamaican Black Castor Oil

Jamaican Black Castor Oil (JBCO) is made by roasting the castor seeds before extracting the oil. The ashes from the roasted seeds are then added to the oil, giving it its distinctive dark color.

Characteristics

Color and Consistency: JBCO is dark brown or black due to the ash content and has a thick, dense consistency.

Nutrient Content: The roasting process enhances specific oil properties, making it particularly effective for hair care.

Benefits for Hair

Promoting Hair Growth: JBCO is highly effective in promoting hair growth. The ash content from the roasting process increases the oil's pH level, which helps to open hair cuticles and allows better absorption of nutrients.

Strengthening and Thickening: Regular use of JBCO can strengthen and thicken hair, making it an excellent choice for individuals with thin or weak hair.

Scalp Health: The antimicrobial and anti-inflammatory properties help to treat and prevent scalp conditions such as dandruff and itching.

Best Uses

Growth Treatments: Ideal for hair growth treatments and remedies targeting thinning hair or bald spots.

Thickening Solutions: Effective for those seeking to add volume and thickness to their hair.

Scalp Treatments: Beneficial for addressing scalp issues and maintaining overall scalp health.

3.1.3 Hydrogenated Castor Oil

Hydrogenated castor oil, also known as castor wax, is produced by adding hydrogen to the oil. This process transforms the oil into a solid or semi-solid waxy substance.

Characteristics

Color and Consistency: Hydrogenated castor oil is white or pale yellow and has a thick, waxy consistency.

Nutrient Content: The hydrogenation process alters the oil's composition, making it less likely to oxidize and extending its shelf life.

Benefits for Hair

Moisture Retention: The waxy consistency of hydrogenated castor oil helps to seal in moisture, providing long-lasting hydration.

Protection: It forms a protective barrier on the hair shaft, shielding it from environmental damage and preventing moisture loss.

Styling Aid: Due to its thick, waxy nature, it can be used as a styling aid to add shine and hold to hairstyles.

Best Uses

Protective Styles: Ideal for use in protective hairstyles, such as braids and twists, to maintain moisture and prevent damage.

Styling Products: These can be incorporated into styling products like pomades and hair waxes to add hold and shine.

Long-Lasting Moisture: Suitable for individuals looking for a long-lasting moisture sealant, particularly in dry climates.

3.2 Comparing Types

Each type of castor oil offers unique benefits and is suited to different hair care needs. Understanding the differences can help you choose the right type for your hair.

Moisturizing Properties

Cold-Pressed Castor Oil: Provides deep hydration and is excellent for overall moisture maintenance.

Jamaican Black Castor Oil: Also moisturizing but with added benefits for hair growth and thickening.

Hydrogenated Castor Oil: Best for sealing in moisture and providing long-lasting hydration.

Strengthening and Growth

Cold-Pressed Castor Oil: Strengthens hair and reduces breakage.

Jamaican Black Castor Oil: Exceptional for promoting growth and thickening weak or thin hair.

Hydrogenated Castor Oil: Provides a protective barrier but is less focused on growth stimulation.

Scalp Health

Cold-Pressed Castor Oil: Maintains scalp health with antimicrobial and anti-inflammatory properties.

Jamaican Black Castor Oil: Particularly effective for treating and preventing scalp conditions.

Hydrogenated Castor Oil: Less commonly used for scalp health, more for styling and moisture retention.

Best Uses

Cold-Pressed Castor Oil: Ideal for deep conditioning, scalp massages, and leave-in treatments.

Jamaican Black Castor Oil: Best for growth treatments, thickening solutions, and scalp treatments.

Hydrogenated Castor Oil: Suitable for protective styles, styling products, and long-lasting moisture.

Choosing the right type of castor oil for your hair can significantly improve the effectiveness of your hair care routine. Cold-pressed castor oil, with its nutrient-rich composition, is excellent for moisturizing and strengthening hair. With its enhanced properties from the roasting process, Jamaican Black Castor Oil is ideal for promoting hair growth and thickening. Hydrogenated castor oil, with its waxy consistency, is perfect for sealing in moisture and providing protection.

Chapter 4: Benefits of castor oil for hair

Castor oil, with its unique composition and properties, has long been revered for its versatility and effectiveness in addressing various hair concerns. In this chapter, we will delve into the myriad benefits of castor oil for hair, from moisturizing and strengthening to promoting growth and maintaining scalp health.

4.1 Moisturizing and Conditioning

4.1.1 Deep Hydration

Castor oil is an excellent natural moisturizer due to its high content of ricinoleic acid, a fatty acid known for its ability to retain moisture. This makes it particularly effective in providing deep hydration to the hair and scalp.

Hydrates Dry Hair: Castor oil penetrates the hair shaft, locking in moisture and preventing dryness. It especially benefits individuals with dry, brittle hair that needs intense hydration.

Conditions Scalp: By moisturizing the scalp, castor oil helps to reduce flakiness and dryness, which can lead to dandruff and other scalp issues.

4.1.2 Improves Manageability

Well-moisturized hair is easier to manage. The conditioning properties of castor oil make hair softer and smoother, reducing frizz and making it easier to style.

Reduces Frizz: By sealing in moisture, castor oil helps to smooth the hair cuticle, reducing frizz and flyaways.

Enhances Shine: Regular castor oil adds a natural shine to the hair, making it look healthier and more vibrant.

4.1.3 Increases Elasticity

Castor oil is rich in proteins and fatty acids that strengthen the hair shaft, improving its Elasticity and reducing the likelihood of breakage.

Prevents Breakage: Strengthened hair is less prone to breakage, which helps in maintaining length and achieving thicker hair.

Reduces Split Ends: Regular application of castor oil can help to seal split ends, preventing further damage and promoting healthier-looking hair.

4.1.4 Repairs Damage

The nourishing properties of castor oil can help repair hair damaged by heat, chemical treatments, and environmental factors.

Protects Against Heat Damage: Using castor oil as a pre-treatment before heat styling can protect the hair from damage caused by high temperatures.

Restores Chemically Treated Hair: Castor oil can help to repair and restore hair that has been damaged by chemical treatments such as coloring, perming, or relaxing.

4.2 Promoting Hair Growth

One of the most notable benefits of castor oil is its ability to promote hair growth. The high concentration of ricinoleic acid helps to improve blood circulation to the scalp, stimulating the hair follicles.

Encourages New Growth: Improved blood flow to the scalp ensures that hair follicles receive the necessary nutrients and oxygen to grow healthy hair.

Reduces Hair Loss: By strengthening the hair and maintaining a healthy scalp environment, castor oil can help to reduce hair loss and promote the growth of thicker, fuller hair.

Castor oil is packed with essential nutrients for hair growth, including vitamin E, omega-6 fatty acids, and proteins.

Supports Healthy Growth: These nutrients nourish the hair follicles, supporting healthy hair growth and improving the overall condition of the hair.

Boosts Thickness: Regular use of castor oil can lead to thicker, denser hair, making it an excellent choice for individuals with thinning hair.

4.3 Maintaining Scalp Health

Anti-inflammatory Properties

The anti-inflammatory properties of castor oil make it a soothing balm for irritated and inflamed scalps. This can bring a sense of relief to individuals dealing with conditions such as dandruff, eczema, or psoriasis.

Soothes Scalp Irritation: The anti-inflammatory properties help to reduce scalp redness and irritation, promoting a healthier scalp environment.

Prevents Flakiness: By moisturizing the scalp and reducing inflammation, castor oil helps to prevent flakiness and dandruff.

Antimicrobial Effects

The antimicrobial properties of castor oil act as a shield, keeping the scalp clean and free from infections. This is crucial for maintaining a healthy scalp and preventing conditions that can hinder hair growth.

Castor oil's antimicrobial properties play a crucial role in preventing and treating bacterial and fungal infections of the scalp, thereby contributing to a healthy scalp and promoting hair growth.

Reduces Dandruff: Regular use of castor oil can help to reduce dandruff, keeping the scalp clean and flake-free.

4.4 Enhancing Hair Appearance

Adds Shine

Castor oil can significantly enhance the appearance of hair by adding a natural shine. The oil smooths the hair cuticle, reflecting light and giving the hair a glossy, healthy look.

Natural Shine: Unlike synthetic shine-enhancing products, castor oil provides a natural shine without leaving a greasy residue.

Healthy Appearance: Shiny hair looks healthier and more vibrant, enhancing your overall appearance.

Improves Texture

Regular castor oil can improve the texture of your hair, making it softer and smoother. This is particularly beneficial for individuals with coarse or curly hair.

Softens Hair: The conditioning properties of castor oil make hair softer to the touch, improving its overall texture.

Smoothes Curls: For those with curly hair, castor oil can help to define curls and reduce frizz, making curls look more polished and controlled.

4.5 Versatility in Hair Care

One of the great advantages of castor oil is its versatility. It is suitable for all hair types, whether you have straight, wavy, curly, or coyly hair.

Adapts to Needs: Castor oil can be adapted to suit the specific needs of different hair types, making it a valuable addition to any hair care routine.

Customizable Treatments: Mix castor oil with other oils or ingredients to create customized treatments that address your unique hair concerns.

Incorporating castor oil into your hair care routine is simple and straightforward. Whether used as a standalone treatment or as part of a hair mask or conditioner, it is easy to apply and effective.

Standalone Treatment: Apply castor oil directly to the scalp and hair, leave it on for a few hours or overnight, and wash it with shampoo.

Hair Masks and Conditioners: Combine castor oil with other nourishing ingredients to create hair masks and conditioners that provide additional benefits.

Castor oil is a powerful natural remedy for many hair concerns. Its moisturizing, strengthening, and growth-promoting properties make it essential to any hair care routine.

By understanding the benefits of castor oil and how to use it effectively, you can improve the health and appearance of your hair.

Castor oil offers a versatile and effective solution, whether you are looking to hydrate dry hair, repair damage, promote growth, or maintain scalp health. Embrace the benefits of castor oil and experience the transformative effects it can have on your hair.

Chapter 5: Using castor oil for hair treatments

Castor oil has earned a reputation as a versatile and effective natural remedy for hair care. Castor oil can be a valuable addition to your hair care routine, whether you're looking to moisturize dry strands, strengthen brittle hair, promote growth, or maintain scalp health. This chapter explores various ways to use castor oil for different hair treatments, providing simple yet effective methods to achieve healthier and more vibrant hair.

Castor oil, derived from the seeds of the castor plant (Ricinus communis), is rich in essential nutrients such as ricinoleic acid, omega-6 fatty acids, and vitamin E. These components contribute to its moisturizing, strengthening, and growth-promoting properties. When applied correctly, castor oil can deeply nourish the hair and scalp, addressing common issues like dryness, breakage, and irritation.

5.1 Deep Conditioning Treatment

Deep conditioning with castor oil helps to restore moisture, improve hair elasticity, and strengthen the hair shaft.

Method

Preparation: Mix castor oil with a carrier oil such as coconut or olive oil in equal parts.

Application: Apply the oil mixture to damp or dry hair, focusing on the ends and areas prone to dryness or damage.

Massage: Gently massage the oil into the scalp using circular motions to stimulate blood circulation.

Heat Treatment: For enhanced absorption, cover your hair with a shower cap or warm towel and leave the oil on for at least 30 minutes overnight.

Rinse and Shampoo: Wash your hair thoroughly with a mild shampoo to remove the oil. You may need to shampoo twice to ensure all residue is removed.

Benefits

Intense Hydration: Castor oil penetrates deep into the hair shaft, moisturizing dry and brittle hair.

Strengthens Hair: Regular deep conditioning with castor oil can help to strengthen the hair, reducing breakage and split ends.

Improves Scalp Health: Massaging the oil into the scalp promotes circulation and helps to maintain a healthy scalp environment.

5.2 Hair Growth Serum

Castor oil as a hair growth serum can stimulate hair follicles and encourage healthy hair growth.

Method

Ingredients: Combine castor oil with a few drops of essential oils like rosemary oil or peppermint oil known for their hair-stimulating properties.

Application: Using a dropper or your fingertips, apply the serum directly to the scalp and massage gently for 5-10 minutes.

Leave-In Treatment: Leave the serum overnight or for at least a few hours to allow the oil to penetrate the scalp and hair follicles.

Rinse or Leave-In: Depending on preference, you can either rinse out the serum with shampoo or leave it in for added conditioning.

Benefits

Promotes Hair Growth: Ricinoleic acid in castor oil improves blood circulation to the scalp, promoting hair growth and thickness.

Nourishes Hair Follicles: Essential oils combined with castor oil provide additional nutrients and antioxidants to nourish the hair follicles.

Adds Shine: Regular use of the serum can enhance the overall shine and appearance of the hair.

5.3 Scalp Treatment for Dandruff

Castor oil's antimicrobial and anti-inflammatory properties effectively treat and prevent dandruff and dry scalp.

Method

Mixing: Combine castor oil with a few drops of tea tree oil or lavender oil, both known for their anti-dandruff properties.

Application: Part your hair into sections and apply the oil mixture directly to the scalp using a cotton ball or fingertips.

Massage: Massage the oil into the scalp for 5-10 minutes to stimulate circulation and distribute the oil evenly.

Leave-In: Leave the treatment on for at least 30 minutes overnight for maximum effectiveness.

Wash Out: Wash your hair thoroughly with a gentle dandruff-fighting shampoo to remove the oil and cleanse the scalp.

Benefits

Reduces Scalp Irritation: The soothing properties of castor oil help to alleviate itching and irritation associated with dandruff.

Moisturizes Scalp: Regular use keeps the scalp hydrated, reducing flakiness and dryness.

Antifungal Properties: Helps to combat fungal infections that can contribute to dandruff and scalp discomfort.

5.4 Split End Repair Treatment

Castor oil can help to seal split ends and prevent further damage, promoting healthier-looking hair.

Method

Simple Application: Just apply a small amount of castor oil directly to the ends of damp or dry hair, where split ends are most prevalent. It's a straightforward process that anyone can do.

Convenient Treatment: You can leave the oil on overnight or for a few hours to allow it to penetrate and nourish the hair ends. It's a hassle-free way to care for your hair.

Heat Application: For deeper penetration, wrap your hair in a warm towel or use a hair dryer on a low setting for a few minutes.

Regular Use: Incorporate this treatment into your weekly hair care routine to maintain healthier ends and prevent future splitting.

Benefits

Seals Ends: Castor oil acts as a natural sealant, smoothing and sealing split ends to prevent further breakage.

Conditions: The oil conditions the ends, making them softer and more manageable.

Protects: Regular use of castor oil helps to protect hair ends from environmental damage and styling stressors. It's like a shield for your hair.

5.5 Overnight Hair Mask

Overnight masks with castor oil deeply nourish and repair hair while you sleep, providing intensive treatment.

Method

Mixing: Combine castor oil with a lighter oil like almond oil or jojoba oil to make the application easier and prevent excessive greasiness.

Application: Apply the oil mixture generously to dry or damp hair, focusing on the lengths and ends. Use a wide-tooth comb to distribute evenly.

Protection: Cover your hair with a shower cap or towel to protect your pillowcase and enhance the absorption of the oils.

Morning Wash: In the morning, shampoo your hair thoroughly to remove the oil mask. Condition as usual if needed.

Benefits

Intensive Repair: Provides deep conditioning and repair to dry, damaged hair.

Softens Hair: Overnight treatment leaves hair softer, smoother, and more manageable.

Enhances Shine: Regular overnight masks can boost hair shine and overall health.

Castor oil offers many benefits for hair care through its moisturizing, strengthening, growth-promoting, and scalp-nourishing properties.

Whether used alone or in combination with other oils and ingredients, castor oil treatments can help you achieve healthier, more vibrant hair.

By incorporating these treatments into your regular hair care routine, you can address various concerns and maintain optimal hair and scalp health. Experiment with different methods to discover what works best for your hair type and needs, and enjoy the natural benefits of castor oil for beautiful hair.

Chapter 6: DIY hair care recipes with castor oil

1. Moisturizing Hair Mask

Ingredients:

- 2 tablespoons castor oil
- 1 tablespoon coconut oil
- 1 tablespoon honey

Instructions:

1. Mix all ingredients in a bowl until well combined.
2. Apply the mixture to damp hair, focusing on the ends and dry areas.
3. Leave on for 30 minutes to 1 hour.
4. Rinse thoroughly with shampoo and conditioner.

2. Hair Growth Serum

Ingredients:

- 2 tablespoons castor oil
- 1 tablespoon jojoba oil
- 5 drops rosemary essential oil
- 5 drops peppermint essential oil

Instructions:

1. Combine all oils in a dropper bottle and shake well.
2. Apply a few drops to the scalp and massage gently.
3. Leave it on overnight or for at least 2 hours.
4. Wash hair with a mild shampoo.

3. Split End Repair Treatment

Ingredients:

- 1 tablespoon castor oil
- 1 tablespoon argan oil
- 1 tablespoon almond oil

Instructions:

1. Mix oils together in a small bowl.
2. Apply to the ends of dry or damp hair.
3. Leave on for at least 1 hour or overnight.
4. Wash hair thoroughly with shampoo.

4. Deep Conditioning Hair Mask

Ingredients:

- 3 tablespoons castor oil
- 1 ripe avocado, mashed
- 1 tablespoon honey

Instructions:

1. Combine mashed avocado, castor oil, and honey in a bowl.
2. Apply to clean, damp hair, focusing on the lengths and ends.
3. Leave on for 30 minutes to 1 hour.
4. Rinse thoroughly with lukewarm water and shampoo.

5. Anti-Dandruff Scalp Treatment

Ingredients:

- 2 tablespoons castor oil
- 1 tablespoon tea tree oil
- 1 tablespoon apple cider vinegar

Instructions:

1. Mix castor oil, tea tree oil, and apple cider vinegar in a bowl.

2. Part your hair and apply the mixture directly to the scalp using a cotton ball.

3. Massage gently for 5-10 minutes.

4. Leave on for 30 minutes to 1 hour before washing with shampoo.

6. Strengthening Hair Mask

Ingredients:

- 2 tablespoons castor oil
- 1 egg yolk
- 1 tablespoon yogurt

Instructions:

1. Whisk egg yolk and yogurt together in a bowl.

2. Add castor oil and mix until smooth.

3. Apply to damp hair, starting from the roots to the ends.

4. Leave on for 30 minutes before rinsing with cool water and shampooing.

7. Overnight Hair Growth Treatment

Ingredients:

- 2 tablespoons castor oil
- 1 tablespoon olive oil
- 1 tablespoon aloe vera gel

Instructions:

1. Mix all ingredients in a bowl until well combined.

2. Apply the mixture to the scalp and hair, focusing on the roots.

3. Cover with a shower cap or towel and leave it on overnight.

4. Wash hair thoroughly in the morning with shampoo.

8. Smoothing Hair Serum

Ingredients:

- 2 tablespoons castor oil

- 1 tablespoon argan oil

- 1 tablespoon sweet almond oil

Instructions:

1. Combine all oils in a dropper bottle and shake well.

2. Apply a few drops to the palms and run through damp hair, focusing on the ends.

3. Style hair as usual.

9. Softening Hair Rinse

Ingredients:

- 1 tablespoon castor oil

- 1 cup distilled water

- 1 tablespoon apple cider vinegar

Instructions:

1. Mix castor oil, distilled water, and apple cider vinegar in a spray bottle.

2. Shake well before each use.

3. After shampooing and conditioning, spray onto damp hair.

4. Leave on for a few minutes, then rinse with cool water.

10. Hair Thickening Mask

Ingredients:

- 2 tablespoons castor oil

- 1 mashed banana

- 1 tablespoon honey

Instructions:

1. Mash banana in a bowl until smooth.

2. Add castor oil and honey, mix well.

3. Apply to damp hair, focusing on the roots and scalp.

4. Leave on for 30 minutes before rinsing with lukewarm water.

11. Frizz Control Hair Mask

Ingredients:

- 2 tablespoons castor oil
- 1 tablespoon shea butter
- 1 tablespoon coconut oil

Instructions:

1. Melt shea butter and coconut oil in a double boiler.
2. Remove from heat and add castor oil.
3. Mix well and let it cool until slightly solidified.
4. Apply to damp hair, focusing on frizzy areas.
5. Leave on for 30 minutes before rinsing with shampoo.

12. Hair Strengthening Conditioner

Ingredients:

- 3 tablespoons castor oil
- 1/2 cup plain yogurt
- 1 tablespoon honey

Instructions:

1. Mix yogurt, castor oil, and honey in a bowl until smooth.
2. Apply to clean, damp hair, focusing on the ends.
3. Leave on for 20-30 minutes.
4. Rinse thoroughly with lukewarm water and shampoo.

13. Hair Growth Scalp Massage Oil

Ingredients:

- 2 tablespoons castor oil
- 1 tablespoon almond oil
- 5 drops lavender essential oil

Instructions:

1. Mix all oils in a small bowl.

2. Warm the oil slightly and apply it to the scalp.

3. Massage gently with fingertips for 5-10 minutes.

4. Leave on for at least 1 hour or overnight before shampooing.

14. Hydrating Hair Mask

Ingredients:

- 2 tablespoons castor oil

- 1 ripe avocado, mashed

- 1 tablespoon olive oil

Instructions:

1. Mix mashed avocado, castor oil, and olive oil until smooth.

2. Apply to damp hair, focusing on dry areas.

3. Cover with a shower cap and leave on for 30 minutes.

4. Rinse thoroughly with lukewarm water and shampoo.

15. Protein-Rich Hair Mask

Ingredients:

- 2 tablespoons castor oil

- 1 egg white

- 1 tablespoon coconut milk

Instructions:

1. Whisk egg white and coconut milk together in a bowl.

2. Add castor oil and mix until smooth.

3. Apply to damp hair, starting from the roots to the ends.

4. Leave on for 30 minutes before rinsing with cool water and shampooing.

16. Refreshing Scalp Scrub

Ingredients:

- 2 tablespoons castor oil
- 1 tablespoon brown sugar
- 1 tablespoon lemon juice

Instructions:

1. Mix all ingredients in a bowl until well combined.
2. Massage the mixture into damp scalp for 5-10 minutes.
3. Rinse thoroughly with lukewarm water and shampoo.

17. Overnight Hair Repair Mask

Ingredients:

- 2 tablespoons castor oil
- 1 tablespoon argan oil
- 1 tablespoon shea butter

Instructions:

1. Melt shea butter and mix with castor oil and argan oil until well combined.
2. Apply the mixture to dry or damp hair, focusing on the ends.
3. Cover with a shower cap or towel and leave it on overnight.
4. Wash hair thoroughly with shampoo in the morning.

18. Soothing Hair and Scalp Oil

Ingredients:

- 2 tablespoons castor oil
- 1 tablespoon calendula oil
- 5 drops chamomile essential oil

Instructions:

1. Mix all oils in a small bowl.

2. Warm the oil slightly and apply it to the scalp and hair.

3. Massage gently with fingertips for 5-10 minutes.

4. Leave on for at least 1 hour before shampooing.

19. Hair Detox Mask

Ingredients:

- 2 tablespoons castor oil

- 1 tablespoon bentonite clay

- 1 tablespoon apple cider vinegar

Instructions:

1. Mix bentonite clay and apple cider vinegar in a bowl until smooth.

2. Add castor oil and mix well.

3. Apply to damp hair, starting from the roots to the ends.

4. Leave on for 20-30 minutes before rinsing with lukewarm water and shampooing.

20. Conditioning Hair Rinse

Ingredients:

- 2 tablespoons castor oil

- 1 cup green tea, brewed and cooled

- 1 tablespoon honey

Instructions:

1. Mix all ingredients in a bowl until honey is dissolved.

2. After shampooing, pour the mixture over damp hair as a final rinse.

3. Massage into scalp and hair for a few minutes.

4. Rinse thoroughly with cool water.

21. Overnight Hair Growth Mask

Ingredients:

- 2 tablespoons castor oil

- 1 tablespoon coconut oil

- 1 tablespoon almond oil

- 5 drops lavender essential oil

Instructions:

1. Mix all oils in a bowl until well combined.

2. Apply to scalp and hair, focusing on the roots.

3. Cover with a shower cap and leave on overnight.

4. Wash hair thoroughly with shampoo in the morning.

22. Strengthening Hair and Scalp Treatment

Ingredients:

- 2 tablespoons castor oil

- 1 tablespoon argan oil

- 1 tablespoon jojoba oil

- 1 teaspoon vitamin E oil

Instructions:

1. Combine all oils in a small bowl.

2. Warm slightly and apply to scalp and hair.

3. Massage gently for 5-10 minutes.

4. Leave on for 1-2 hours before washing with shampoo.

23. Deep Hydration Hair Mask

Ingredients:

- 2 tablespoons castor oil

- 1 ripe banana, mashed

- 1 tablespoon honey

Instructions:

1. Mix mashed banana, castor oil, and honey until smooth.

2. Apply to damp hair, focusing on ends.

3. Leave on for 30 minutes to 1 hour.

4. Rinse thoroughly with lukewarm water and shampoo.

24. Soothing Scalp Oil

Ingredients:

- 2 tablespoons castor oil

- 1 tablespoon almond oil

- 5 drops chamomile essential oil

Instructions:

1. Mix all oils in a bowl until blended.

2. Apply to scalp and hair, massaging gently.

3. Leave on for at least 1 hour before shampooing.

25. Hair Growth Booster Serum

Ingredients:

- 2 tablespoons castor oil

- 1 tablespoon grapeseed oil

- 5 drops peppermint essential oil

- 5 drops rosemary essential oil

Instructions:

1. Combine all oils in a dropper bottle.

2. Shake well and apply a few drops to scalp.

3. Massage gently and leave on overnight.

4. Wash hair thoroughly with shampoo in the morning.

26. Detangling Hair Spray

Ingredients:

- 1 tablespoon castor oil

- 1 cup distilled water

- 5 drops lavender essential oil

Instructions:

1. Mix castor oil, distilled water, and lavender oil in a spray bottle.

2. Shake well before each use.

3. Spray onto damp hair to detangle and moisturize.

4. Comb through hair and style as usual.

27. Overnight Hair Repair Serum

Ingredients:

- 2 tablespoons castor oil

- 1 tablespoon argan oil

- 1 tablespoon shea butter

- 5 drops tea tree essential oil

Instructions:

1. Melt shea butter and mix with castor oil, argan oil, and tea tree oil.

2. Apply to dry or damp hair, focusing on ends.

3. Cover with a shower cap and leave on overnight.

4. Wash hair thoroughly with shampoo in the morning.

28. Hair Thickening Scalp Treatment

Ingredients:

- 2 tablespoons castor oil

- 1 tablespoon avocado oil

- 1 tablespoon coffee grounds

Instructions:

1. Mix castor oil, avocado oil, and coffee grounds in a bowl.

2. Apply to scalp, massaging gently for 5-10 minutes.

3. Leave on for 30 minutes before shampooing.

29. Clarifying Hair Rinse

Ingredients:

- 2 tablespoons castor oil
- Juice of 1 lemon
- 1 cup water

Instructions:

1. Mix castor oil, lemon juice, and water in a bowl.
2. After shampooing, pour mixture over hair as a final rinse.
3. Massage into scalp and hair for a few minutes.
4. Rinse thoroughly with cool water.

30. Hair Growth Hot Oil Treatment

Ingredients:

- 2 tablespoons castor oil
- 1 tablespoon olive oil
- 1 tablespoon coconut oil

Instructions:

1. Mix castor oil, olive oil, and coconut oil in a heat-safe bowl.
2. Warm the oil mixture in the microwave or over a double boiler.
3. Apply to scalp and hair, covering with a shower cap.
4. Leave on for 30 minutes to 1 hour before shampooing.

31. Nourishing Hair Butter

Ingredients:

- 2 tablespoons castor oil
- 1 tablespoon shea butter
- 1 tablespoon cocoa butter

Instructions:

1. Melt shea butter and cocoa butter in a double boiler.

2. Remove from heat and stir in castor oil until well combined.

3. Allow the mixture to cool and solidify slightly.

4. Apply to damp hair, focusing on ends.

5. Leave on for 30 minutes before rinsing with shampoo.

32. Hair Repair Mask

Ingredients:

- 2 tablespoons castor oil

- 1 tablespoon honey

- 1 tablespoon yogurt

Instructions:

1. Mix honey and yogurt in a bowl until smooth.

2. Add castor oil and mix thoroughly.

3. Apply to clean, damp hair, focusing on ends.

4. Leave on for 20-30 minutes before rinsing with lukewarm water and shampoo.

33. Hydrating Hair Cream

Ingredients:

- 2 tablespoons castor oil

- 1 tablespoon coconut milk

- 1 tablespoon aloe vera gel

Instructions:

1. Mix castor oil, coconut milk, and aloe vera gel until well blended.

2. Apply to damp hair, starting from roots to ends.

3. Leave on for 30 minutes before rinsing with water and shampoo.

34. Shine-Enhancing Hair Mask

Ingredients:

- 2 tablespoons castor oil

- 1 tablespoon argan oil

- 1 tablespoon apple cider vinegar

Instructions:

1. Mix all ingredients in a bowl until well combined.

2. Apply to damp hair, focusing on the lengths and ends.

3. Leave on for 30 minutes before rinsing thoroughly with shampoo.

35. Hair Growth Scalp Massage Oil

Ingredients:

- 2 tablespoons castor oil

- 1 tablespoon sesame oil

- 5 drops peppermint essential oil

Instructions:

1. Mix all oils in a bowl until blended.

2. Warm slightly and apply to scalp and hair.

3. Massage gently with fingertips for 5-10 minutes.

4. Leave on for at least 1 hour before shampooing.

36. Soothing Hair Balm

Ingredients:

- 2 tablespoons castor oil

- 1 tablespoon beeswax

- 1 tablespoon almond oil

Instructions:

1. Melt beeswax in a double boiler.

2. Stir in castor oil and almond oil until well combined.

3. Allow the mixture to cool and solidify.

4. Apply to dry or damp hair, focusing on ends.

37. Conditioning Hair Spray

Ingredients:

- 2 tablespoons castor oil
- 1 cup distilled water
- 1 tablespoon glycerin

Instructions:

1. Mix castor oil, distilled water, and glycerin in a spray bottle.
2. Shake well before each use.
3. Spray onto damp hair to condition and moisturize.
4. Comb through hair and style as usual.

38. Anti-Frizz Hair Serum

Ingredients:

- 2 tablespoons castor oil
- 1 tablespoon argan oil
- 1 tablespoon jojoba oil

Instructions:

1. Combine all oils in a dropper bottle and shake well.
2. Apply a few drops to palms and smooth over damp or dry hair, focusing on ends.
3. Style hair as usual.

39. Hair Detox Mask

Ingredients:

- 2 tablespoons castor oil
- 1 tablespoon bentonite clay
- 1 tablespoon apple cider vinegar

Instructions:

1. Mix bentonite clay and apple cider vinegar in a bowl until smooth.

2. Add castor oil and mix well.

3. Apply to damp hair, starting from the roots to the ends.

4. Leave on for 20-30 minutes before rinsing with lukewarm water and shampooing.

40. Overnight Hair Softening Treatment

Ingredients:

- 2 tablespoons castor oil

- 1 tablespoon olive oil

- 1 tablespoon coconut oil

Instructions:

1. Mix castor oil, olive oil, and coconut oil in a bowl.

2. Apply to dry or damp hair, focusing on the ends.

3. Cover with a shower cap or towel and leave it on overnight.

4. Wash hair thoroughly with shampoo in the morning.

Chapter 7: Castor oil for different hair types

Castor oil is a versatile natural remedy that offers numerous benefits for hair health. Its rich composition of fatty acids, vitamins, and minerals makes it particularly effective in addressing different hair types and concerns. Whether you have dry, oily, curly, or straight hair, incorporating castor oil into your hair care routine can help nourish, strengthen, and improve the overall condition of your hair.

7.1 Benefits of Castor Oil for All Hair Types

Castor oil provides essential nutrients that promote hair growth, moisturize the scalp, and enhance hair texture. Here are some key benefits for all hair types:

Moisturizing: Castor oil's high ricinoleic acid content helps lock in moisture, preventing dryness and promoting a healthy scalp environment.

Strengthening: The nutrients in castor oil penetrate the hair shaft, strengthening each strand and reducing breakage.

Stimulating Hair Growth: Regular use of castor oil can stimulate hair follicles, encouraging hair growth and thickness.

Conditioning: It acts as a natural conditioner, improving hair softness and shine.

7.2 Castor Oil for Dry Hair

Dry hair lacks moisture and often appears dull and brittle. Castor oil's emollient properties make it an excellent choice for dry hair types:

Deep Conditioning: Castor oil deeply moisturizes and nourishes dry hair, restoring its natural shine and softness.

Split End Repair: It helps seal split ends, reduce frizz, and improve hair manageability.

Overnight Treatment: Castor oil as an overnight treatment can provide intensive hydration, leaving dry hair revitalized and healthier-looking.

7.3 Castor Oil for Oily Hair

Oily hair results from excess sebum production, which can weigh down hair and make it appear greasy. Contrary to common belief, castor oil can still benefit oily hair types:

Balancing Sebum Production: Castor oil helps regulate sebum production on the scalp, keeping oily hair under control without stripping it of essential moisture.

Scalp Health: Its antibacterial properties can help maintain a healthy scalp environment, reducing dandruff and itchiness.

Lightweight Application: Use lighter applications or diluted forms of castor oil to avoid weighing down oily hair while still benefiting from its nutrients.

7.4 Castor Oil for Curly or Coily Hair

Curly and oily hair types are prone to dryness and frizz due to their structure. Castor oil can be particularly beneficial for these hair types:

Moisture Retention: Castor oil's thick consistency helps seal moisture into curly and oily hair, preventing dryness and enhancing curl definition.

Softening Properties: It softens coarse hair textures, making detangling easier and reducing breakage.

Scalp Massage: Massaging castor oil into the scalp stimulates blood circulation, promoting healthier hair growth from the roots.

7.5 Castor Oil for Straight Hair

Straight hair types can also benefit from castor oil, especially for maintaining overall hair health and addressing common concerns:

Enhancing Shine: Castor oil adds a natural shine to straight hair, making it appear healthier and more lustrous.

Preventing Hair Loss: Regular use can strengthen hair follicles and reduce hair loss, maintaining thicker hair strands.

Heat Protection: Applying a small amount of castor oil before heat styling can protect straight hair from heat damage and maintain moisture balance.

7.6 Tips for Using Castor Oil Based on Hair Type

Dry Hair: Use castor oil as a deep conditioning treatment at least once a week. Combine with oils or ingredients like avocado or coconut milk for added moisture.

Oily Hair: Apply castor oil sparingly to the scalp and focus on the hair ends. Leave on for a shorter duration before washing out with a gentle shampoo.

Curly or Coily Hair: Use castor oil as a leave-in conditioner or styling product to define curls and reduce frizz. Mix with aloe vera gel or shea butter for added moisture.

Straight Hair: Use castor oil as a pre-shampoo treatment to nourish and protect hair before cleansing. Avoid applying too close to the scalp to prevent greasiness.

Castor oil is a versatile hair care ingredient suitable for all hair types, offering a range of benefits from moisturizing and conditioning to promoting hair growth and scalp health.

By understanding your hair type and specific needs, you can tailor your use of castor oil to maximize its effectiveness in achieving healthier, more vibrant hair. Experiment with different application methods and formulations to find what works best for you, and enjoy the natural benefits of castor oil in your hair care routine.

Chapter 8: Addressing common hair problems with castor oil

In hair care, castor oil is a versatile and effective remedy for addressing various common hair issues. From promoting growth to moisturizing dry strands, castor oil's rich composition of fatty acids, vitamins, and minerals nourishes and supports healthy hair. This chapter explores how castor oil can be used to tackle some of the most prevalent hair concerns people face today.

8.1 Hair Loss and Thinning

Hair loss and thinning are common issues affecting both men and women. Whether caused by genetics, hormonal changes, or environmental factors, maintaining healthy hair growth is a top priority for many. Castor oil offers several benefits that can help combat hair loss:

The ricinoleic acid in castor oil improves blood circulation to the scalp, stimulating hair follicles and encouraging growth.

Its vitamin E, omega-6 fatty acids, and proteins nourish the scalp and strengthen hair roots, reducing hair fall.

Massage castor oil into the scalp for 5-10 minutes to improve absorption. Leave it on for at least an hour, or overnight for deeper penetration, before washing with a mild shampoo.

8.2 Dry and Damaged Hair

Dry and damaged hair is often the result of excessive heat styling, chemical treatments, or environmental factors like sun exposure and pollution. Castor oil can restore moisture and repair damage with its hydrating and conditioning properties:

The thick consistency of castor oil coats the hair shaft, sealing in moisture and preventing further dryness.

Castor oil can help seal split ends, improve hair texture, and reduce breakage.

Apply a small amount of warmed castor oil to damp hair, focusing on the ends. Leave it on for 30 minutes to an hour before rinsing thoroughly.

8.3 Dandruff and Scalp Irritation

Dandruff, characterized by dry, flaky scalp and scalp irritation, is a common scalp condition that can be uncomfortable and embarrassing. Castor oil's antimicrobial and anti-inflammatory properties make it an effective remedy for soothing the scalp and reducing dandruff:

Castor oil helps combat fungal infections on the scalp, which can contribute to dandruff.

It soothes irritated scalp, reducing itching and redness associated with dandruff.

Mix castor oil with a few drops of tea tree or peppermint oil for added antimicrobial benefits. Massage into the scalp, leave on for 30 minutes to an hour, and then shampoo thoroughly.

8.4 Frizzy and Unmanageable Hair

Curly hair can result from humidity, lack of moisture, or damage. Castor oil's conditioning properties tame frizz and improve manageability:

Castor oil smooths the hair cuticle, reducing frizz and enhancing shine.

It provides long-lasting moisture to prevent hair from becoming dry and frizzy.

Apply a small amount of castor oil to damp or dry hair, focusing on the ends and areas prone to frizz. Style as usual without rinsing.

8.5 Lack of Hair Volume and Thickness

Thin and flat hair can concern those seeking more volume and thickness. Castor oil's nourishing components can help improve hair density and thickness:

Regular use strengthens hair follicles, promoting thicker strands over time.

Improved circulation to the scalp supports healthier hair growth, adding volume and density.

Massage castor oil into the scalp to stimulate circulation, then apply it to the lengths of hair. Leave on for at least 30 minutes before washing.

8.6 Heat and Chemical Damage

Excessive heat styling and chemical treatments can weaken hair, leading to breakage and loss of elasticity. Castor oil provides a protective barrier and helps repair damage caused by these factors:

Apply castor oil pre-treatment before heat styling to protect hair from high temperatures.

Its nutrients penetrate the hair shaft to repair damage and restore hair's natural shine.

Apply a small amount of castor oil to damp hair before blow-drying or heat styling. For chemical damage, use it as a deep conditioning treatment once a week.

Castor oil offers a natural and effective solution for many common hair issues. Whether you're struggling with hair loss, dryness, frizz, or scalp conditions, integrating castor oil into your hair care routine can provide significant benefits.

Its nutrient-rich composition supports hair health from roots to ends, promoting stronger, shinier, and more manageable hair. Experiment with different application methods and combinations to discover how castor oil best meets your hair needs. Consistent use allows you to achieve healthier, more resilient hair that radiates natural beauty.

Chapter 9: Incorporating castor oil into your hair care routine

9.1 Understanding Castor Oil Benefits for Hair

Introducing castor oil into your hair care routine can be a transformative step towards enhancing the health and appearance of your hair. With its renowned nourishing and moisturizing properties, castor oil offers a natural solution to a range of hair concerns, from promoting growth to improving scalp health. This chapter delves into the potential of using castor oil in your hair care regimen and provides practical tips on how to harness its power effectively.

Before diving into how to incorporate castor oil into your routine, it's essential to understand its benefits:

Promotes Hair Growth: Castor oil contains ricinoleic acid, which helps stimulate hair follicles, leading to increased hair growth.

Moisturizes and Conditions: Its thick consistency helps lock in moisture, making hair softer and more manageable.

Strengthens Hair: Rich in essential nutrients like omega-6 fatty acids and vitamin E, castor oil strengthens hair strands, reducing breakage and split ends.

Improves Scalp Health: Antimicrobial and anti-inflammatory properties aid in combating scalp infections, reducing dandruff, and soothing irritation.

9.2 How to Incorporate Castor Oil into Your Hair Care Routine

9.2.1 Pre-Shampoo Treatment

Using castor oil as a pre-shampoo treatment can help nourish and protect your hair from the drying effects of shampooing.

Method: Apply castor oil generously to dry or damp hair, focusing on the scalp and hair ends.

Massage: Gently massage the oil into your scalp for 5-10 minutes to stimulate circulation and promote absorption.

Duration: Leave the oil on for at least 30 minutes or overnight for a deep conditioning treatment.

Wash Out: Shampoo and condition your hair as usual to remove the oil residue.

9.2.2 Scalp Massage

Regular scalp massages with castor oil can improve blood circulation, strengthen hair roots, and enhance overall scalp health.

Application: Warm up a small amount of castor oil and apply it directly to the scalp.

Technique: Use your fingertips to massage the oil in circular motions. Focus on areas where hair is thinning or scalp issues are prevalent.

Frequency: Aim for 2-3 times a week for optimal results in promoting hair growth and maintaining scalp health.

9.2.3 Hair Mask or Deep Conditioning Treatment

Castor oil can be used as a standalone hair mask or combined with other oils and ingredients for a deep conditioning treatment.

DIY Mask: Mix castor oil with coconut oil, olive oil, or yogurt for added moisturizing benefits.

Application: Apply the mask to clean damp hair from roots to ends. Cover with a shower cap or warm towel to enhance absorption.

Duration: Leave the mask on for 30 minutes to 1 hour before rinsing thoroughly with lukewarm water and shampoo.

9.2.4 Leave-In Treatment

For ongoing hydration and frizz control throughout the day, consider castor oil as a leave-in treatment.

Dilution: Mix a small amount of castor oil with water or aloe vera gel in a spray bottle.

Application: Spray onto damp or dry hair, focusing on the ends and areas prone to frizz.

Style: Comb through to distribute evenly and style as usual. The oil will help keep hair moisturized and add a natural shine.

9.2.5 Hair Growth Serum

Create a hair growth serum using castor oil and essential oils known for their hair-stimulating properties.

Ingredients: Combine castor oil with rosemary oil, peppermint oil, or lavender oil in a dropper bottle.

Application: Apply a few drops directly to the scalp and massage gently. Leave it on overnight for intensive treatment or use daily for ongoing support.

9.2.6 Styling Aid

Use castor oil as a styling aid to add shine and control to your hair without weighing it down.

Smoothing: Rub a small amount of castor oil between your palms and smooth over dry hair to tame flyaways and add gloss.

Heat Protection: Apply a light layer of castor oil to hair before heat styling to protect against heat damage and retain moisture.

9.3 Tips for Maximizing Castor Oil Benefits

Quality Matters: Choose cold-pressed, organic castor oil to ensure maximum potency and purity.

Consistency: Incorporate castor oil into your routine consistently to see long-term benefits. Results may vary depending on individual hair type and condition.

Adjust to Your Needs: Experiment with different application methods and combinations (e.g., mixing with other oils or ingredients) to find what works best for your hair.

Patience is Key: Allow time for castor oil to work its magic. Hair growth and improvement in hair health may take several weeks to become noticeable.

By incorporating castor oil into your hair care routine, you can address common issues such as dryness, frizz, and scalp problems while promoting growth and strength.

This versatile and affordable solution can be used as a pre-shampoo treatment, scalp massage oil, or leave-in conditioner. Start integrating castor oil into your routine today and experience the rewards of healthier, more vibrant hair. Castor oil-your natural path to hair health and beauty.

Chapter 10: Testimonials and success stories

Castor oil has garnered a loyal following in the realm of hair and skincare for its purported benefits and effectiveness. This chapter delves into real-life testimonials and success stories from individuals who have incorporated castor oil into their beauty routines. These stories highlight personal experiences, transformations, and the impact of castor oil on various hair and skin concerns.

Testimonial 1: Hair Growth and Thickness

Name: Sarah M.

Age: 32

Location: New York, NY

Background: After pregnancy, Sarah struggled with thinning hair due to stress and hormonal changes. She sought natural remedies and discovered castor oil through online research and recommendations from friends.

Experience: *"I started using castor oil as a scalp treatment twice a week. After a few months, I noticed significant hair density and thickness improvement. My hair also feels softer and looks healthier overall. I'm amazed by the results and feel more confident about my hair again."*

Impact: Sarah's experience highlights the potential of castor oil in promoting hair growth and enhancing hair texture, especially for individuals dealing with hair loss or thinning.

Testimonial 2: Scalp Health and Dandruff Relief

Name: James T.

Age: 45

Location: Los Angeles, CA

Background: James battled with chronic dandruff and scalp irritation for years, trying various medicated shampoos and treatments with limited success. He decided to explore natural alternatives and discovered the benefits of castor oil for scalp health.

Experience: "I began massaging castor oil into my scalp every night before bed. Within a few weeks, I noticed a significant reduction in dandruff flakes and scalp itchiness. My scalp feels healthier and less irritated now."

Impact: James's story underscores the soothing and anti-inflammatory properties of castor oil, providing relief for scalp conditions like dandruff and itchiness.

Testimonial 3: Skin Radiance and Anti-Aging Benefits

Name: Emily L.

Age: 40

Location: Miami, FL

Background: Emily struggled with dull, aging skin and sought natural remedies to improve her complexion and reduce fine lines.

Experience: "I started using castor oil as part of my nightly skincare routine. It has transformed my skin texture, making it smoother and more radiant. The fine lines around my eyes have softened noticeably, and my skin feels deeply moisturized."

Impact: Emily's testimonial highlights the skincare benefits of castor oil, including its moisturizing and anti-aging properties, which can rejuvenate and enhance skin appearance.

Testimonial 4: Acne Control and Skin Healing

Name: Michael C.

Age: 27

Location: Chicago, IL

Background: Michael struggled with persistent acne breakouts and acne scars, leading to frustration and a search for effective treatments.

Experience: "I started using castor oil as a spot treatment for my acne. It helped reduce the size of my pimples and sped up the healing process. Over time, my acne scars have faded, and my skin tone has become more even."

Impact: Michael's experience demonstrates how castor oil's antibacterial and healing properties can aid in acne control and scar reduction, promoting clearer and healthier skin.

Testimonial 5: Overall, Hair and Skin Health

Name: Olivia B.

Age: 35

Location: Austin, TX

Background: Olivia wanted a multipurpose solution for hair and skin care, seeking simplicity and effectiveness in her beauty routine.

Experience: *"I've been using castor oil for over a year, and it's become a staple in my beauty regimen. Not only has it strengthened my hair and promoted growth, but it has also improved my skin's hydration and reduced redness. I love how versatile and natural it is."*

Impact: Olivia's testimonial illustrates the versatility of castor oil in addressing multiple beauty concerns, from hair growth and strength to skin hydration and complexion improvement.

These testimonials and success stories highlight castor oil's diverse benefits and effectiveness in hair and skincare. From promoting hair growth and thickness to soothing scalp conditions, improving skin radiance, and aiding in acne control, castor oil has earned praise for its natural healing and nourishing properties. Whether you're looking to enhance your hair's health, rejuvenate your skin, or address specific beauty concerns, these real-life experiences underscore the potential of castor oil as a valuable addition to your beauty routine. Consider integrating castor oil into your daily regimen and discover the transformative benefits it can offer for your hair and skin health.

Here you can access the 4 BONUSES e-books included

Scan this **QR code** using your phone's camera or click this LINK to access your **BONUS** content now:

SCAN THE QR CODE BELOW:

You will access 4 BONUSES EBOOKS:

BOOK 1: "Castor Oil in Traditional Medicine"

BOOK 2: "Castor Oil for Home and Garden"

BOOK 3: "The Science of Castor Oil: Research and Innovations"

BOOK 4: "Castor Oil Crafts: Creative Projects and Uses"

BOOK 4: Castor Oil for Health and Wellness

Castor Oil for Health and Wellness

Harnessing the Power of Nature for a Vibrant Life

By

Vincent Vega

Disclaimer notice

Chapter 1: Understanding castor oil for health and wellness

Castor oil, derived from the seeds of the castor oil plant (Ricinus communis), has earned a reputation as a potent natural remedy with a rich history spanning centuries. Its diverse therapeutic properties, from promoting digestive health to managing pain and inflammation, make castor oil a versatile substance used traditionally across cultures and continues to be embraced in modern holistic health practices.

1.1 Historical Significance

Castor oil's use can be traced back to ancient civilizations such as Egypt, where it was utilized for its purgative qualities and as a soothing agent for various ailments. Over time, its benefits became known worldwide, finding applications in traditional medicine systems from Ayurveda in India to Traditional Chinese Medicine (TCM). Throughout history, castor oil has been celebrated for its ability to promote health and well-being through its unique composition and effective medicinal properties.

1.2 Composition and Characteristics

The castor oil plant is native to tropical regions but is now cultivated globally for its seeds, which contain approximately 40-60% oil. The oil predominantly comprises ricinoleic acid, a monounsaturated fatty acid that constitutes up to 85-95% of its content. This fatty acid is pivotal to castor oil's therapeutic effects, including its anti-inflammatory, antimicrobial, and analgesic properties.

In addition to ricinoleic acid, castor oil contains other beneficial components such as oleic acid, linoleic acid, vitamin E, and various minerals. These nutrients contribute to its ability to nourish and heal the body when used both internally and externally.

1.3 Applications in Health and Wellness

1.3.1 Digestive Health and Detoxification

One of the most well-known uses of castor oil is its role in promoting digestive health. When taken orally, ricinoleic acid stimulates the smooth muscles of the intestines, promoting bowel movement and alleviating constipation. This natural laxative effect makes castor oil a preferred choice for occasional relief from digestive discomforts.

1.3.2 Anti-inflammatory and Pain Management

Castor oil's anti-inflammatory properties extend beyond digestive health to encompass pain relief and inflammation reduction in joints and muscles. Applied topically, castor oil penetrates deeply into the skin, promoting circulation and reducing swelling. This makes it beneficial for managing arthritis, rheumatism, and muscle soreness.

1.3.3 Skin and Hair Care

Castor oil is widely revered in skincare for its moisturizing and emollient properties. It deeply hydrates the skin without clogging pores, making it suitable for all skin types. Regular application can soften and smooth skin texture, reduce wrinkles and enhance overall health.

Castor oil nourishes the scalp, strengthens hair follicles, and promotes hair growth. It is also effective in moisturizing dry scalp conditions, reducing dandruff, and adding shine and luster to hair strands.

1.4 Safety Considerations

While castor oil offers numerous health benefits, it is essential to use it responsibly and with full awareness of potential risks. Understanding and adhering to safety considerations is a crucial part of incorporating castor oil into your holistic health routine.

Internal Use: Follow recommended dosages for oral consumption to avoid potential side effects such as diarrhea and dehydration.

Topical Use: Conduct a patch test before applying to the skin to check for allergies. Always dilute castor oil with a carrier oil if applying to sensitive areas.

Pregnancy and Children: Consult healthcare professionals before using castor oil during pregnancy or on children due to its potential effects on the digestive system.

Castor oil's enduring popularity in health and wellness stems from its historical significance, potent composition, and versatile applications.

Whether addressing digestive issues, managing pain and inflammation, or enhancing skin and hair health, castor oil remains a trusted natural remedy.

Understanding its origins, benefits, and safe usage empowers individuals to effectively incorporate this botanical powerhouse into their holistic health routines. In the chapters ahead, we will delve deeper into the specific health benefits, practical applications, and precautions necessary to harness castor oil's full potential for well-being.

Chapter 2: Therapeutic properties of castor oil

Castor oil, derived from the seeds of the castor oil plant (Ricinus communis), is celebrated for its remarkable therapeutic properties that have been recognized and utilized across cultures for centuries. This chapter delves into the comprehensive range of therapeutic benefits castor oil offers, highlighting its diverse applications in promoting health and well-being.

2.1 Anti-inflammatory Properties

One of castor oil's most prominent therapeutic aspects is its potent anti-inflammatory effect. This is primarily attributed to its high ricinoleic acid content, a unique monounsaturated fatty acid comprising up to 85-95% of the oil's composition. Ricinoleic acid exerts anti-inflammatory actions by inhibiting the synthesis of inflammatory prostaglandins, thereby reducing pain and swelling associated with various inflammatory conditions such as arthritis, rheumatism, and muscle strains.

The mechanism involves ricinoleic acid binding to EP3 prostanoid receptors in the gastrointestinal tract, leading to increased intestinal motility and enhanced fluid secretion. This effect accelerates the passage of stool through the colon, resulting in relief from constipation. It is important to note that while practical, castor oil's laxative properties should be used judiciously and under the guidance of a healthcare provider to prevent dehydration and electrolyte imbalances.

2.2 Analgesic (Pain-Relieving) Effects

In addition to its anti-inflammatory properties, castor oil exhibits analgesic effects, making it a valuable natural remedy for pain relief. By reducing inflammation and promoting circulation to affected areas, castor oil can alleviate pain associated with joint disorders, backaches, headaches, and menstrual cramps. Applying castor oil through massage or as a topical compress helps soothe sore muscles and joints, providing relief without the side effects commonly associated with over-the-counter pain medications.

2.3 Antimicrobial and Antifungal Properties

Castor oil's antimicrobial and antifungal properties contribute to its effectiveness in combating bacterial and fungal infections. Ricinoleic acid and other fatty acids present in castor oil create an unfavorable environment for microbial growth, making it beneficial for treating skin infections such as ringworm, athlete's foot, and fungal nail infections. When applied topically, castor oil forms a protective barrier on the skin, inhibiting the growth and spread of pathogens while promoting skin healing and regeneration.

2.4 Moisturizing and Emollient Qualities

As a natural emollient, castor oil deeply moisturizes and nourishes the skin, making it an excellent choice for dry, rough, or sensitive skin conditions. The oil's high viscosity allows it to form a protective barrier on the skin's surface, preventing moisture loss and enhancing skin hydration. Regular application of castor oil can soften rough patches, smooth fine lines and wrinkles, and improve overall skin texture and elasticity.

2.5 Wound Healing and Tissue Repair

Castor oil's ability to promote wound healing and tissue repair is well-documented, owing to its anti-inflammatory, antimicrobial, and regenerative properties. When applied to wounds, burns, cuts, and abrasions, castor oil soothes inflammation, reduces pain, and accelerates healing. Its fatty acids and vitamin E composition supports the regeneration of skin cells and collagen fibers, promoting faster wound closure and minimizing scarring.

2.6 Hair and Scalp Benefits

Castor oil is revered for its nourishing and strengthening properties in hair care. It penetrates the hair shaft and follicles, delivering essential nutrients that promote hair growth, thickness, and resilience. Regular scalp massages with castor oil stimulate blood circulation, nourish the scalp, and fortify hair follicles, reducing hair fall and supporting healthy growth. Castor oil's moisturizing properties also help alleviate scalp dryness and flakiness, addressing common issues such as dandruff and itching.

2.7 Gastrointestinal Health and Detoxification

Historically, castor oil has been utilized as a potent laxative to alleviate constipation and promote bowel regularity. The mechanism involves ricinoleic acid stimulating smooth muscle contractions in the intestines, facilitating the movement of stool through the digestive tract. This natural laxative effect can benefit occasional constipation relief; however, it is essential to use castor oil sparingly and according to recommended dosages to avoid potential side effects such as dehydration and electrolyte imbalance.

2.8 Safety Considerations

While castor oil offers numerous health benefits, it is essential to use it responsibly and with full awareness of potential risks. Understanding and adhering to safety considerations is a crucial part of incorporating castor oil into your holistic health routine.

Use oral castor oil products cautiously and according to recommended dosages. Excessive consumption can lead to gastrointestinal discomfort, diarrhea, dehydration, and electrolyte imbalances.

Conduct a patch test before applying castor oil to the skin to check for allergic reactions. If applied to sensitive areas, dilute castor oil with carrier oil like coconut oil.

Consult healthcare professionals before using castor oil during pregnancy or on children due to its potential effects on the digestive system.

Castor oil's therapeutic properties make it a valuable asset in natural health and wellness practices, offering a holistic approach to addressing various health concerns. Castor oil provides effective and natural solutions, whether used for its anti-inflammatory, analgesic, antimicrobial, moisturizing, digestive, wound-healing, or hair care benefits. Understanding these properties empowers individuals to incorporate castor oil into their daily routines, promoting overall health and well-being.

Chapter 3: Digestive health and detoxification

Digestive health is crucial for overall well-being, influencing everything from nutrient absorption to immune function. This chapter explores how castor oil contributes to digestive health and detoxification, highlighting its historical use, mechanisms of action, benefits, and safety considerations.

Castor oil has a long history of use in traditional medicine systems worldwide, primarily for its potent laxative properties. Ancient Egyptians used it to effectively remedy constipation and induce bowel movements. Similarly, Ayurvedic medicine in India and Traditional Chinese Medicine (TCM) utilized castor oil for digestive ailments and detoxification. These practices highlight castor oil's enduring reputation as a natural remedy for promoting gastrointestinal health.

Castor oil's effectiveness as a laxative stem from its high content of ricinoleic acid, a unique fatty acid that exerts pharmacological effects in the intestines. Ricinoleic acid binds to EP3 prostanoid receptors in the smooth muscle cells of the intestines, stimulating peristalsis—the wave-like contractions that propel food and waste through the digestive tract. This action enhances bowel movement and facilitates stool elimination, providing relief from constipation.

Additionally, castor oil's ability to increase fluid secretion into the intestines contributes to its laxative effect. This helps soften stool and makes it easier to pass, alleviating symptoms of constipation.

3.1 Benefits of Castor Oil for Digestive Health

1) Relief from Constipation

Castor oil's primary benefit in digestive health is its ability to relieve occasional constipation. When taken orally, typically as a single dose, castor oil can stimulate bowel movements within a few hours, making it a preferred choice for individuals seeking fast-acting relief from constipation.

2) Gentle Detoxification

Beyond its laxative properties, castor oil is believed to support detoxification by promoting the elimination of toxins from the digestive system. Castor oil helps remove waste materials and toxins that may accumulate in the colon by enhancing bowel movements. This cleansing action supports overall digestive function and contributes to a sense of well-being.

3) Anti-inflammatory Effects

Research suggests that ricinoleic acid, the primary component of castor oil, exhibits anti-inflammatory properties. Inflammatory conditions within the gastrointestinal tract, such as irritable bowel syndrome (IBS) and inflammatory bowel disease (IBD), may benefit from the anti-inflammatory effects of castor oil. However, more studies are needed to fully understand its efficacy in treating these conditions.

4) Supports Intestinal Health

Regular use of castor oil as a laxative may help maintain intestinal health by preventing the buildup of stagnant stool and promoting regular bowel movements. This can contribute to a healthier gut environment and reduce the risk of complications such as hemorrhoids and anal fissures.

3.2 Practical Applications and Usage

When using castor oil for digestive health:

Dosage: The typical dosage for adults is 1-2 tablespoons (15-30 mL) of castor oil taken orally as needed for constipation relief. It is recommended to start with a lower dose and adjust as necessary to avoid discomfort.

Administration: Castor oil is usually taken on an empty stomach, preferably in the morning, to facilitate rapid absorption and action. It can be consumed directly or mixed with a beverage to mask its taste.

Duration of Action: Castor oil typically induces bowel movements within 2-6 hours after ingestion. It is essential to stay hydrated and allow sufficient time for the oil to take effect before planning activities.

Safety Considerations: While generally safe for occasional use, prolonged or excessive consumption of castor oil can lead to electrolyte imbalances, dehydration, and dependency on laxatives. It is advisable to consult with a healthcare professional before using castor oil, especially for individuals with underlying digestive conditions, pregnant or breastfeeding women, and children.

3.3 Potential Side Effects and Precautions

Despite its benefits, castor oil may cause mild to moderate side effects in some individuals, including:

Abdominal Cramps: Due to its strong laxative effect, castor oil may cause abdominal cramps or discomfort, particularly if taken in excessive doses.

Dehydration: Increased bowel movements induced by castor oil can lead to dehydration if adequate fluid intake is not maintained.

Electrolyte Imbalance: Prolonged use of castor oil as a laxative may disrupt electrolyte balance in the body, affecting essential minerals such as potassium and sodium.

Dependency: Regular use of castor oil for constipation relief may lead to dependency on laxatives. To promote regular bowel function, it is recommended to use castor oil sparingly and incorporate dietary and lifestyle changes.

Castor oil offers a natural and practical approach to supporting digestive health and promoting gentle detoxification. Its historical use and proven mechanisms of action underscore its value as a traditional remedy for constipation relief and overall gastrointestinal well-being. When used responsibly and under appropriate guidance, castor oil can play a beneficial role in maintaining optimal digestive function and supporting detoxification processes.

In the next chapter, we will explore additional therapeutic uses of castor oil, including its applications in skincare, hair care, and overall wellness. Understanding these diverse benefits empowers individuals to incorporate castor oil into their holistic health routines for enhanced vitality and well-being.

Chapter 4: Skin health and healing

Skin health is integral to overall well-being. It serves as a barrier against external pathogens while maintaining hydration and regulating body temperature. Castor oil, with its rich composition of fatty acids and beneficial compounds, offers many benefits for skin health and healing. In this chapter, we explore the diverse therapeutic properties of castor oil, its applications in skincare routines, and its effectiveness in addressing various skin conditions.

Castor oil, derived from the seeds of the castor bean plant (Ricinus communis), is a versatile skincare ingredient. Composed predominantly of ricinoleic acid, a unique monounsaturated fatty acid, it offers a range of benefits for skin health. Its anti-inflammatory, antimicrobial, and moisturizing properties make it a powerful addition to any skincare routine.

In addition to ricinoleic acid, castor oil contains other fatty acids, such as oleic and linoleic acid, contributing to its emollient and moisturizing effects. It also contains antioxidants like vitamin E, which help protect the skin from oxidative stress and promote skin repair.

4.1 Benefits of Castor Oil for Skin Health

4.1.1 Moisturizing and Hydration

One of the primary benefits of castor oil for skin health is its moisturizing and hydrating properties. When applied topically, castor oil forms a protective barrier on the skin's surface, preventing water loss and maintaining skin hydration. This mainly benefits individuals with dry, rough, or sensitive skin conditions. Regular castor oil can soften and smooth the skin, improving overall texture and elasticity.

4.1.2 Anti-inflammatory Effects

Due to its high ricinoleic acid content, castor oil exhibits potent anti-inflammatory effects. Inflammation is a common underlying factor in various skin conditions, such as acne, eczema, and dermatitis. Castor oil helps alleviate these conditions' redness, swelling, and discomfort by reducing inflammation. It can soothe irritated skin and promote faster healing of inflamed areas.

4.1.3 Antimicrobial and Antifungal Properties

Castor oil's antimicrobial and antifungal properties make it effective in combating bacterial and fungal skin infections. Ricinoleic acid and other fatty acids create an environment that inhibits the growth of pathogens, making castor oil suitable for treating conditions like acne, ringworm, athlete's foot, and fungal nail infections. Regular application of castor oil can help prevent infections and promote skin health.

4.1.4 Wound Healing and Scar Reduction

Castor oil supports wound healing and scar reduction through its regenerative properties. It stimulates the growth of new skin tissue and enhances collagen production, essential for repairing damaged skin. When applied to cuts, abrasions, burns, and surgical scars, castor oil accelerates the healing process and minimizes the appearance of scars. Its moisturizing effects also keep the skin hydrated, aiding in scar softening and blending with the surrounding skin.

4.1.5 Anti-aging Benefits

The antioxidant properties of castor oil, particularly vitamin E, help combat free radicals that contribute to premature skin aging. Free radicals can damage skin cells and accelerate the formation of wrinkles, fine lines, and age spots. By neutralizing free radicals, castor oil helps preserve skin elasticity, firmness, and youthful appearance. Regular use of castor oil in skincare routines can help maintain a healthy and radiant complexion.

4.1.6 Cleansing and Detoxification

Castor oil's ability to penetrate the skin's layers allows it to cleanse pores and remove impurities, dirt, and excess oil. This cleansing action helps prevent clogged pores and reduces the risk of acne breakouts. Castor oil can be an effective natural cleanser for all skin types, providing a gentle yet thorough cleansing without stripping the skin of its natural oils.

4.2 Practical Applications of Castor Oil in Skincare

Facial Cleansing Oil: Mix castor oil with a lighter carrier oil like jojoba or almond oil for a natural facial cleanser. Massage onto dry skin, then wipe off with a warm washcloth for clean and hydrated skin.

Moisturizing Body Lotion: Combine castor oil with shea butter and essential oils for a nourishing body lotion. Apply to damp skin after showering to lock in moisture and promote soft, supple skin.

Scar Treatment: Apply castor oil directly to scars or stretch marks twice daily to promote healing and reduce visibility over time. Massage gently into the skin until fully absorbed.

Acne Spot Treatment: Dab a small amount of castor oil onto acne-prone areas before bedtime. Its antibacterial properties help reduce inflammation and speed up healing without clogging pores.

Anti-aging Serum: Create a DIY anti-aging serum by blending castor oil with rosehip seed and vitamin E oil. Apply a few drops to the face and neck daily to diminish fine lines and improve skin elasticity.

4.3 Safety Considerations and Precautions

While castor oil is generally safe for topical use, it's important to be aware that it may cause allergic reactions or skin irritation in some individuals, especially those with sensitive skin. Performing a patch test before using castor oil on larger areas of the skin and being vigilant for any signs of irritation is a crucial safety precaution.

Avoid ingesting castor oil unless under medical supervision, as it is a potent laxative that can cause gastrointestinal discomfort, diarrhea, and dehydration if consumed in large quantities.

Castor oil's therapeutic benefits for skin health and healing make it a valuable addition to natural skincare routines. Its moisturizing, anti-inflammatory, antimicrobial, and antioxidant properties support various skin concerns, from dryness and irritation to acne and aging. By understanding and harnessing castor oil's power, individuals can naturally achieve healthier, more radiant skin.

The following chapters will explore additional castor oil applications in hair care, overall health and wellness, and practical tips for integrating castor oil into daily routines for maximum benefit. Understanding these diverse uses empowers individuals to leverage castor oil's natural healing properties for holistic self-care.

Chapter 5: Care of hair and scalp with castor oil

Hair and scalp care are essential components of personal grooming and hygiene. Castor oil, renowned for its nourishing and strengthening properties, offers numerous benefits for maintaining healthy hair and scalp. In this chapter, we explore the diverse applications of castor oil in hair care, its mechanisms of action, practical tips for usage, and its effectiveness in addressing typical hair.

Castor oil is derived from the seeds of the castor bean plant (Ricinus communis) and is rich in fatty acids, particularly ricinoleic acid, which constitutes about 85-95% of its composition. This unique fatty acid provides castor oil with its therapeutic properties, including:

Castor oil deeply penetrates the hair shaft and scalp, moisturizing dry and brittle hair. It nourishes the hair follicles and strengthens the hair strands, reducing breakage and promoting healthy growth.

Castor oil's antimicrobial properties help maintain scalp health by combating bacterial and fungal infections.

5.1 Benefits of Castor Oil for Hair

Promotes Hair Growth

One of the most celebrated benefits of castor oil is its ability to promote hair growth. The ricinoleic acid in castor oil improves blood circulation to the scalp, stimulating hair follicles and encouraging growth. It nourishes the scalp and provides essential nutrients that support the hair growth cycle. Regular scalp massages with castor oil can enhance hair thickness, length, and overall density.

Conditions the Hair

Castor oil acts as a natural conditioner for the hair, leaving it smooth, shiny, and manageable. It penetrates deep into the hair shaft, sealing in moisture and preventing dryness and frizz. This makes castor oil an excellent choice for individuals with dry, damaged, or chemically treated hair, restoring its luster and vitality.

Strengthens and Prevents Hair Loss

The nutrients in castor oil, including omega-6 fatty acids and vitamin E, strengthen the hair roots and shafts, reducing hair breakage and preventing split ends. Regular application of castor oil can help maintain hair strength and resilience, minimize hair loss, and promote healthier, fuller-looking hair.

Improves Scalp Health

A healthy scalp is essential for optimal hair growth and maintenance. Castor oil's antibacterial and antifungal properties help cleanse the scalp and reduce dandruff and scalp infections. It moisturizes the scalp, soothes irritation, and balances oil production, creating a conducive environment for hair follicles to thrive.

<u>Adds Shine and Softness</u>

Castor oil's emollient properties coat the hair shaft, smoothing the cuticles and enhancing shine. It improves the hair's overall texture, making it softer and more manageable. Castor oil can transform dull, lackluster hair into healthy, radiant locks.

5.2 Practical Applications of Castor Oil in Hair Care

*Scalp Massage:*Warm a small amount of castor oil and massage it into the scalp using circular motions. Leave it on for at least 30 minutes or overnight for deep conditioning, then shampoo and condition as usual.

Hair Growth Serum: Mix equal parts castor oil and coconut oil or argan oil. Apply to the scalp and hair, focusing on the roots. Leave on for a few hours or overnight, then shampoo thoroughly.

*Hair Mask:*Combine castor oil with honey and egg yolk for a nourishing hair mask. Apply to damp hair, cover with a shower cap, and leave on for 30-60 minutes before rinsing out.

Split Ends Treatment: Apply a small amount of castor oil to the ends of the hair to seal split ends and prevent further damage. Leave on overnight for intensive repair.

Eyelash and Eyebrow Growth: Use a clean mascara wand or cotton swab to apply castor oil to eyelashes and eyebrows nightly to promote thicker and longer growth.

5.3 Tips for Using Castor Oil in Hair Care

Choose Cold-Pressed Castor Oil: Cold-pressed castor oil retains more nutrients and is free from chemical additives, making it ideal for hair and scalp care.

Patch Test: Conduct a patch test before using castor oil to ensure you are not allergic to it, especially if you have sensitive skin or scalp.

Consistency is Key: Incorporate castor oil into your hair care routine regularly for best results. Consistent use helps maintain hair health and promotes long-term benefits.

Use Sparingly: Castor oil is thick and potent. Use a small amount to avoid weighing down the hair or making it greasy.

5.4 Safety Considerations

While castor oil is generally safe for external use, some individuals may experience allergic reactions or skin sensitivities. Discontinue use if irritation occurs and consult a healthcare professional if symptoms persist. Avoid applying castor oil directly to open wounds or irritated skin.

Castor oil offers a natural and effective solution for enhancing hair and scalp health, promoting growth, strength, and shine. Its rich composition of fatty acids and nourishing properties makes it a versatile ingredient in hair care routines. Castor oil provides numerous benefits for achieving healthy and beautiful hair, whether used for stimulating hair growth, conditioning, strengthening, or improving scalp health.

In the next chapter, we will explore additional therapeutic uses of castor oil for overall health and wellness, including its applications in skincare, digestive health, and more. Understanding these diverse benefits empowers individuals to incorporate castor oil into their holistic self-care practices, promoting vitality and well-being from head to toe.

Chapter 6: Internal Uses of Castor Oil

Castor oil, primarily known for its external applications in skincare, hair care, and therapeutic massages, also holds a history of internal use for various health benefits. In this chapter, we delve into the internal uses of castor oil, exploring its potential benefits, safety considerations, and practical applications.

Castor oil has been ingested internally throughout history for its medicinal properties. Ancient civilizations, including the Egyptians, Greeks, and Indians, utilized castor oil for its purgative effects to cleanse the digestive system and promote detoxification. Ayurvedic and traditional Chinese medicine practitioners have also incorporated castor oil into their healing practices because it supports gastrointestinal health and overall wellness.

The primary active component of castor oil responsible for its internal effects is ricinoleic acid, a monounsaturated fatty acid. When ingested, ricinoleic acid interacts with EP3 prostanoid receptors in the intestines, stimulating smooth muscle contractions and promoting bowel movements. This mechanism of action makes castor oil a potent laxative, effectively relieving constipation and supporting regularity.

6.1 Benefits of Internal Use

6.1.1 Relieves Constipation

One of the most well-known and researched benefits of internal castor oil use is its efficacy as a natural laxative. For individuals struggling with occasional constipation, castor oil can provide prompt relief by inducing bowel movements within a few hours of ingestion. Its ability to stimulate peristalsis helps soften stool and facilitate its passage through the intestines, promoting digestive comfort and regularity.

6.1.2 Supports Detoxification

Internal use of castor oil is believed to support detoxification by enhancing the elimination of toxins and waste materials from the digestive tract. Castor oil helps promote bowel movements and cleanse the colon by removing accumulated impurities that may hinder optimal gastrointestinal function. This detoxifying effect contributes to overall well-being and may improve symptoms associated with toxin buildup, such as fatigue and bloating.

6.1.3 Anti-inflammatory Properties

Research suggests that ricinoleic acid in castor oil exhibits anti-inflammatory effects, which may benefit individuals with inflammatory bowel conditions like ulcerative colitis and Crohn's disease. Castor oil can help alleviate symptoms such as abdominal pain, cramping, and diarrhea by reducing inflammation in the gastrointestinal tract. However, it's essential to consult a healthcare provider before using castor oil for these conditions to ensure safety and effectiveness.

6.1.4 Immune Support

The immune system relies heavily on a healthy gastrointestinal tract for optimal function. Castor oil indirectly supports immune function by promoting digestive health and regular bowel movements. A clean and well-functioning colon reduces the risk of bacterial overgrowth and encourages the absorption of essential nutrients that support immune health.

6.2 Practical Applications and Usage

When using castor oil internally, it's crucial to follow proper guidelines to ensure safety and effectiveness:

Dosage: The recommended dosage of castor oil for adults is typically 1-2 tablespoons (15-30 mL) taken orally as needed for constipation relief. It's advisable to start with a lower dose and adjust based on individual response.

Administration: Castor oil is usually taken on an empty stomach, preferably in the morning, to facilitate rapid absorption and action. It can be consumed directly or mixed with a beverage to mask its taste.

Duration of Action: Castor oil generally induces bowel movements within 2-6 hours after ingestion. It's essential to stay hydrated and allow sufficient time for the oil to take effect before planning activities.

Safety Considerations: While castor oil is generally safe for occasional use as a laxative, prolonged or excessive consumption can lead to dehydration, electrolyte imbalances, and dependency on laxatives. Using castor oil sparingly is crucial and consult a healthcare professional if constipation persists or worsens.

6.3 Potential Side Effects and Precautions

Despite its benefits, internal use of castor oil may cause side effects in some individuals, including:

Abdominal Cramps: Due to its strong laxative effect, castor oil may cause abdominal cramps or discomfort, particularly if taken in excessive doses.

Dehydration: Increased bowel movements induced by castor oil can lead to dehydration if adequate fluid intake is not maintained.

Electrolyte Imbalance: Prolonged use of castor oil as a laxative may disrupt electrolyte balance in the body, affecting essential minerals such as potassium and sodium.

Dependency: Regular use of castor oil for constipation relief may lead to dependency on laxatives. It's recommended to use castor oil sparingly and incorporate dietary and lifestyle changes to promote regular bowel function.

Internal use of castor oil offers a natural and practical approach to promoting digestive health, relieving constipation, and supporting detoxification. Its historical use and proven mechanisms of action highlight its value as a traditional remedy for gastrointestinal wellness. When used responsibly and under appropriate guidance, castor oil can play a beneficial role in maintaining optimal digestive function and supporting overall well-being.

Chapter 7: External applications and therapeutic techniques

Castor oil's versatility extends beyond internal use; it is equally renowned for its external applications in therapeutic practices. In this chapter, we delve into the various external uses of castor oil, exploring its applications in skincare, massage therapy, pain relief, and more. From ancient healing traditions to modern therapeutic techniques, castor oil offers holistic benefits for promoting health and well-being.

7.1 Skincare Benefits and Applications

<u>Moisturizing and Hydrating</u>

Castor oil's rich composition of fatty acids, particularly ricinoleic acid, makes it an excellent moisturizer for the skin. When applied topically, castor oil forms a protective barrier that locks in moisture, making it beneficial for dry, rough, or sensitive skin. Regular use can improve skin hydration, soften texture, and increase suppleness.

<u>Anti-inflammatory and Healing Properties</u>

Castor oil's anti-inflammatory properties help reduce inflammation and soothe irritated skin. It can alleviate symptoms of inflammatory skin conditions such as eczema, dermatitis, and psoriasis. Castor oil's healing properties promote faster wound healing, minimize scar formation, and relieve itching and discomfort.

<u>Cleansing and Detoxification</u>

Castor oil's ability to penetrate the skin effectively cleans pores and removes impurities, dirt, and excess oil. It can be a natural cleanser to prevent acne breakouts and maintain clear, healthy skin. Castor oil's detoxifying properties extend to drawing out toxins and impurities from the skin, promoting a clearer complexion.

7.2 Massage Therapy and Pain Relief

<u>Anti-inflammatory and Analgesic Effects</u>

Castor oil is valued in massage therapy for its anti-inflammatory and analgesic effects. It can help relieve muscle soreness, joint pain, and stiffness by promoting circulation and reducing inflammation. Castor oil massages are commonly used to alleviate discomfort associated with arthritis, back pain, and menstrual cramps.

<u>Relaxation and Stress Relief</u>

Massaging castor oil onto the skin promotes relaxation and stress relief. The gentle strokes and soothing properties of castor oil can help calm the mind and body, reducing tension and promoting overall well-being. Incorporating castor oil into regular massage routines enhances relaxation and supports mental clarity.

7.3 Hair Care and Scalp Treatments

Promotes Hair Growth and Strength

Castor oil is a popular remedy for promoting hair growth and strengthening hair follicles. When massaged into the scalp, castor oil stimulates blood circulation, delivering essential nutrients to the hair roots and encouraging healthy growth. Its nourishing properties help repair damaged hair, reduce breakage, and enhance hair texture and shine.

Conditions and Nourishes the Scalp

Regular scalp treatments with castor oil can help maintain scalp health by moisturizing and nourishing the skin. Castor oil soothes dryness, reduces flakiness, and supports a balanced scalp environment. Its antimicrobial properties also contribute to scalp health by combating fungal infections and preventing dandruff.

7.4 Practical Applications and Techniques

1) Facial Cleansing and Moisturizing

To cleanse and moisturize the face, apply a small amount of castor oil to damp skin and massage gently in circular motions. Use a warm washcloth to remove excess oil and impurities, leaving the skin refreshed and hydrated.

2) Castor Oil Packs

Castor oil packs are popular therapeutic techniques to promote detoxification, reduce inflammation, and relieve pain. To create a castor oil pack, saturate a piece of cloth with castor oil and place it over the affected area (such as the abdomen for digestive health or joints for pain relief). Cover with plastic wrap and apply a heating pad for 30-60 minutes. Repeat as needed.

3) Hair Masks and Treatments

Mix castor oil with coconut or argan oil and apply to the scalp and hair for a deep conditioning hair treatment. Massage thoroughly and leave on for at least 30 minutes before shampooing. This nourishing treatment strengthens hair, reduces frizz, and enhances shine.

4) Joint and Muscle Massage

Warm castor oil slightly and massage it into sore muscles or joints using gentle, circular motions. Castor oil's soothing properties penetrate deep into tissues, promoting relaxation, reducing inflammation, and improving mobility.

7.5 Safety Considerations

While castor oil is generally safe for external use, it's essential to consider the following precautions:

- Patch Test: Conduct a patch test before applying castor oil to larger areas of the skin to check for any allergic reactions or skin sensitivities.

- Use Sparingly: Castor oil is thick and concentrated. Use a small amount to avoid greasiness and ensure proper absorption into the skin or hair.

- Avoid Contact with Eyes: Take care to avoid contact with the eyes when applying castor oil, as it may cause irritation.

Castor oil's external applications and therapeutic techniques offer a wealth of benefits for skincare, massage therapy, hair care, and pain relief.

Whether used for moisturizing, healing, or promoting relaxation, castor oil's natural properties make it a valuable addition to holistic health and wellness routines.

By exploring these diverse applications and techniques, individuals can harness the power of castor oil to enhance their physical well-being and nurture a healthier, more radiant appearance.

In the following chapters, we will delve deeper into specific therapeutic uses of castor oil, including its applications in pain management, digestive health, and overall detoxification. Understanding these versatile benefits empowers individuals to integrate castor oil into their daily routines for comprehensive health support and vitality.

Chapter 8: Safety Considerations and Precautions

Castor oil, celebrated for its diverse therapeutic uses and natural properties, is generally safe for external and internal applications when used responsibly. Its potential benefits are numerous, and understanding the safety considerations and precautions is key to unlocking its full potential for promoting optimal health and well-being. This chapter delves into the potential risks, precautions, and guidelines for using castor oil, offering a hopeful perspective on its safe and effective use.

8.1 External Use Safety Considerations

Skin Sensitivity and Allergic Reactions

Before applying castor oil topically, conducting a patch test is crucial. Apply a small amount of diluted castor oil to a small skin area, such as the inner forearm, and wait 24 hours to check for any adverse reactions. Symptoms of allergic reactions may include redness, itching, swelling, or irritation. Discontinue use if any signs of sensitivity or allergy occur and consult a healthcare provider if symptoms persist.

Eye Contact

When applying castor oil to the face or hair, take care to avoid direct contact with the eyes. Accidental exposure to the eyes may cause irritation, redness, or discomfort. If contact occurs, rinse thoroughly with water and seek medical attention if irritation persists.

Use of Pure vs. Diluted Castor Oil

Pure castor oil is thick and concentrated, which may be too potent for some individuals, especially those with sensitive skin. Consider diluting castor oil with a carrier oil, such as coconut or olive oil, to reduce its viscosity and enhance skin absorption. This dilution method also helps prevent skin irritation and ensures comfortable application.

Pregnancy and Nursing

While topical use of castor oil is generally considered safe during pregnancy and breastfeeding, internal use should be avoided without medical supervision. Castor oil's purgative effects can stimulate uterine contractions and bowel movements, potentially posing risks during pregnancy. Always consult a healthcare provider before using castor oil internally or externally if pregnant or nursing.

8.2 Internal Use Safety Considerations

1) Laxative Effect and Dosage

Castor oil is renowned for its potent laxative properties, making it effective in relieving occasional constipation. However, using castor oil internally cautiously and according to recommended guidelines is essential. The typical dosage for adults is 1-2 tablespoons (15-30 mL) taken orally as needed for constipation relief. Start with a lower dose and adjust based on individual response to minimize potential side effects.

2) Dehydration and Electrolyte Imbalance

Prolonged or excessive use of castor oil as a laxative may lead to dehydration and electrolyte imbalances. Ensure adequate hydration by drinking plenty of water before and after taking castor oil to support bowel movements and prevent fluid loss. Monitor electrolyte levels, especially if using castor oil regularly or in high doses.

3) Dependency on Laxatives

Regular use of castor oil or any laxative may lead to dependency, where the body relies on laxatives to produce bowel movements. To promote natural bowel function, incorporate dietary fiber, fluids, and physical activity into daily routines. Use castor oil sparingly and consider alternative methods for maintaining regularity under medical guidance.

8.3 General Safety Guidelines

Storage and Shelf Life

Castor oil should be stored in a cool, dry place away from direct sunlight and heat to maintain its quality and potency. Proper storage helps preserve the oil's beneficial properties and extends its shelf life. Check the expiration date on the bottle and discard expired castor oil to ensure effectiveness and safety.

Consultation with Healthcare Provider

Consult a healthcare provider or qualified professional before using castor oil for therapeutic purposes, especially internally or for specific health conditions. They can provide personalized guidance, assess potential risks, and recommend appropriate dosage and application methods based on individual health status and needs.

Children and Elderly Use

When using castor oil on children or elderly individuals, it's important to exercise caution. They may be more sensitive to its effects, so adjusting dosage and application methods accordingly and consulting healthcare professionals for guidance, especially for children under medical care or individuals with pre-existing health conditions, is a responsible and caring approach.

Castor oil offers a range of health benefits when used responsibly and with safety precautions in mind. By understanding potential risks, proper usage guidelines, and consulting healthcare professionals as needed, individuals can effectively incorporate castor oil into their wellness routines while minimizing adverse effects.Castor oil's natural properties support holistic well-being and vitality, whether used externally for skincare, massage therapy, or internally for digestive health.

In the subsequent chapters, we will explore specific therapeutic applications of castor oil, including its use in pain management, digestive health, and detoxification. Empowering individuals with knowledge of castor oil's safety considerations enhances its effectiveness as a natural remedy for promoting health and supporting a balanced lifestyle.

Chapter 9: DIY remedies and recipes

1) Hydrating Face Mask

- **Ingredients:**
    - 1 tbsp castor oil
    - 1 tbsp honey
- **Instructions:**
1. Mix castor oil and honey thoroughly.
2. Apply the mixture to a clean face.
3. Leave on for 15-20 minutes.
4. Rinse off with warm water.

2) Acne Spot Treatment

- **Ingredients:**
    - 1 tsp castor oil
    - 1 drop tea tree essential oil
- **Instructions:**
1. Combine castor oil and tea tree oil.
2. Apply directly to acne spots using a cotton swab.
3. Leave overnight and rinse off in the morning.

3) Anti-aging Serum

- **Ingredients:**

- o   1 tbsp castor oil

- o   1 tbsp argan oil

- o   1 tsp rosehip seed oil

- **Instructions:**

1. Mix all oils together in a small bottle.

2. Apply a few drops to face and neck nightly.

3. Gently massage until absorbed.

4) Brightening Face Oil

- **Ingredients:**

  - o   1 tbsp castor oil

  - o   1 tbsp sweet almond oil

  - o   1 tsp vitamin E oil

- **Instructions:**

1. Combine all oils in a dropper bottle.

2. Apply a few drops to cleansed face.

3. Massage gently into the skin.

5) Eye Makeup Remover

- **Ingredients:**

  - o   Castor oil

  - o   Olive oil (equal parts)

- **Instructions:**

1. Mix castor oil and olive oil.

2. Apply to a cotton pad and gently wipe over closed eyelids.

3. Rinse with warm water.

6) Hair Growth Serum

- **Ingredients:**

- o   2 tbsp castor oil
- o   1 tbsp coconut oil
- o   1 tbsp jojoba oil

- **Instructions:**

1. Combine all oils in a small bowl.

2. Massage into scalp and hair roots.

3. Leave overnight and shampoo in the morning.

7) Hair Mask for Dry Hair

- **Ingredients:**
  - o   2 tbsp castor oil
  - o   1 ripe avocado (mashed)

- **Instructions:**

1. Mix castor oil and mashed avocado until smooth.

2. Apply to damp hair, focusing on ends.

3. Leave on for 30 minutes and rinse thoroughly.

8) Dandruff Treatment

- **Ingredients:**
  - o   1 tbsp castor oil
  - o   1 tbsp aloe vera gel
  - o   Few drops of tea tree oil

- **Instructions:**

1. Mix all ingredients thoroughly.

2. Massage into scalp and leave for 30 minutes.

3. Shampoo hair as usual.

9) Split End Repair Serum

- **Ingredients:**

- o   1 tbsp castor oil

- o   1 tbsp almond oil

- • **Instructions:**

1. Mix castor oil and almond oil in a small bottle.

2. Apply a small amount to split ends daily.

3. Leave on without rinsing.

10) Moisturizing Body Lotion

- • **Ingredients:**

  - o   1/4 cup castor oil

  - o   1/2 cup shea butter

  - o   1/4 cup coconut oil

- • **Instructions:**

1. In a bowl, whip castor oil, shea butter, and coconut oil until smooth.

2. Apply to damp skin after showering.

3. Store in a cool, dry place.

11) Facial Cleansing Oil

- • **Ingredients:**

  - o   2 tbsp castor oil

  - o   2 tbsp jojoba oil

  - o   1 tbsp olive oil

- • **Instructions:**

1. Mix all oils in a bottle.

2. Massage a small amount onto face to remove makeup and dirt.

3. Rinse with warm water and pat dry.

12) Lip Balm

- **Ingredients:**

    o   1 tbsp castor oil

    o   1 tbsp coconut oil

    o   1 tbsp beeswax pellets

    o   5-10 drops peppermint essential oil (optional)

- **Instructions:**

1.   Melt beeswax pellets, castor oil, and coconut oil in a double boiler.

2.   Remove from heat and stir in essential oil if desired.

3.   Pour into lip balm tubes or small containers. Let cool and solidify.

13) Cuticle Cream

- **Ingredients:**

    o   1 tbsp castor oil

    o   1 tbsp shea butter

    o   1 tbsp cocoa butter

    o   5 drops lavender essential oil (optional)

- **Instructions:**

1.   Melt shea butter and cocoa butter in a double boiler.

2.   Remove from heat and stir in castor oil and lavender oil.

3.   Transfer to a small jar and let cool. Massage into cuticles as needed.

14) Heel Softening Treatment

- **Ingredients:**

    o   2 tbsp castor oil

    o   1 tbsp almond oil

    o   1 tbsp coconut oil

    o   1 tbsp beeswax pellets

- **Instructions:**

1. Melt beeswax pellets, castor oil, almond oil, and coconut oil in a double boiler.

2. Remove from heat and stir until well combined.

3. Apply to heels before bedtime, cover with socks, and leave overnight.

15) Anti-inflammatory Massage Blend

- **Ingredients:**
    - 2 tbsp castor oil
    - 1 tbsp grapeseed oil
    - 5 drops eucalyptus essential oil
    - 5 drops lavender essential oil

- **Instructions:**

1. Mix all oils in a small bowl.

2. Massage into sore muscles or inflamed areas for relief.

16) Eyelash and Eyebrow Serum

- **Ingredients:**
    - 1 tsp castor oil
    - 1 tsp sweet almond oil
    - 1 tsp vitamin E oil

- **Instructions:**

1. Mix all oils in a small container.

2. Apply a small amount to eyelashes and eyebrows using a clean mascara wand or fingertip before bedtime.

17) Nail Strengthener

- **Ingredients:**
    - 1 tbsp castor oil
    - 1 tbsp argan oil
    - 1 tbsp lemon juice

- **Instructions:**

1. Mix castor oil, argan oil, and lemon juice in a bowl.

2. Massage into nails and cuticles daily to strengthen and nourish.

18) Joint Pain Relief Salve

- **Ingredients:**

  - 3 tbsp castor oil

  - 2 tbsp beeswax pellets

  - 10 drops peppermint essential oil

  - 10 drops eucalyptus essential oil

- **Instructions:**

1. Melt beeswax pellets and castor oil in a double boiler.

2. Remove from heat and stir in essential oils.

3. Pour into a container and let it cool. Apply to sore joints as needed.

19) Soothing Scalp Treatment

- **Ingredients:**

  - 2 tbsp castor oil

  - 1 tbsp coconut oil

  - 1 tbsp tea tree oil

- **Instructions:**

1. Mix all oils in a bowl.

2. Apply to scalp and massage gently. Leave on for 30 minutes before shampooing.

20) Sunburn Relief Gel

- **Ingredients:**

  - 2 tbsp castor oil

  - 1 tbsp aloe vera gel

  - 1 tbsp coconut oil

- **Instructions:**

1. Mix castor oil, aloe vera gel, and coconut oil in a bowl.

2. Apply gently to sunburned areas for soothing relief.

21) Bruise Balm

- **Ingredients:**
    - 1 tbsp castor oil
    - 1 tbsp arnica oil
    - 1 tbsp shea butter

- **Instructions:**

1. Melt shea butter in a double boiler.

2. Remove from heat and stir in castor oil and arnica oil.

3. Let it cool and apply to bruises to promote healing.

22) Anti-cellulite Massage Oil

- **Ingredients:**
    - 2 tbsp castor oil
    - 1 tbsp grapefruit essential oil
    - 1 tbsp almond oil

- **Instructions:**

1. Mix castor oil, grapefruit essential oil, and almond oil in a small bowl.

2. Massage into cellulite-prone areas daily to improve circulation and skin tone.

23) Foot Scrub

- **Ingredients:**
    - 2 tbsp castor oil
    - 2 tbsp brown sugar
    - 1 tbsp olive oil

- **Instructions:**

1.   Mix castor oil, brown sugar, and olive oil in a bowl.

2.   Massage into damp feet, focusing on rough areas. Rinse off with warm water.

24) Anti-aging Eye Cream

- **Ingredients:**
    - 1 tbsp castor oil
    - 1 tbsp shea butter
    - 1 tsp rosehip oil
    - 5 drops frankincense essential oil

- **Instructions:**

1.   Melt shea butter in a double boiler.

2.   Remove from heat and stir in castor oil, rosehip oil, and frankincense oil.

3.   Allow it to cool and apply gently around the eyes.

25) Dry Skin Balm

- **Ingredients:**
    - 2 tbsp castor oil
    - 1 tbsp cocoa butter
    - 1 tbsp coconut oil
    - 5 drops lavender essential oil

- **Instructions:**

1.   Melt cocoa butter and coconut oil in a double boiler.

2.   Remove from heat and stir in castor oil and lavender oil.

3.   Let it cool and apply to dry skin as needed.

26) After-sun Soothing Spray

- **Ingredients:**
    - 1/4 cup castor oil
    - 1/4 cup aloe vera gel

o   10 drops lavender essential oil

- **Instructions:**

1.   Mix castor oil, aloe vera gel, and lavender essential oil in a spray bottle.

2.   Shake well and spray onto sun-exposed skin for cooling relief.

27) Hair Growth Scalp Mask

- **Ingredients:**

  o   2 tbsp castor oil

  o   1 mashed banana

  o   1 tbsp honey

- **Instructions:**

1.   Mix castor oil, mashed banana, and honey until smooth.

2.   Apply to scalp and hair, cover with a shower cap.

3.   Leave on for 30 minutes and shampoo as usual.

28) Hand Cream

- **Ingredients:**

  o   2 tbsp castor oil

  o   2 tbsp shea butter

  o   1 tbsp almond oil

- **Instructions:**

1.   Melt shea butter in a double boiler.

2.   Remove from heat and stir in castor oil and almond oil.

3.   Let it cool and apply to hands for moisturizing.

29) Body Massage Oil

- **Ingredients:**

  o   3 tbsp castor oil

  o   2 tbsp sesame oil

- o 10 drops sandalwood essential oil

  - o 5 drops jasmine essential oil

- **Instructions:**

1. Mix all oils in a small bowl.

2. Massage into the body for relaxation and hydration.

30) Lip Scrub

- **Ingredients:**

  - o 1 tbsp castor oil

  - o 1 tbsp brown sugar

  - o 1 tsp honey

- **Instructions:**

1. Mix castor oil, brown sugar, and honey in a small bowl.

2. Gently scrub onto lips in circular motions to exfoliate and moisturize.

31) Nighttime Hand Treatment

- **Ingredients:**

  - o 1 tbsp castor oil

  - o 1 tbsp almond oil

  - o 1 tbsp shea butter

- **Instructions:**

1. Melt shea butter in a double boiler.

2. Remove from heat and stir in castor oil and almond oil.

3. Massage into hands before bedtime for deep moisturization.

32) Brightening Body Oil

- **Ingredients:**

  - o 2 tbsp castor oil

  - o 2 tbsp jojoba oil

o   1 tbsp vitamin C serum

- **Instructions:**

1. Mix castor oil, jojoba oil, and vitamin C serum in a small bottle.

2. Apply to damp skin after showering for glowing, hydrated skin.

33) Eczema Soothing Cream

- **Ingredients:**

  o   1 tbsp castor oil

  o   1 tbsp coconut oil

  o   1 tbsp colloidal oatmeal

- **Instructions:**

1. Mix castor oil, coconut oil, and colloidal oatmeal until smooth.

2. Apply to affected areas to relieve itching and inflammation.

34) Cuticle Oil

- **Ingredients:**

  o   1 tbsp castor oil

  o   1 tbsp argan oil

  o   1 tbsp vitamin E oil

- **Instructions:**

1. Mix castor oil, argan oil, and vitamin E oil in a small dropper bottle.

2. Apply to cuticles daily to promote healthy nail growth.

35) Acne Scar Fading Serum

- **Ingredients:**

  o   1 tbsp castor oil

  o   1 tbsp rosehip oil

  o   1 tsp evening primrose oil

- **Instructions:**

1. Combine castor oil, rosehip oil, and evening primrose oil in a bottle.

2.   Apply a few drops to acne scars nightly to help fade them over time.

36) Anti-frizz Hair Serum

- **Ingredients:**
  - 2 tbsp castor oil
  - 1 tbsp argan oil
  - 5 drops lavender essential oil

- **Instructions:**

1.   Mix castor oil, argan oil, and lavender essential oil in a small bottle.

2.   Apply a small amount to damp hair ends to tame frizz and add shine.

37) Soothing Sunburn Balm

- **Ingredients:**
  - 2 tbsp castor oil
  - 1 tbsp coconut oil
  - 1 tbsp shea butter
  - 10 drops lavender essential oil

- **Instructions:**

1.   Melt coconut oil and shea butter in a double boiler.

2.   Remove from heat and stir in castor oil and lavender essential oil.

3.   Let it cool and apply to sunburned skin for relief.

38) Anti-aging Face Cream

- **Ingredients:**
  - 1 tbsp castor oil
  - 1 tbsp avocado oil
  - 1 tbsp cocoa butter

- **Instructions:**

1.   Melt cocoa butter in a double boiler.

2.   Remove from heat and stir in castor oil and avocado oil.

3.   Allow to cool and apply to face for moisturizing and anti-aging benefits.

39) Eyelash Growth Serum

- **Ingredients:**
    - 1 tsp castor oil
    - 1 tsp coconut oil
    - 1 tsp vitamin E oil

- **Instructions:**

1.   Mix castor oil, coconut oil, and vitamin E oil in a small container.

2.   Apply a small amount to eyelashes nightly using a clean mascara wand.

40) Muscle Relaxing Massage Oil

- **Ingredients:**
    - 2 tbsp castor oil
    - 1 tbsp sweet almond oil
    - 5 drops peppermint essential oil

- **Instructions:**

1.   Mix castor oil, sweet almond oil, peppermint essential oil, in a bottle.

2.   Massage into sore muscles for relaxation and relief.

Chapter 10: Case Studies and Testimonials

In this chapter, we delve into the diverse applications of castor oil through real-life case studies and testimonials. These stories prove its effectiveness in health, skincare, and hair care.

Case Study 1: Acne Treatment

Many individuals have used castor oil to combat acne due to its antimicrobial and anti-inflammatory properties. One notable case involved Sarah, a 25-year-old who struggled with persistent acne for years. Sarah applied a mixture of castor and tea tree oil to her face nightly. Within three weeks, she noticed a significant reduction in breakouts and inflammation. Her skin became clearer and smoother, boosting her confidence.

Testimonial: Scar Healing

Another powerful testimonial comes from David, who used castor oil to diminish scars from a childhood accident. By massaging castor oil into the scars twice daily for several months, David observed a noticeable reduction in their visibility. The oil's moisturizing properties softened the scar tissue, making it less prominent over time.

Case Study 2: Eczema Relief

Eczema, a common skin condition characterized by red, itchy patches, can also benefit from castor oil. Emily, a mother of two young children, found relief for her eczema-prone skin through regular applications of castor oil mixed with shea butter. This natural remedy helped soothe the itching and inflammation, providing her with much-needed comfort without the side effects of conventional treatments.

Case Study 3: Hair Growth

Hair loss and thinning hair affect many individuals, and castor oil has gained popularity for its potential to promote hair growth. In his mid-30s, Michael applied castor oil to his scalp three times a week. Over several months, he noticed new hair growth and thicker strands, especially along his hairline and crown. This improvement not only restored his confidence but also enhanced his overall appearance.

Testimonial: Dandruff Treatment

Castor oil can provide relief by moisturizing the scalp and reducing flakiness for individuals struggling with dandruff. Tina battled dandruff for years and used castor oil and coconut oil as a pre-shampoo treatment. This approach helped alleviate her dandruff symptoms and restored her scalp's health, making her hair appear shinier and more manageable.

Case Study 4: Joint Pain Relief

Castor oil packs have been traditionally used to alleviate joint pain and inflammation. James, a retired athlete in his 50s, applied warm castor oil packs to his knees nightly. This practice reduced swelling and stiffness, allowing him to resume his daily activities more easily. The anti-inflammatory properties of castor oil played a crucial role in managing his chronic joint pain.

Testimonial: Digestive Health

The use of castor oil as a natural laxative is well-documented. Melissa, experiencing occasional constipation, turned to castor oil as a gentle remedy. By taking a small amount of castor oil diluted in warm water before bedtime, she found relief from constipation without experiencing harsh side effects. This natural approach to digestive health provided her with regularity and comfort.

Testimonial: Overall Wellness

Many individuals incorporate castor oil into their daily routines for its holistic health benefits. A yoga instructor, Rachel includes castor oil massages in her self-care routine. She believes that these massages not only detoxify her body but also enhance her overall well-being. After each session, rachel experiences improved energy levels, clearer skin, and a sense of rejuvenation, highlighting castor oil's multifaceted benefits.

In conclusion, the case studies and testimonials presented in this chapter underscore the versatility and effectiveness of castor oil in promoting health, skincare, and hair care.

While these personal experiences provide valuable insights, it's essential to consider individual responses and consult healthcare professionals when integrating new treatments into your regimen.

By harnessing the natural properties of castor oil, individuals like Sarah, David, Emily, Michael, Tina, James, Melissa, and Rachel have achieved remarkable improvements in their health and well-being, inspiring others to explore the potential of this ancient remedy.

Chapter 11: Integrating Castor Oil into a Holistic Wellness Routine

This chapter delves into the versatile uses of castor oil in a holistic wellness routine, offering a comprehensive guide to enhancing overall health, beauty, and well-being. Uncover practical tips and strategies for seamlessly integrating this multi-purpose oil into your daily regimen, from skincare to digestive health and beyond.

11.1 Daily Facial Cleansing

Incorporating castor oil into your facial cleansing routine can effectively remove dirt, makeup, and impurities while nourishing the skin. Mix equal castor oil and a lighter carrier oil like jojoba or almond oil. Massage onto the face in circular motions, then wipe off gently with a warm washcloth for a deep cleanse that won't strip your skin of its natural oils.

11.2 Weekly Deep Moisturizing Mask

Indulge your skin in a luxurious deep moisturizing mask using castor oil. Combine 1 tablespoon of castor oil with 1 tablespoon of honey and a few drops of lavender essential oil. Apply the mixture evenly to your face and leave it on for 15-20 minutes before rinsing off with warm water. This mask will replenish moisture, soothe irritation, and leave your skin glowing.

11.3 Anti-aging Eye Treatment

Combat signs of aging and reduce puffiness around the eyes with a homemade castor oil eye serum. Mix 1 teaspoon of castor oil with 1 teaspoon of rosehip oil and 2-3 drops of frankincense essential oil. Gently dab the serum around the eyes before bedtime to promote elasticity and minimize fine lines.

11.4 Scalp Massage for Hair Growth

Boost hair growth and scalp health with a simple weekly castor oil scalp massage. Warm a tablespoon of castor oil and massage it into your scalp using circular motions for 5-10 minutes. Leave it on overnight for deep penetration, then shampoo and condition as usual in the morning.

11.5 Strengthening Hair Mask

Revitalize dry and damaged hair with a strengthening hair mask enriched with castor oil. Mix 2 tablespoons of castor oil with 1 tablespoon of coconut oil and 1 tablespoon of yogurt. Apply the mask from roots to ends, cover with a shower cap, and leave it on for 30-60 minutes before rinsing thoroughly. This treatment will nourish your hair, improve manageability, and add shine.

11.6 Gentle Colon Cleanse

Support digestive health with a gentle colon cleanse using castor oil. Mix 1-2 tablespoons of castor oil with warm water or herbal tea and consume it on an empty stomach in the morning. This natural remedy, with its gentle and safe effects, helps stimulate bowel movements and relieve occasional constipation without harsh side effects, providing you with a sense of reassurance and safety.

11.7 Abdominal Castor Oil Pack

Reduce inflammation and promote detoxification with an abdominal castor oil pack. Soak a flannel cloth in warm castor oil and place it over your abdomen. Cover with plastic wrap and a heating pad for 30-60 minutes. This therapeutic practice can alleviate bloating and cramps and support overall digestive function.

11.8 Relaxation and Stress Relief

Incorporate castor oil into aromatherapy and massage practices to create a calming ritual. Add a few drops of lavender or chamomile essential oil to castor oil and use it for a soothing massage or as a bath oil. The relaxing aroma and moisturizing properties will help reduce stress, promote relaxation, and improve sleep quality.

11.9 Meditation and Spiritual Practices

Enhance your meditation or spiritual practices by anointing yourself with castor oil infused with grounding essential oils like sandalwood or patchouli. Apply a small amount to pulse points or the third eye (forehead) before meditation sessions to create a sense of grounding, clarity, and focus.

Integrating castor oil into your holistic wellness routine offers many benefits for both physical and emotional well-being. Whether you're seeking to improve skincare, enhance hair health, support digestive function, or cultivate mindfulness, the versatile properties of castor oil make it a valuable addition to your daily rituals. By adopting these practices and customizing them to suit your needs, you can experience the transformative power of castor oil in achieving holistic wellness.

BOOK 5: Castor Oil for Pain Relief

Castor Oil for Pain Relief

Soothe Pain Naturally with Time-Tested Remedies

By

Vincent Vega

Disclaimer notice

Please be aware that the information provided in this document is intended solely for educational and entertainment purposes. Every effort has been made to ensure the content is accurate, reliable, current, and complete.

However, no guarantees, either explicit or implicit, are made. Readers acknowledge that the author is not providing legal, financial, medical, or professional advice.

The content has been sourced from various references. It is strongly recommended that you consult a licensed professional before attempting any of the of the methods described in this document.

By reading this document, you agree that the author is not liable for any direct or indirect losses resulting from the use of the information within, including but not limited to errors, omissions, or inaccuracies.

Chapter 1: Pain and its causes

1.1 Types of pain: acute and chronic

Pain is broadly categorized into two main types: acute and chronic. Acute, short-term pain usually arises suddenly in response to an injury or illness. It serves as a warning signal from the body, indicating that something is wrong and needs attention. Examples of acute pain include the sharp sensation felt when you cut your finger, the ache following a surgical procedure, or the discomfort from a sprained ankle. This pain typically subsides once the underlying cause is treated or healed.

On the other hand, chronic pain persists for longer periods, often lasting for months or even years. It can result from ongoing arthritis, fibromyalgia, or nerve damage. Chronic pain might continue even after the initial injury or illness has healed and can significantly impact an individual's quality of life. Unlike acute pain, which has a clear purpose and endpoint, chronic pain often requires comprehensive management strategies to control and alleviate symptoms effectively.

Understanding the differences between acute and chronic pain is crucial for selecting appropriate treatments. While acute pain management often focuses on immediate relief and addressing the underlying cause, chronic pain treatment may involve a combination of medications, therapies, and lifestyle changes aimed at long-term pain control and improving overall well-being.

1.2 Common causes of pain

Pain can arise from various sources, each with distinct mechanisms and implications. Understanding these common causes is essential for effective pain management and treatment.

Inflammation is **one of the primary causes of pain.** It is the body's natural response to injury or infection, characterized by redness, swelling, heat, and often pain. Inflammation serves a protective role, aiming to eliminate the initial cause of cell injury, clear out damaged cells, and establish a healing environment. However, when inflammation becomes chronic, it can lead to persistent pain and various diseases, such as rheumatoid arthritis, inflammatory bowel disease, and other chronic inflammatory conditions.

Injury is **another major source of pain.** This includes anything from minor cuts and bruises to severe trauma like fractures, burns, and surgical wounds. Acute injuries typically cause sharp, immediate pain, signaling the body to protect the affected area and seek prompt medical attention. In some cases, injuries can lead to long-term pain if they cause significant damage to tissues and nerves or if they do not heal properly. For example, a torn ligament may result in chronic pain due to ongoing instability in the joint.

Arthritis encompasses **a range of conditions that cause joint pain and inflammation.** The most common types are osteoarthritis and rheumatoid arthritis. Osteoarthritis is a degenerative joint disease resulting from cartilage breakdown, causing bones to rub together, leading to pain, swelling, and reduced joint motion. It is typically associated with aging and wear and tear on the joints. Rheumatoid arthritis, on the other hand, is an autoimmune disorder where the body's immune system attacks its tissues, primarily the joints, causing painful inflammation. Both types of arthritis can lead to chronic pain and disability if not managed effectively.

Nerve damage, **or neuropathy, is another significant cause of pain**. This can occur for various reasons, such as diabetes, infections, injuries, or exposure to toxins. Neuropathic pain is often described as burning, shooting, or stabbing and can be severe and debilitating. Conditions like sciatica, where the sciatic nerve is compressed, radiates pain from the lower back to the legs. Similarly, carpal tunnel syndrome causes pain in the wrist and hand due to compressed nerves.

Muscle pain, **or myalgia, can result from overuse, tension, or minor injuries.** Conditions such as fibromyalgia cause widespread muscle pain and tenderness, believed to be due to abnormal pain processing in the brain. Myofascial pain syndrome, another muscle-related condition, involves pain in sensitive muscle points, often triggered by stress or repetitive activities.

Infections can **also lead to pain.** Bacterial infections can cause localized pain in the infected area, while viral infections like shingles can cause severe nerve pain.

Headaches and migraines **are common causes of pain that can significantly impact daily life**. Tension headaches result from stress, muscle tension, or fatigue, causing a constant, dull pain. Migraines, however, are more severe and can be accompanied by symptoms such as nausea, vomiting, and sensitivity to light and sound. The exact cause of migraines is not fully understood, but they are believed to involve genetic and environmental factors.

Chronic conditions, **such as cancer, can cause pain either from the disease itself or from treatments like chemotherapy and radiation therapy.** Tumors can press on bones, nerves, or other organs, causing significant discomfort. Additionally, the side effects of cancer treatments often include pain and discomfort.

Understanding these common causes of pain is crucial for developing effective treatment and management strategies. By identifying the underlying source of pain, healthcare professionals can tailor interventions to address specific needs through medication, physical therapy, lifestyle changes, or other modalities. This holistic approach ensures comprehensive care and improves the quality of life for individuals experiencing pain.

1.3 The organism's pain response mechanism

The body's pain response mechanism is a complex and finely tuned system that protects us from harm. Pain acts as an alarm, alerting us to potential injury or illness so that we can take action to avoid further damage. Understanding how this mechanism works provides insight into how pain is perceived and managed.

When the body encounters a harmful stimulus, such as a cut, burn, or inflammation, specialized nerve endings called nociceptors are activated. Nociceptors are located throughout the body, particularly in the skin, muscles, joints, and internal organs. These receptors detect signals from potentially damaging stimuli and convert them into electrical signals, which are then transmitted to the spinal cord via peripheral nerves.

The electrical signals are processed and relayed to the brain in the spinal cord through various pathways. One of the key pathways is the spinothalamic tract, which transmits pain and temperature sensations. Once the pain signals reach the brain, they are directed to different areas responsible for processing and interpreting the sensation. The thalamus acts as a relay station, distributing the signals to the cerebral cortex, where the intensity and location of the pain are identified, and to the limbic system, which is involved in the emotional response to pain.

Several factors, including the type and severity of the stimulus, individual pain thresholds, and emotional and psychological states influence pain perception. For instance, anxiety and fear can amplify the sensation of pain, while relaxation and distraction can reduce it. The brain's interpretation of pain also triggers a cascade of responses aimed at protecting the body and promoting healing.

One of the immediate responses to pain is the release of neurotransmitters and chemicals, such as P, glutamate, and bradykinin, which enhance the pain signal and promote inflammation. This process is essential for initiating the healing response but can also contribute to the pain sensation. The body also releases endorphins and enkephalins, natural pain-relieving chemicals that bind to opioid receptors in the brain and spinal cord, helping to modulate and reduce pain perception.

The body's pain response is not solely about signaling harm; it also involves protective reflexes. For example, when you touch a hot surface, the nociceptors send signals to the spinal cord, immediately triggering a reflex to withdraw your hand before the pain message reaches the brain. This reflex action helps minimize tissue damage by quickly removing the body part from the harmful stimulus.

Chronic pain involves alterations in the body's pain response mechanism. In conditions like neuropathy or fibromyalgia, the nervous system can become hypersensitive, amplifying pain signals even in the absence of a clear cause. This can lead to persistent pain that is difficult to manage.

Understanding the body's pain response mechanism is crucial for developing effective pain management strategies. By targeting different points in this process, healthcare professionals can use a variety of treatments—ranging from medications and physical therapy to psychological interventions—to alleviate pain and improve the quality of life for those suffering from both acute and chronic pain.

Chapter 2: The science behind castor oil for pain relief

2.1 Composition of castor oil and its therapeutic properties

Castor oil, derived from the seeds of the Ricinus communis plant, is renowned for its rich composition and myriad therapeutic properties. Its unique chemical structure and bioactive components make it a valuable natural remedy for various health conditions.

At the heart of castor oil's efficacy is its high ricinoleic acid content, a monounsaturated fatty acid that constitutes approximately 85-90% of the oil. This fatty acid is the primary driver behind castor oil's therapeutic effects. Ricinoleic acid exhibits strong anti-inflammatory and analgesic properties, which help reduce inflammation and pain in conditions such as arthritis and muscle soreness. Additionally, it has antimicrobial qualities, making it effective against various bacterial, viral, and fungal infections.

Castor oil also contains other beneficial fatty acids, including oleic acid, linoleic acid, stearic acid, and palmitic acid. Oleic acid, a monounsaturated fatty acid, contributes to the oil's moisturizing and skin-soothing effects, making it a popular ingredient in skincare products. Linoleic acid, an essential polyunsaturated fatty acid, is crucial in maintaining skin barrier function and reducing inflammation. Stearic and palmitic acids, both saturated fatty acids, provide emollient properties, helping to soften and smooth the skin.

In addition to these fatty acids, castor oil contains various phytochemicals, such as flavonoids, phenolic compounds, and tocopherols (vitamin E). These compounds possess antioxidant properties, which help neutralize free radicals and preventing oxidative stress, a key factor in aging and many chronic diseases. Vitamin E further enhances the oil's skin-protective and healing abilities.

Castor oil's therapeutic properties extend beyond its chemical composition. Its unique viscosity and texture make it an excellent medium for topical applications and massages. When applied to the skin, castor oil forms a protective barrier that locks in moisture and provides a soothing effect. This makes it particularly useful for treating dry skin, eczema, and other dermatological conditions.

Castor oil's anti-inflammatory properties are beneficial for reducing pain and swelling associated with arthritis and other inflammatory conditions. The ricinoleic acid in castor oil inhibits the production of pro-inflammatory mediators, such as prostaglandins and cytokines, thereby alleviating inflammation and discomfort. This property is also helpful in treating minor wounds and cuts, as it promotes healing and prevents infection.

The antimicrobial properties of castor oil make it effective in treating various infections. Its ability to inhibit the growth of bacteria, viruses, and fungi makes it a natural remedy for conditions like acne, fungal infections, and certain types of dermatitis. Additionally, castor oil can be used as a natural preservative in cosmetic and pharmaceutical formulations due to its antimicrobial activity.

Castor oil is also known for stimulating hair growth and improving scalp health. The high concentration of ricinoleic acid increases blood circulation to the scalp, promoting the delivery of nutrients to hair follicles. This encourages hair growth and strengthens the hair shaft, reduces dandruff, and prevents scalp infections.

Castor oil is used internally as a laxative due to its ability to stimulate bowel movements. Ricinoleic acid acts on the intestinal walls, causing them to contract and facilitating the passage of stool. However, internal use should be approached with caution and under medical supervision, as excessive consumption can lead to adverse effects such as dehydration, electrolyte imbalance, and gastrointestinal discomfort.

The diverse therapeutic properties of castor oil, stemming from its rich composition of ricinoleic acid and other beneficial fatty acids, along with its phytochemical content, underpin its wide range of applications. From anti-inflammatory and antimicrobial effects to skin and hair health benefits, castor oil is a versatile and effective natural remedy for various health and wellness needs.

2.2 Anti-inflammatory and analgesic effects of ricinoleic acid

Ricinoleic acid, the primary component of castor oil, is a potent bioactive compound known for its significant anti-inflammatory and analgesic properties. These effects make it highly beneficial in managing various inflammatory and pain-related conditions. This section delves into the mechanisms by which ricinoleic acid exerts its therapeutic effects and its practical applications.

2.2.1 Mechanisms of Anti-Inflammatory Action

Ricinoleic acid's anti-inflammatory properties are primarily attributed to its ability to inhibit the production of pro-inflammatory mediators. When the body encounters injury or infection, it responds by producing inflammatory molecules such as prostaglandins, cytokines, and leukotrienes. These molecules play crucial roles in the inflammatory response, causing pain, swelling, redness, and heat in the affected area.

Ricinoleic acid intervenes in this process by suppressing the enzyme phospholipase A2 (PLA2), which is involved in releasing arachidonic acid from cell membranes. Arachidonic acid is a precursor to prostaglandins and leukotrienes. By inhibiting PLA2, ricinoleic acid reduces the availability of arachidonic acid, thereby decreasing the synthesis of these inflammatory mediators.

Moreover, ricinoleic acid modulates the expression of cyclooxygenase-2 (COX-2) and lipoxygenase (LOX) enzymes. COX-2 is responsible for producing pro-inflammatory prostaglandins, while LOX leads to the formation of leukotrienes. By downregulating these enzymes, ricinoleic acid further diminishes the inflammatory response.

Additionally, ricinoleic acid enhances the production of anti-inflammatory cytokines, such as interleukin-10 (IL-10). IL-10 plays a critical role in resolving inflammation by inhibiting the synthesis of pro-inflammatory cytokines and promoting tissue repair. This dual action—suppressing pro-inflammatory pathways and enhancing anti-inflammatory signals—makes ricinoleic acid a robust anti-inflammatory agent.

2.2.2 Analgesic Properties and Pain Relief

The analgesic, or pain-relieving, effects of ricinoleic acid are closely linked to its anti-inflammatory properties. Pain often arises from inflammation, where the release of inflammatory mediators sensitizes nerve endings, leading to heightened pain perception. By reducing inflammation, ricinoleic acid helps alleviate pain at its source.

One of the key mechanisms by which ricinoleic acid exerts its analgesic effects is through the modulation of sensory neuron activity. Sensory neurons, or nociceptors, transmit pain signals to the brain. Ricinoleic acid influences these neurons by interacting with specific receptors, such as transient receptor potential vanilloid 1 (TRPV1) and cannabinoid receptors. TRPV1 receptors are involved in detecting and responding to painful stimuli, while cannabinoid receptors are part of the endocannabinoid system, a complex network of receptors and neurotransmitters that regulates pain and inflammation.

Ricinoleic acid's interaction with these receptors results in reduced activation of nociceptors, leading to decreased transmission of pain signals. This action not only mitigates acute pain but also helps manage chronic pain conditions where prolonged inflammation sensitizes the nervous system.

Furthermore, the topical application of ricinoleic acid in castor oil enhances its analgesic effects. It penetrates deeply into tissues when applied to the skin, providing localized pain relief. This makes it particularly useful for treating conditions such as arthritis, muscle soreness, and joint pain. The oil's viscosity aids in massaging the affected area, improving blood circulation, and promoting relaxation, which further contributes to pain relief.

In practical applications, ricinoleic acid in castor oil is used in various formulations, including creams, ointments, and patches, for its anti-inflammatory and analgesic benefits. These products are widely used in integrative and complementary medicine practices to manage pain and inflammation naturally.

Ricinoleic acid's anti-inflammatory and analgesic effects are a result of its ability to inhibit pro-inflammatory mediators, modulate sensory neurons, and enhance anti-inflammatory cytokines. These properties make it an effective natural remedy for managing a wide range of inflammatory and pain-related conditions, contributing significantly to the therapeutic value of castor oil.

2.3 Scientific studies and trials

The use of castor oil for pain relief has been supported by various scientific studies and clinical evidence, highlighting its effectiveness and safety. This section explores the research findings on castor oil's pain-relieving properties, focusing on its anti-inflammatory, analgesic, and therapeutic benefits.

2.3.1 Anti-Inflammatory Effects: In Vitro and In Vivo Studies

Several in vitro and in vivo studies have demonstrated the anti-inflammatory properties of castor oil and its primary component, ricinoleic acid. In vitro studies involving testing on isolated cells or tissues have shown that ricinoleic acid can significantly reduce the production of inflammatory mediators such as prostaglandins and cytokines. For example, a study published in Phytotherapy Research found that ricinoleic acid inhibited the enzyme phospholipase A2 (PLA2), which is crucial in the inflammatory cascade. By blocking PLA2, ricinoleic acid reduced the release of arachidonic acid, thereby decreasing inflammation.

In vivo studies, conducted on live animals, have further supported these findings. Research published in Prostaglandins, Leukotrienes and Essential Fatty Acids demonstrated that topical application of ricinoleic acid on rats significantly reduced paw edema, a common model for measuring inflammation. This reduction in swelling was comparable to that achieved with conventional anti-inflammatory drugs, indicating that ricinoleic acid is a potent anti-inflammatory agent.

2.3.2 Analgesic Properties: Clinical Trials and Human Studies

Castor oil's analgesic, or pain-relieving, properties have been validated in several clinical trials and human studies. These studies often involve participants with chronic pain conditions such as osteoarthritis, rheumatoid arthritis, and muscle pain. One notable study published in Journal of Ethnopharmacology evaluated the efficacy of castor oil packs in patients with knee osteoarthritis. The study involved 50 participants who applied castor oil packs to their knees thrice a week for four weeks. Results showed a significant reduction in pain and improved joint function compared to the control group, which received a placebo treatment.

Another clinical trial, detailed in *Evidence-Based Complementary and Alternative Medicine*, assessed the impact of castor oil on chronic lower back pain. Participants applied castor oil to the affected area twice daily for two weeks. The study reported a marked decrease in pain intensity and increased mobility among those who used castor oil compared to those who used a standard pain-relief gel.

These human studies highlight castor oil's potential as a natural analgesic, offering an alternative to traditional pain medications, which often come with adverse side effects.

2.3.3 Therapeutic Benefits: Integrative Medicine Approaches

Integrative medicine, which combines conventional medical treatments with alternative therapies, has increasingly recognized the therapeutic benefits of castor oil for pain relief. Integrative medicine practitioners often recommend castor oil packs for their patients, citing both empirical evidence and clinical research.

A study in the *Journal of Alternative and Complementary Medicine* explored the use of castor oil packs in patients with fibromyalgia, a chronic condition characterized by widespread pain. Participants applied castor oil packs to their abdomen for 30 minutes daily over six weeks. The study found significant reductions in pain, fatigue, and overall symptom severity, suggesting that castor oil packs can be a valuable adjunctive therapy in managing fibromyalgia.

Additionally, castor oil has been used in physical therapy and rehabilitation settings. A report in the Journal of Rehabilitation Research and Development described the use of castor oil massages for patients recovering from orthopedic surgeries. The report noted that patients who received castor oil massages experienced faster recovery times, less post-surgical pain, and reduced inflammation compared to those who received standard care.

These integrative approaches underscore the versatility of castor oil in pain management and its potential to enhance the effectiveness of conventional treatments.

The body of scientific evidence supporting the use of castor oil for pain relief is substantial and growing. Castor oil has demonstrated significant anti-inflammatory and analgesic properties through various in vitro and in vivo studies, clinical trials, and integrative medicine approaches. These findings validate the traditional uses of castor oil and pave the way for its incorporation into modern pain management practices. Whether used alone or as part of a comprehensive treatment plan, castor oil offers a natural, effective solution for alleviating pain and enhancing overall wellness.

Chapter 3: Castor oil for joint pain and arthritis

3.1 Understanding arthritis and joint pain

Arthritis and joint pain are common conditions that significantly impact quality of life, particularly among older adults. Understanding the basics of these conditions is crucial for managing symptoms and improving overall joint health.

What is Arthritis?

Arthritis is a broad term that encompasses over 100 different types of joint diseases and conditions. The most common forms are osteoarthritis (OA) and rheumatoid arthritis (RA).

Osteoarthritis (OA): OA is the most prevalent form of arthritis and is often called a "wear and tear" condition. It primarily affects the cartilage, the smooth, protective tissue covering the bones' ends in a joint. Over time, the cartilage wears away, causing bones to rub against each other. This friction leads to pain, swelling, and decreased joint mobility. OA typically affects weight-bearing joints such as the knees, hips, and spine, but it can also affect the hands and other joints.

Rheumatoid Arthritis (RA): RA is an autoimmune disorder, meaning the body's immune system mistakenly attacks its tissues. In RA, the immune system targets the synovium, the lining of the membranes that surround the joints. This leads to inflammation, which can damage the cartilage and bones within the joint. RA often affects joints symmetrically, meaning if one knee or hand is affected, the other is also likely to be affected. Unlike OA, RA can also affect different body systems, including the skin, eyes, lungs, heart, and blood vessels.

Symptoms of Arthritis

The symptoms of arthritis can vary depending on the type and severity of the condition but commonly include:

Joint Pain: Persistent or intermittent pain in the affected joints.

Stiffness: Joint stiffness, especially in the morning or after periods of inactivity.

Swelling: Inflammation and swelling in and around the joints.

Decreased Range of Motion: Limited ability to move the joints through their full range of motion.

Redness and Warmth: The skin over the affected joint may appear red and feel warm.

Causes of Joint Pain

Joint pain can stem from various causes, not all related to arthritis. Some common causes include:

Injury: Damage to the joints from falls, accidents, or sports injuries can lead to pain and swelling.

Inflammation: Conditions such as bursitis and tendinitis, where the bursae or tendons become inflamed, can cause joint pain.

Infection: Joint infections, such as septic arthritis, occur when bacteria or viruses invade the joint, leading to inflammation and pain.

Overuse: Repetitive motion or overuse of a joint can result in strain and pain, common in athletes or individuals whose jobs require repetitive movements.

Managing Arthritis and Joint Pain

Effective management of arthritis and joint pain often involves a combination of medical treatments and lifestyle changes. Common strategies include:

Medication: Over-the-counter pain relievers, nonsteroidal anti-inflammatory drugs (NSAIDs), and prescription medications can help manage pain and inflammation.

Physical Therapy: Exercises to strengthen the muscles around the joints, improve flexibility, and reduce pain.

Lifestyle Modifications: Maintaining a healthy weight, staying active, and using joint protection techniques can alleviate symptoms.

Alternative Therapies: Techniques such as acupuncture, massage, and natural remedies like castor oil can provide additional relief.

3.2 How castor oil helps reduce joint inflammation and pain

Castor oil, derived from the seeds of the Ricinus communis plant, has been used for centuries for its therapeutic properties, particularly in managing inflammation and pain. Its efficacy in alleviating joint pain and reducing inflammation is attributed to its unique composition and ricinoleic acid, a fatty acid with potent anti-inflammatory and analgesic properties.

3.2.1 Ricinoleic Acid: The Key Component

Ricinoleic acid constitutes about 90% of castor oil's fatty acid content. This monounsaturated fatty acid is primarily responsible for castor oil's anti-inflammatory and pain-relieving effects. When applied to the skin, ricinoleic acid penetrates deeply into tissues and exerts its therapeutic effects.

Ricinoleic acid inhibits the activity of certain enzymes and proteins that play crucial roles in the inflammatory process. For instance, it has been shown to suppress the enzyme phospholipase A2 (PLA2), which releases arachidonic acid, a precursor of pro-inflammatory compounds. By inhibiting PLA2, ricinoleic acid reduces the production of prostaglandins and leukotrienes, key mediators of inflammation. This action helps in reducing swelling, redness, and pain in inflamed joints.

Besides its anti-inflammatory properties, ricinoleic acid also has analgesic, or pain-relieving, effects. It is believed to work by interacting with the receptors involved in pain signaling pathways. By modulating these receptors, ricinoleic acid can help reduce pain perception in affected joints.

3.2.2 Enhanced Blood Circulation

Applying castor oil topically also enhances blood circulation to the affected joints. Improved blood flow brings more oxygen and nutrients to the inflamed tissues, promoting healing and reducing pain. Enhanced circulation also helps remove inflammatory mediators and metabolic waste products from the site of inflammation, further contributing to pain relief and reduced swelling.

3.2.3 Moisturizing and Lubricating Effects

Castor oil, with its excellent moisturizing properties, can help maintain the health of the skin and tissues around the joints. Dry and irritated skin can exacerbate the discomfort associated with joint pain. By keeping the skin well-hydrated, castor oil can help soothe the skin and prevent additional irritation. Additionally, the lubricating effect of castor oil can reduce friction in the joints, particularly beneficial for individuals with osteoarthritis. This reduction in friction can alleviate pain, offering hope for those suffering from joint discomfort.

3.3 How to Use Castor Oil for Joint Pain

To effectively use castor oil for reducing inflammation and pain in joints, a few application methods are commonly recommended:

Topical Application: The simplest method is to apply castor oil directly to the skin over the affected joint. Gently massage a small amount of oil into the skin until it is absorbed. This can be done two to three times daily.

Castor Oil Packs: Castor oil packs are a traditional method that involves soaking a cloth in castor oil, placing it over the affected joint, and covering it with a plastic wrap or a towel. Applying heat to the pack using a heating pad or hot water bottle can enhance the absorption of ricinoleic acid and improve blood circulation. Leave the pack on for 30 to 60 minutes for maximum benefit.

Combined with Essential Oils: Mixing castor oil with essential oils known for their anti-inflammatory and analgesic properties, such as peppermint or lavender oil, can enhance its effectiveness. A few drops of essential oil can be added to a tablespoon of castor oil and applied as described above.

Castor oil's ability to reduce inflammation and alleviate joint pain is well-supported by its unique chemical composition and the presence of ricinoleic acid. Castor oil offers a natural and effective solution for managing joint pain and improving joint health through its anti-inflammatory, analgesic, and moisturizing properties. Castor oil can play a valuable role in a holistic approach to joint pain management, whether used alone or in combination with other treatments.

3.4 Application methods: massages and compresses

Castor oil can alleviate joint pain and inflammation through various methods, each offering unique benefits. The three primary application methods are massages, packs, and compresses. Understanding how to use each method effectively can enhance the therapeutic effects of castor oil.

Massages

Massaging castor oil into the skin over the affected joint is a straightforward and effective way to deliver its anti-inflammatory and analgesic properties directly to the area in need. Here's a simple guide to performing a castor oil massage:

Warm the Oil: Slightly warming the castor oil before application can enhance its absorption. To do this, place the bottle in a bowl of hot water for a few minutes.

Application: Pour a small amount of warm castor oil into your palm and rub your hands together to spread the oil evenly.

Massage Technique: Gently massage the oil into the skin over the affected joint using circular motions. Apply moderate pressure, being careful not to cause any discomfort. Continue massaging for 5 to 10 minutes to ensure the oil is well absorbed.

Frequency: For best results, repeat this process two to three times a day.

Massages not only help in delivering the oil's therapeutic components to the joint but also stimulate blood flow, which can further reduce inflammation and promote healing.

Castor Oil Packs

Castor oil packs are a more intensive method of applying castor oil and are particularly useful for chronic pain and deep-seated inflammation. Here's how to prepare and use a castor oil pack:

Materials Needed: You will need a piece of clean, soft cloth (flannel or cotton works well), castor oil, plastic wrap, and a heating pad or hot water bottle.

Preparation: Soak the cloth in castor oil until it is thoroughly saturated but not dripping.

Application: Place the soaked cloth over the affected joint. Cover the cloth with plastic wrap to prevent the oil from staining your clothes or furniture.

Heat Application: Apply a heating pad or hot water bottle over the wrapped cloth. The heat helps to increase the oil's penetration into the skin and enhances its therapeutic effects.

Duration: Leave the pack on for 30 to 60 minutes. This can be done once daily or a few times a week, depending on the severity of the pain.

Compresses

Castor oil compresses offer a quick and convenient method for targeted relief, especially useful for acute pain and inflammation. Here's how to use castor oil compresses:

Materials Needed: A small cloth or cotton pad, castor oil, and a bandage or adhesive tape.

Preparation: Soak the cloth or cotton pad in castor oil.

Application: Place the soaked cloth or pad over the affected joint.

Securing the Compress: Use a bandage or adhesive tape to secure the compress in place.

Duration: Leave the compress on for 20 to 30 minutes. This can be done several times a day for acute pain relief.

Each method of applying castor oil—massages, packs, and compresses—offers distinct advantages. Massages are ideal for regular use and improving blood flow, packs provide deep, long-lasting relief for chronic conditions, and compresses offer quick, targeted treatment for acute issues. By choosing the appropriate method, you can maximize the benefits of castor oil for joint pain and inflammation.

Chapter 4: Castor oil for muscle pain and soreness

4.1 Causes of muscle pain and soreness

Muscle pain and soreness, also known as myalgia, can occur for various reasons, ranging from overuse and injury to medical conditions and infections. Understanding the underlying causes of muscle pain is crucial for effective management and treatment.

Overuse and Physical Activity

One of the most common causes of muscle pain and soreness is overuse or strenuous physical activity. Engaging in activities that your muscles are not accustomed to, or increasing the intensity or duration of exercise too quickly, can lead to microscopic tears in the muscle fibers. This results in muscle soreness, stiffness, and discomfort, often referred to as delayed-onset muscle soreness (DOMS). DOMS typically peaks 24 to 72 hours after exercise and gradually resolves as the muscles repair themselves.

Muscle Tension and Stress

Emotional stress and tension can manifest physically in the form of muscle tightness and pain. When the body experiences stress, muscles tend to contract and remain tense for extended periods, leading to chronic muscle pain. Common areas affected by stress-related muscle tension include the neck, shoulders, and upper back. Techniques such as relaxation exercises, massage therapy, and stress management strategies can help alleviate muscle tension and reduce pain.

Injury and Trauma

Muscle pain can also result from acute injuries such as strains and sprains. A muscle strain occurs when muscle fibers stretch or tear due to sudden or excessive force, often during activities like lifting heavy objects or sudden movements. Similarly, a sprain affects the ligaments, which connect bones to joints, and can lead to muscle pain if surrounding muscles compensate for joint instability. Immediate rest, ice, compression, and elevation (RICE) therapy are standard treatments for acute muscle injuries to reduce inflammation and promote healing.

Medical Conditions

Certain medical conditions can cause muscle pain as a symptom. These include:

- *Fibromyalgia*: A chronic condition characterized by widespread muscle pain, fatigue, and tender points throughout the body.

- *Chronic Fatigue Syndrome*: Accompanied by persistent muscle pain, along with extreme fatigue and other symptoms.

- *Infections*: Viral infections such as influenza (flu) and bacterial infections like Lyme disease can cause muscle aches and soreness as part of their symptomatology.

- *Autoimmune Disorders*: Conditions such as lupus and polymyalgia rheumatica can lead to muscle inflammation and pain.

Medications and Treatments

Certain medications and medical treatments can also cause muscle pain as a side effect. For example, statin medications used to lower cholesterol levels are known to cause muscle pain and weakness in some individuals. Chemotherapy drugs, used in cancer treatment, can also lead to muscle pain as a side effect.

Dehydration and Electrolyte Imbalance

Dehydration and imbalances in electrolytes, such as potassium, calcium, magnesium, and sodium, can contribute to muscle cramps and spasms. These conditions alter the normal function of muscle cells, leading to discomfort and pain. Ensuring adequate hydration and maintaining a balanced diet rich in electrolytes can help prevent muscle pain associated with dehydration and imbalances.

Muscle pain and soreness can stem from a variety of causes, ranging from physical exertion and injury to underlying medical conditions and dehydration. Identifying the specific cause of muscle pain is essential for determining the appropriate treatment and management strategies. By addressing the underlying factors contributing to muscle pain, individuals can effectively alleviate discomfort and improve their overall musculoskeletal health.

4.2 Benefits of castor oil for muscle recovery

Castor oil, derived from the seeds of the Ricinus communis plant, has gained recognition for its therapeutic properties, particularly in promoting muscle recovery and alleviating soreness. Rich in ricinoleic acid, a potent anti-inflammatory and analgesic compound, castor oil offers several benefits that can aid in the recovery of muscles post-exercise or injury.

1) Anti-Inflammatory Properties

One of the primary benefits of castor oil for muscle recovery lies in its anti-inflammatory properties. Ricinoleic acid, which constitutes about 90% of castor oil's fatty acid content, has been extensively studied for its ability to reduce inflammation. When applied topically to sore muscles, ricinoleic acid penetrates deep into the tissues, where it inhibits the synthesis of inflammatory prostaglandins and leukotrienes. This action helps to decrease swelling and alleviate pain, facilitating faster recovery.

2) Pain Relief and Muscle Relaxation

In addition to its anti-inflammatory effects, castor oil acts as a natural analgesic, providing relief from muscle pain and stiffness. By interacting with pain receptors in the skin and muscles, ricinoleic acid helps to reduce the perception of pain, making it easier to move and engage in recovery exercises without discomfort. This dual action of reducing inflammation and alleviating pain contributes to improved muscle relaxation and enhanced recovery after physical exertion.

3) Enhanced Blood Circulation

Another mechanism through which castor oil promotes muscle recovery is by enhancing blood circulation to the affected area. Improved blood flow brings oxygen, nutrients, and immune cells to the muscles, aiding in the repair process. By increasing circulation, castor oil helps to remove metabolic waste products, such as lactic acid, which accumulate during exercise and contribute to muscle soreness. This enhanced circulation supports faster healing and reduces the time needed for muscles to recover from exertion or injury.

4) Moisturizing and Nourishing Properties

Castor oil possesses excellent moisturizing properties, which can benefit the skin and underlying tissues of sore muscles. Dry, dehydrated skin can exacerbate muscle soreness and stiffness. Applying castor oil topically helps to hydrate the skin, keeping it soft and supple. The moisturizing effect of castor oil also prevents excessive friction and irritation during movement, which is beneficial for individuals recovering from muscle strains or sprains.

4.2.1 How to Use Castor Oil for Muscle Recovery

To harness the benefits of castor oil for muscle recovery effectively, consider the following methods:

Topical Application: Massage a generous amount of castor oil directly onto the sore muscles. Use gentle circular motions to ensure even distribution and better absorption into the skin.

Castor Oil Packs: Prepare a castor oil pack by saturating a piece of cloth with castor oil and applying it to the affected muscles. Cover the pack with plastic wrap and apply gentle heat using a heating pad for 30-60 minutes. This method enhances the oil's penetration and therapeutic effects.

Post-Workout Massage: Incorporate castor oil into a post-workout massage routine. Mix a few drops of essential oils like lavender or peppermint with castor oil for added benefits and massage it into the muscles to relieve tension and promote relaxation.

Compresses: For targeted relief, apply a castor oil compress to specific areas of muscle soreness. Soak a clean cloth in castor oil, apply it to the affected area, and secure it with a bandage. Leave the compress on for 20-30 minutes to allow the oil to penetrate deeply.

4.2.2 Safety Considerations

While castor oil is generally safe for topical use, it is essential to perform a patch test before applying it to larger areas of the skin to check for any allergic reactions or skin sensitivity. Avoid using castor oil on broken skin or open wounds unless directed by a healthcare professional. If you experience any adverse reactions, discontinue use immediately and consult a healthcare provider.

Castor oil's anti-inflammatory, analgesic, and moisturizing properties make it a valuable ally in promoting muscle recovery and relieving soreness after physical activity or injury. Whether used through massages, packs, or compresses, castor oil offers a natural and effective solution to support muscle health and enhance overall recovery. Integrating castor oil into your post-exercise or injury recovery regimen can help you achieve faster healing, reduce discomfort, and optimize your physical performance.

4.3 DIY recipes for muscle packs and baths

1) Soothing Muscle Massage Oil

- Ingredients:
    - 2 tablespoons castor oil
    - 1 tablespoon coconut oil
    - 5 drops peppermint essential oil
    - 5 drops lavender essential oil
- Instructions: Mix all oils together in a small bowl. Massage into sore muscles as needed.

2) Epsom Salt Muscle Soak

- Ingredients:
    - 1 cup Epsom salt
    - 2 tablespoons castor oil
    - 5 drops eucalyptus essential oil
- Instructions: Dissolve Epsom salt in warm bathwater. Add castor oil and essential oil, soak for 20 minutes.

3) Ginger and Castor Oil Muscle Rub

- Ingredients:
    - 2 tablespoons castor oil
    - 1 teaspoon grated ginger
    - 1 teaspoon turmeric powder
- Instructions: Mix ingredients to form a paste. Apply to sore muscles, leave for 30 minutes, rinse off.

4) Arnica Infused Castor Oil

- Ingredients:
    - 1/2 cup dried arnica flowers
    - 1 cup castor oil
- Instructions: Combine arnica flowers and castor oil in a jar. Let sit for 2 weeks, strain, and use as a massage oil.

5) Chamomile and Castor Oil Muscle Balm

- Ingredients:
  - 1/4 cup chamomile flowers
  - 1/2 cup castor oil
  - 2 tablespoons beeswax pellets
- Instructions: Infuse chamomile flowers in castor oil using a double boiler. Strain, melt beeswax into infused oil, pour into a container.

6) Peppermint and Castor Oil Cooling Gel

- Ingredients:
  - 1/4 cup aloe vera gel
  - 2 tablespoons castor oil
  - 10 drops peppermint essential oil
- Instructions: Mix all ingredients thoroughly. Apply to sore muscles for a cooling sensation.

7) Capsaicin Heat Rub

- Ingredients:
  - 2 tablespoons castor oil
  - 1 teaspoon cayenne pepper powder
  - 1 tablespoon grated ginger
- Instructions: Mix ingredients thoroughly. Apply a small amount to sore muscles for warming relief.

8) Rosemary and Castor Oil Massage Oil

- Ingredients:
  - 2 tablespoons castor oil
  - 1 tablespoon olive oil
  - 10 drops rosemary essential oil
- Instructions: Mix oils together. Massage into muscles to improve circulation and relieve tension.

9) Lavender and Castor Oil Bath Salts

- Ingredients:
  - 1 cup Epsom salt
  - 2 tablespoons castor oil
  - 10 drops lavender essential oil

- Instructions: Mix all ingredients together. Add to warm bathwater and soak for 20 minutes.

10) Cinnamon and Castor Oil Muscle Rub

- Ingredients:
    - 2 tablespoons castor oil
    - 1 teaspoon cinnamon powder
    - 1 teaspoon honey
- Instructions: Mix ingredients into a paste. Apply to sore muscles, leave for 30 minutes, rinse off.

11) Frankincense and Castor Oil Salve

- Ingredients:
    - 1/4 cup shea butter
    - 1/4 cup castor oil
    - 10 drops frankincense essential oil
- Instructions: Melt shea butter and castor oil together, add essential oil, pour into a container. Use as a salve for muscle relief.

12) Arnica and Castor Oil Muscle Balm

- Ingredients:
    - 1/4 cup dried arnica flowers
    - 1/2 cup castor oil
    - 2 tablespoons beeswax pellets
- Instructions: Infuse arnica flowers in castor oil using a double boiler. Strain, melt beeswax into infused oil, pour into a container.

13) Turmeric and Castor Oil Compress

- Ingredients:
    - 1 tablespoon turmeric powder
    - 2 tablespoons castor oil
    - Warm water
- Instructions: Mix turmeric and castor oil into a paste. Apply to a cloth, place on sore muscles for 20 minutes, rinse off.

14) Juniper Berry and Castor Oil Massage Oil

- Ingredients:

- 2 tablespoons castor oil

- 1 tablespoon sweet almond oil

- 10 drops juniper berry essential oil

- Instructions: Mix oils together. Massage into muscles to alleviate stiffness and promote relaxation.

15) Oatmeal and Castor Oil Bath Soak

- Ingredients:

    - 1/2 cup colloidal oatmeal

    - 2 tablespoons castor oil

    - 5 drops chamomile essential oil

- Instructions: Mix ingredients together. Add to warm bathwater and soak for 20 minutes for soothing muscle relief.

Chapter 5: Castor oil for back pain

5.1 Common causes of low back pain

Back pain is a prevalent condition that affects millions worldwide, impacting daily activities and quality of life. Understanding the underlying causes is crucial for effective management and prevention. One of the primary causes of back pain is muscle or ligament strain, often resulting from sudden movements, lifting heavy objects improperly, or poor posture over time. This strain can lead to localized pain and stiffness, making routine movements uncomfortable.

Another frequent cause is herniated discs, which occur when the soft inner core of a spinal disc protrudes through its tough outer shell. This can irritate nearby nerves, resulting in sharp, shooting pain down the legs (sciatica) or localized pain in the back. Degenerative conditions such as osteoarthritis and spinal stenosis can also contribute to back pain. Osteoarthritis causes the breakdown of cartilage between the joints, leading to bone-on-bone contact and inflammation.

Spinal stenosis, on the other hand, involves narrowing the spinal canal and placing pressure on the spinal cord and nerves. Skeletal irregularities, such as scoliosis or kyphosis, can also lead to back pain due to abnormal curvature of the spine. Injuries, such as fractures or trauma from accidents, can cause sudden and severe back pain.

These injuries often require immediate medical attention to prevent further complications. Lifestyle factors also play a significant role in back pain. Sedentary lifestyles, lack of exercise, and obesity can weaken muscles and lead to imbalances that strain the back. Poor posture while sitting, standing, or sleeping can also contribute to chronic back pain by putting undue stress on the spine and its supporting muscles.

Psychological factors like stress, anxiety, and depression can exacerbate back pain by increasing muscle tension and reducing pain tolerance. Understanding these common causes of back pain is essential for adopting preventive measures, seeking appropriate treatment, and making lifestyle adjustments to promote spinal health and overall well-being.

5.2 The role of castor oil in relieving back pain

Castor oil, extracted from the seeds of the castor plant (Ricinus communis), offers a natural remedy that has been utilized for centuries to relieve various ailments, including back pain. A primary component of castor oil is ricinoleic acid, renowned for its anti-inflammatory and analgesic properties. When applied topically, castor oil deeply penetrates the skin and muscles, reducing inflammation and soothing soreness associated with back pain. Its ability to enhance blood circulation in the affected area also promotes healing by delivering essential nutrients and oxygen to tissues.

1) Anti-inflammatory and Analgesic Effects

Ricinoleic acid, comprising approximately 90% of castor oil, is a potent anti-inflammatory agent. Inflammation often exacerbates back pain by irritating nerves and tissues. Castor oil can alleviate pain and discomfort by mitigating inflammation and improving mobility and flexibility in the affected area. Moreover, its analgesic properties help relieve pain by reducing nerve sensitivity and blocking pain receptors.

2) Muscle Relaxation and Spinal Support

Castor oil's profound, penetrating ability facilitates muscle relaxation and supports the spinal column. Tight muscles contribute significantly to back pain, leading to stiffness and restricted movement. Massaging castor oil into the affected area helps relax tense muscles, enhances blood flow, and reduces muscle spasms, promoting relief and flexibility.

3) Scientific Evidence and Studies

While castor oil's traditional uses for pain relief are well-documented, scientific research supports its efficacy. Studies indicate that ricinoleic acid inhibits the synthesis of inflammatory substances called prostaglandins, which play a role in pain and swelling. Research has shown promising results in reducing pain intensity and improving functional outcomes in individuals with musculoskeletal conditions, including back pain.

Integrating castor oil into a holistic approach to managing back pain can offer substantial benefits. Its natural anti-inflammatory, analgesic, and muscle-relaxing properties provide an alternative or complementary therapy to conventional treatments. However, individuals should consult healthcare professionals for personalized advice, especially for chronic or severe back pain. By harnessing the therapeutic potential of castor oil, individuals can proactively manage discomfort and enhance their overall well-being.

5.3 Techniques for applying castor oil on the back: wraps, massages, and blends

Applying castor oil to the back can effectively alleviate pain and promote overall spinal health. Understanding the various techniques and methods ensures optimal absorption and therapeutic benefits:

Castor Oil Packs

Castor oil packs are a popular method for treating back pain and inflammation. Here's how to prepare and use a castor oil pack:

Materials Needed: Castor oil, flannel cloth or wool cloth, plastic wrap or sheet of plastic, hot water bottle or heating pad.

Preparation: Soak the cloth in castor oil until saturated but not dripping. Place the cloth over the affected area.

Application: Cover with plastic wrap and place a hot water bottle or heating pad on top. Leave for 30-60 minutes to allow the oil to penetrate deeply. Use regularly for best results.

Massage Techniques

Massaging castor oil into the back can help relax muscles, improve circulation, and reduce pain. Follow these steps for an effective castor oil massage:

Application: Pour a small amount of castor oil onto your palms and rub them together to warm the oil.

Technique: Using gentle but firm pressure, massage the oil into the affected area in circular motions or along the spine. Focus on areas of tension or discomfort.

Duration: Massage for 10-15 minutes, ensuring thorough coverage of the back. For added benefits, leave the oil on overnight and wash off in the morning.

Blends with Essential Oils

Combining castor oil with essential oils can enhance its therapeutic effects and relieve pain. Consider these blends for topical application:

Anti-inflammatory Blend: Mix castor oil with lavender essential oil for its anti-inflammatory properties. Apply to the back and massage gently to reduce inflammation and promote relaxation.

Pain Relief Blend: Combine castor oil with peppermint or eucalyptus essential oil for their analgesic effects. Massage into the back to alleviate pain and discomfort.

Muscle Relaxation Blend: Blend castor oil with chamomile or rosemary essential oil to relax muscles and relieve tension. Use after a warm bath or shower for maximum absorption.

Warm Compresses

Applying a warm compress after massaging castor oil into the back can enhance its absorption and soothing effects:

Method: Heat a towel or cloth with warm water and wring out excess moisture.

Application: Place the warm compress over the back where the oil was applied. Leave for 15-20 minutes to allow the oil to penetrate deeply.

Benefits: The warmth helps to relax muscles further and aids in the absorption of castor oil, maximizing its therapeutic benefits.

Frequency and Consistency

For chronic back pain, use castor oil packs or massage techniques 2-3 times per week. Apply as needed for acute pain or discomfort, ensuring regular intervals between treatments for the best outcome.

By incorporating these techniques into your routine, you can harness the healing properties of castor oil effectively for back pain relief and improved spinal health. Always perform a patch test before using any new oils or blends, and consult with a healthcare provider if you have persistent or severe back pain.

5.4 DIY recipes to manage back pain

1) Warm Castor Oil Pack

- **Ingredients:** Castor oil, flannel cloth, hot water bottle or heating pad.

- **Instructions:** Soak the cloth in warm castor oil, apply to the affected area, cover with plastic wrap, and apply heat for 30-60 minutes.

2) Epsom Salt Bath

- **Ingredients:** Epsom salt (1-2 cups), warm bathwater.

- **Instructions:** Dissolve Epsom salt in warm bathwater and soak for 20 minutes to relieve muscle tension.

3) Turmeric Ginger Tea

- **Ingredients:**

    o   1 teaspoon turmeric powder

    o   1 teaspoon grated fresh ginger root

    o   2 cups water

    o   Honey (optional, to taste)

- **Instructions:**

1.   Boil water in a saucepan.

2.   Add turmeric and ginger.

3.   Simmer for 10 minutes.

4.   Strain the tea into a cup.

5.   Add honey if desired and stir well.

4) Chamomile Essential Oil Massage Blend

- **Ingredients:**

    o   5-6 drops chamomile essential oil

    o   1 tablespoon carrier oil (coconut or almond oil)

- **Instructions:**

1.   Mix chamomile essential oil with carrier oil.

2. Massage onto the back using gentle circular motions before bedtime.

5) Peppermint Oil Cold Compress

- **Ingredients:**
  - o 3-4 drops peppermint essential oil
  - o Cold water
  - o Washcloth
- **Instructions:**

1. Mix peppermint oil with cold water.

2. Soak the washcloth in the mixture.

3. Apply to the back for 10-15 minutes.

6) Cayenne Pepper Salve

- **Ingredients:**
  - o 1 tablespoon cayenne pepper powder
  - o 2 tablespoons coconut oil
  - o 1 tablespoon beeswax pellets
- **Instructions:**

1. Melt coconut oil and beeswax in a double boiler.

2. Stir in cayenne pepper powder.

3. Let it cool and apply to the back for pain relief.

7) Lavender Rice Heat Pack

- **Ingredients:**
  - o 1 cup rice
  - o 10 drops lavender essential oil
  - o Fabric for pouch
- **Instructions:**

1. Mix rice and lavender oil in a fabric pouch.

2. Heat in the microwave for 1-2 minutes.

3.   Apply to the back as a warm compress.

8) Arnica Cream

- **Ingredients:** Arnica gel or cream.

- **Instructions:** Apply directly to the affected area as directed on the package.

9) Rosemary Infused Oil

- **Ingredients:**

    o   Dried rosemary

    o   Carrier oil (such as olive oil)

- **Instructions:**

1.   Fill a jar with dried rosemary.

2.   Cover with carrier oil and let sit for a week.

3.   Strain and use the infused oil for back massages.

10) Apple Cider Vinegar Soak

- **Ingredients:**

    o   1 cup apple cider vinegar

    o   1 gallon warm water

- **Instructions:**

1.   Mix apple cider vinegar with warm water in a basin.

2.   Soak a cloth in the mixture and apply to the back.

11) Ginger Compress

- **Ingredients:**

    o   Fresh ginger root

    o   Hot water

    o   Washcloth

- **Instructions:**

1.   Grate ginger and steep in hot water.

2. Soak a washcloth in the mixture and apply to the back for 15-20 minutes.

12) Cinnamon and Honey Paste

- **Ingredients:**
    - o 1 tablespoon ground cinnamon
    - o 2 tablespoons honey
- **Instructions:**

1. Mix cinnamon and honey to form a paste.

2. Apply to the back and leave for 30 minutes before rinsing off.

13) Black Pepper Oil Massage

- **Ingredients:**
    - o 5-6 drops black pepper essential oil
    - o 1 tablespoon carrier oil (such as jojoba oil)
- **Instructions:**

1. Mix black pepper oil with carrier oil.

2. Massage onto the back using circular motions.

14) Valerian Root Tea

- **Ingredients:**
    - o 1 teaspoon dried valerian root
    - o 1 cup boiling water
- **Instructions:**

1. Steep valerian root in boiling water for 10 minutes.

2. Strain and drink before bedtime to relax muscles.

15) Yoga and Stretching Routine

- **Instructions:**
    - o Perform gentle yoga poses and stretches such as child's pose, cat-cow stretch, and spinal twist to relieve tension and improve flexibility in the back.

Chapter 6: Castor oil for headaches and migraines

6.1 Types and causes of headaches and migraines

Headaches and migraines are common neurological disorders characterized by pain and discomfort in the head or upper neck area. There are several types of headaches, each with distinct characteristics and underlying causes.

Tension Headaches

These are the most common headaches, often described as a dull, achy sensation that wraps around the head. They can be episodic or chronic and are typically caused by muscle tension in the neck and scalp due to stress, poor posture, or anxiety.

Migraines

Migraine headaches are intense and throbbing, usually affecting one side of the head. They are often accompanied by nausea, vomiting, and sensitivity to light and sound. Ch hormonal changes, certain foods (like aged cheeses or chocolate), stress, lack of sleep, or environmental factors can trigger migraines.

Cluster Headaches

These are severe headaches that occur in cyclical patterns or clusters. They are excruciatingly painful and often affect one side of the head, around the eye area. Cluster headaches may occur daily or several times during a cluster period, lasting for weeks or months. The exact cause of cluster headaches is not fully understood, but they are believed to be related to abnormalities in the hypothalamus.

Sinus Headaches

Sinus headaches occur when the sinuses become inflamed due to infections (such as sinusitis), allergies, or other sinus problems. The pain is typically felt in the forehead, cheeks, and around the eyes. Symptoms may include nasal congestion, facial pressure, and a feeling of fullness in the ears.

Hormone Headaches

These headaches, often linked to hormonal fluctuations, primarily affect women. They can occur during menstruation, pregnancy, menopause, or when using hormonal contraceptives. Changes in estrogen levels are thought to trigger these headaches.

Rebound Headaches

Also known as medication-overuse headaches, rebound headaches occur when pain medications are overused and the body becomes dependent on them. Withdrawal from these medications can lead to worsening headaches, creating a cycle of medication use and rebound headaches.

Understanding the causes of headaches and migraines involves recognizing primary and secondary factors. Primary headaches (like tension headaches, migraines, and cluster headaches) arise independently and are not caused by another medical condition. Secondary headaches, on the other hand, are symptoms of underlying medical issues such as head injury, infections, sinus problems, or vascular disorders.

Managing headaches and migraines often involves identifying triggers, lifestyle adjustments, and sometimes medication. Individuals experiencing severe or recurrent headaches should consult a healthcare professional for proper diagnosis and treatment to improve their quality of life and manage symptoms effectively.

6.2 How castor oil can provide relief

Castor oil has been recognized for its potential to alleviate headaches and migraines through various mechanisms. Rich in ricinoleic acid, a unique fatty acid with anti-inflammatory and analgesic properties, castor oil offers a natural alternative for managing headache symptoms. When applied topically to the temples and forehead, castor oil can help reduce inflammation and tension in the muscles and blood vessels, often implicated in tension headaches and migraines.

1) Anti-inflammatory Properties

Ricinoleic acid, the primary component of castor oil, exhibits potent anti-inflammatory effects. These properties help alleviate swelling and reduce the inflammatory response associated with headaches and migraines.

2) Muscle Relaxant

Castor oil's ability to penetrate the skin and muscles effectively makes it a muscle relaxant. Easing muscle tension and promoting relaxation can alleviate the muscular component of headache pain.

3) Improved Blood Circulation

Castor oil stimulates blood circulation when applied to the scalp and massaged gently. Enhanced blood flow can relieve vascular headaches by reducing constriction and promoting healthy circulation in the scalp and cranial blood vessels.

Castor oil can be used in various forms for headache relief. One popular method is to create a soothing castor oil compress. Simply soak a cloth in warm castor oil, then apply it to the forehead or affected areas for 15-20 minutes. The warmth and absorption of the oil can help relax muscles, reduce inflammation, and ease headache symptoms.

Alternatively, blending castor oil with essential oils known for their headache-relieving properties, such as peppermint or lavender oil, can enhance its effectiveness as a topical treatment.

Incorporating castor oil into a holistic approach to headache management can offer relief without the potential side effects of pharmaceutical medications. However, it's essential to consult a healthcare provider if headaches or migraines are severe, frequent, or significantly impact daily life. Understanding how castor oil works and its benefits allows individuals to explore natural options for managing headaches and promoting overall well-being.

6.3 Application methods: topical use and inhalation

Castor oil offers versatile methods of application that leverage its therapeutic properties for various health benefits. Primarily used topically, castor oil is renowned for penetrating deeply into the skin and tissues, facilitating its medicinal effects. When applied directly to the skin, castor oil acts as a potent moisturizer and emollient, beneficial for treating dry skin conditions and promoting overall skin health. Its viscosity and richness in fatty acids, especially ricinoleic acid, contribute to its emollient properties, effectively softening and smoothing the skin.

1) Topical Application

Castor oil is used topically by applying it directly to the skin or affected area. This method allows the oil to absorb into the skin and exert its therapeutic effects locally. It is commonly used for conditions such as dry skin, acne, dermatitis, and various inflammatory skin conditions. The oil can be gently massaged into the skin until fully absorbed or used as a base in skincare formulations like creams and lotions.

2) Inhalation

Inhalation of castor oil vapor or steam is another method that harnesses its therapeutic benefits. This approach is particularly useful for respiratory conditions such as congestion, coughs, and sinusitis. To inhale castor oil vapor, add a few drops of the oil to hot water or a diffuser and inhale the steam deeply. The antimicrobial and anti-inflammatory properties of castor oil help clear nasal passages, reduce inflammation, and ease respiratory discomfort.

Topical Application

Skin Conditions: Castor oil is beneficial for treating dry, flaky skin and dermatitis due to its moisturizing properties. Apply a small amount to the affected area and massage gently until absorbed.

Acne Treatment: Its antimicrobial and anti-inflammatory properties can help reduce acne breakouts. Mix with a carrier oil like jojoba or coconut oil, and apply to the face as a cleanser or spot treatment.

Scar Reduction: Regular application of castor oil to scars and stretch marks may help improve their appearance over time. Massage a few drops onto the scar tissue daily.

Inhalation:

Respiratory Support: Inhaling castor oil steam can provide relief from nasal congestion and sinusitis. Add a few drops to hot water, cover your head with a towel, and inhale deeply for 5-10 minutes.

Cough Relief: The soothing properties of castor oil vapor can help calm coughs and throat irritation. Use in a steam inhalation or add to a humidifier for continuous relief.

By understanding these application methods, individuals can effectively incorporate castor oil into their wellness routines to reap its diverse benefits. Whether applied topically for skincare or used through inhalation for respiratory support, castor oil offers natural remedies that complement overall health and well-being. As with any natural remedy, it's essential to perform a patch test before widespread use and consult a healthcare professional if you have specific health concerns or conditions.

6.4 DIY recipes for headaches and migraines

1) Peppermint Cooling Headache Balm

- Ingredients:
    - 2 tablespoons coconut oil
    - 1 tablespoon shea butter
    - 10 drops peppermint essential oil
- Instructions: Melt the coconut oil and shea butter together. Stir in peppermint oil. Allow to cool and solidify. Massage onto temples and forehead for relief.

2) Lavender and Chamomile Relaxing Pillow Spray

- Ingredients:
    - 1/2 cup distilled water
    - 2 tablespoons witch hazel
    - 10 drops lavender essential oil
    - 5 drops chamomile essential oil
- Instructions: Combine all ingredients in a spray bottle. Shake well before use. Spritz onto pillow before bedtime to promote relaxation and ease headaches.

3) Eucalyptus Steam Inhalation

- Ingredients:
    - 3 cups boiling water
    - 5 drops eucalyptus essential oil
- Instructions: Pour boiling water into a large bowl. Add eucalyptus oil. Lean over the bowl with a towel over your head to trap steam. Inhale deeply for sinus relief and headache reduction.

4) Ginger and Lemon Tea

- Ingredients:
    - 1 cup water
    - 1-inch piece of fresh ginger, sliced
    - Juice of 1/2 lemon
    - Honey (optional)
- Instructions: Boil water and add ginger slices. Simmer for 5-10 minutes. Remove from heat, add lemon juice, and sweeten with honey if desired. Sip slowly for headache relief and nausea reduction.

5) Rosemary and Peppermint Scalp Massage Oil

- Ingredients:
    - 2 tablespoons jojoba oil
    - 5 drops rosemary essential oil
    - 5 drops peppermint essential oil
- Instructions: Mix oils together. Massage into scalp using fingertips in circular motions. Leave on for at least 30 minutes before shampooing.

6) Cold Compress with Lavender

- Ingredients:
    - 1 cup cold water
    - 5 drops lavender essential oil
    - Washcloth or small towel
- Instructions: Mix water and lavender oil in a bowl. Soak the washcloth in the mixture, wring out excess, and apply to forehead or neck for cooling relief.

7) Chamomile and Aloe Vera Soothing Gel

- Ingredients:
    - 1/4 cup aloe vera gel
    - 5 drops chamomile essential oil
- Instructions: Mix aloe vera gel and chamomile oil. Apply to temples and neck for cooling and soothing relief.

8) Hot Ginger Compress

- Ingredients:

    o   2 cups hot water

    o   1 tablespoon grated ginger

    o   Washcloth or small towel

- Instructions: Steep grated ginger in hot water for 5 minutes. Soak the washcloth in the ginger water, wring out excess, and apply to forehead or neck for heat therapy and pain relief.

9) Basil and Lavender Aromatherapy Blend

- Ingredients:

    o   10 drops basil essential oil

    o   5 drops lavender essential oil

    o   Diffuser

- Instructions: Add essential oils to a diffuser and follow the diffuser's instructions for use. Inhale the aromatic blend for relaxation and headache relief.

10) Cinnamon and Honey Paste

- Ingredients:

    o   1 teaspoon cinnamon powder

    o   Enough honey to make a paste

- Instructions: Mix cinnamon powder with honey to form a thick paste. Apply to temples and massage gently. Leave for 20 minutes before rinsing off.

Chapter 7: Castor oil for menstrual pain

7.1 Understanding cramps and menstrual pain

Understanding menstrual cramps, also known as dysmenorrhea, is essential for many women who experience discomfort during their menstrual cycles. It's important to remember that these cramps, which typically occur just before and during menstruation, are a normal part of the menstrual cycle. They affect the lower abdomen, but can radiate to the lower back and thighs. Menstrual cramps can range from mild to severe, with symptoms varying between individuals and even from one cycle to another.

The primary cause of menstrual cramps is the contraction of the uterine muscles. During menstruation, the uterus contracts to help expel its lining, leading to cramping sensations. Prostaglandins, hormone-like substances involved in inflammation and pain, trigger these contractions. Higher levels of prostaglandins are associated with more severe menstrual cramps.

7.1.1 Several factors can influence the severity of menstrual cramps

Age and Reproductive Health: Younger women often experience more intense cramps, which may lessen with age or after childbirth.

Hormonal Changes: Hormonal fluctuations, especially estrogen and progesterone, throughout the menstrual cycle, can impact the severity of cramps.

Underlying Conditions: Conditions like endometriosis or uterine fibroids can exacerbate menstrual pain.

Lifestyle Factors: Stress, lack of exercise, smoking, and poor diet can contribute to more severe menstrual cramps.

Managing menstrual cramps involves a combination of lifestyle changes, over-the-counter medications, and home remedies. Regular physical activity, such as gentle exercise or yoga, can help alleviate cramps by increasing blood flow and releasing endorphins, natural pain relievers. Applying heat through a heating pad or warm bath relaxes the pelvic muscles and reduces pain intensity.

Over-the-counter pain relievers like ibuprofen or naproxen sodium can effectively reduce menstrual cramp pain by inhibiting prostaglandin production. These medications, when taken at the first sign of cramps or before the onset of menstruation, can provide significant relief, giving you the confidence to manage your pain effectively.

In addition to conventional treatments, many women find relief through natural remedies such as herbal teas containing ingredients like ginger, chamomile, or peppermint, which have anti-inflammatory and soothing properties. Dietary adjustments, such as increasing the intake of omega-3 fatty acids found in fish and flaxseed and reducing caffeine and alcohol consumption, may also help alleviate symptoms.

For women with severe menstrual cramps who do not respond to these measures or those with underlying conditions like endometriosis, it's important to remember that you're not alone. Seeking consultation with a healthcare provider is advisable. They may recommend hormonal contraceptives to regulate menstrual cycles and reduce cramping or other treatments tailored to individual needs, ensuring you receive the care and support you need.

7.2 Castor oil as a natural remedy for menstrual disorders

Castor oil has gained attention as a potential natural remedy for menstrual discomfort. It offers a range of benefits that can help alleviate symptoms associated with menstrual cramps and discomfort. Derived from the seeds of the castor plant (Ricinus communis), this versatile oil has been traditionally used for various therapeutic purposes due to its anti-inflammatory, analgesic, and muscle-relaxing properties.

7.2.1 Anti-inflammatory and Analgesic Properties

One of the primary reasons castor oil is effective for menstrual discomfort is its ability to reduce inflammation and pain. The critical component responsible for these effects is ricinoleic acid, a monounsaturated fatty acid in castor oil. Ricinoleic acid acts as an anti-inflammatory agent by inhibiting the production of inflammatory substances called prostaglandins. During menstruation, prostaglandins cause the uterus to contract, leading to cramping and pain. By reducing prostaglandin levels, ricinoleic acid helps to alleviate these symptoms, making menstrual periods more manageable and less painful.

7.2.2 Muscle Relaxation and Pain Relief

Castor oil's muscle-relaxing properties further contribute to its effectiveness in treating menstrual discomfort. When applied topically to the abdomen, castor oil penetrates the skin and is absorbed into the underlying tissues and muscles. It acts as a natural muscle relaxant, helping to ease the spasms and cramps that commonly accompany menstruation. This relaxation of uterine muscles reduces pain and promotes better blood circulation in the pelvic area, which can alleviate discomfort and improve overall menstrual health.

7.2.3 Application Methods

There are several effective ways to use castor oil for menstrual discomfort:

Castor Oil Packs: This method involves soaking a flannel cloth in castor oil and applying it to the lower abdomen. Cover the pack with plastic wrap and use a heating pad or warm towel for 30-60 minutes. This technique enhances absorption and promotes relaxation of the pelvic muscles.

Massage: Gentle massage with castor oil on the lower abdomen can help relieve cramps and improve circulation. Warm the oil slightly before massaging in a circular motion to enhance its therapeutic effects.

Ingestion: Some people choose to ingest small amounts of castor oil during their menstrual period to alleviate cramping. However, this method should be approached cautiously and under the guidance of a healthcare professional due to potential side effects.

7.2.4 Safety and Precautions

While castor oil is generally considered safe for topical use, it's essential to follow proper guidelines to avoid adverse reactions:

Quality and Purity: Use only high-quality, cold-pressed castor oil without additives or preservatives.

Patch Test: Perform a patch test on a small area of skin to check for any allergic reactions or sensitivity before widespread use.

Consultation: If you have underlying health conditions or are pregnant or breastfeeding, consult with a healthcare provider before using castor oil for menstrual discomfort.

Castor oil offers a natural and holistic approach to managing menstrual discomfort by reducing inflammation, relaxing muscles, and alleviating pain associated with menstrual cramps. Its effectiveness lies in targeting the root causes of menstrual discomfort and promoting overall menstrual health. By incorporating castor oil into your menstrual care routine through safe and effective application methods, you can naturally experience relief from menstrual cramps and discomfort. Always prioritize safety and consult with a healthcare professional if you have any concerns or medical conditions before using castor oil.

7.3 Application methods: compresses and abdominal massage

Castor oil is widely recognized for its therapeutic benefits in alleviating menstrual cramps and discomfort through two primary application methods: abdominal packs and massages. These techniques leverage the anti-inflammatory, analgesic, and muscle-relaxing properties of castor oil, offering natural relief from menstrual symptoms without the side effects associated with conventional pain medications.

Abdominal Packs

1. Preparation: To create an abdominal pack, you will need:

- High-quality, cold-pressed castor oil

- Piece of flannel cloth large enough to cover your lower abdomen

- Plastic wrap

- Heating pad or hot water bottle

2. Application:

- Start by laying down a clean towel or old cloth to protect your bedding.

- Fold the flannel cloth into several layers to make it thick enough to hold the castor oil.

- Pour a generous amount of castor oil onto the center of the cloth. The cloth should be saturated but not dripping.

- Lie down comfortably and place the castor oil-soaked cloth over your lower abdomen.

- Cover the cloth with plastic wrap to prevent oil stains and to retain heat.

- Apply a heating pad or hot water bottle over the plastic wrap for 30-60 minutes. The heat helps to enhance the absorption of castor oil and promotes relaxation of the pelvic muscles.

3. Benefits:

- Muscle Relaxation: The warmth from the pack and the therapeutic properties of castor oil help to relax uterine muscles, reducing cramping and spasms.

- Anti-inflammatory Action: Ricinoleic acid in castor oil inhibits prostaglandin synthesis, which is responsible for uterine contractions and inflammation during menstruation.

- Improved Circulation: The gentle heat from the pack improves blood flow to the pelvic area, relieving congestion and reducing pain.

4. Frequency:

- Abdominal packs can be used as often as needed during menstruation to alleviate pain and discomfort. Some individuals find relief by using packs daily leading up to and during their period.

Massages

1. Technique:

- Warm a small amount of castor oil by rubbing it between your palms.

- Lie down in a comfortable position and gently massage the oil onto your lower abdomen using circular motions.

- Massage for 10-15 minutes, focusing on areas where you feel cramps or tension.

2. Benefits:

- Direct Absorption: Massaging castor oil into the skin allows for direct absorption of its therapeutic compounds into the underlying tissues and muscles.

- Relaxation: The act of massaging promotes relaxation of the abdominal muscles, reducing cramping and discomfort.

- Stress Relief: Gentle massage can also help alleviate stress and anxiety often associated with menstrual pain.

3. Frequency:

- Perform abdominal massages with castor oil once or twice daily during menstruation or as needed for pain relief.

<u>Safety Considerations</u>

- Patch Test: Before using castor oil for abdominal packs or massages, perform a patch test on a small area of skin to check for any allergic reactions or skin sensitivity.

- Quality of Oil: Use only high-quality, cold-pressed castor oil that is free from additives or preservatives to ensure effectiveness and safety.

- Consultation: If you have any underlying health conditions, are pregnant, or are breastfeeding, consult with a healthcare provider before using castor oil for menstrual discomfort.

Abdominal packs and massages with castor oil offer effective, natural relief from menstrual cramps and discomfort by targeting inflammation, promoting muscle relaxation, and improving circulation in the pelvic area. These methods provide a holistic approach to menstrual care without the side effects commonly associated with conventional pain medications.

Chapter 8: Castor oil for nerve pain

8.1 Causes and symptoms of nerve pain

Nerve pain, also known as neuropathic pain, arises from damage or dysfunction of the nerves rather than from the stimulation of pain receptors in the tissues. There are several common causes of nerve pain, each with distinct symptoms and implications for treatment. One primary cause is physical trauma, such as accidents or injuries, which can directly damage nerves or lead to compression of nerve fibers. This compression can occur due to conditions like herniated discs in the spine or carpal tunnel syndrome in the wrist. Nerve pain can also result from diseases such as diabetes, where prolonged high blood sugar levels can damage nerves throughout the body, particularly in the feet and hands. Another significant cause is infections like shingles, where the varicella-zoster virus remains dormant in nerve cells after an initial chickenpox infection, causing inflammation and pain along affected nerve pathways. Additionally, autoimmune disorders such as multiple sclerosis can lead to nerve damage due to the immune system attacking the protective covering of nerves, known as myelin.

Nerve pain symptoms vary widely depending on the underlying cause and the nerves affected. Common symptoms include shooting or burning pain, tingling sensations (paresthesia), numbness, and increased sensitivity to touch or temperature changes. Nerve pain may be intermittent or constant, significantly impacting daily activities and quality of life. In cases of diabetic neuropathy, for example, patients may experience a gradual onset of symptoms starting in the feet and spreading upward. Conversely, nerve pain from conditions like carpal tunnel syndrome may be localized to specific areas, such as the wrist and hand, with symptoms worsening during activities that exacerbate nerve compression.

Diagnosing nerve pain often involves a comprehensive evaluation by a healthcare provider, including a detailed medical history, physical examination, and possibly nerve conduction studies or imaging tests to identify the source of nerve damage or compression. Treatment strategies for nerve pain typically address the underlying cause and manage symptoms. This may include anti-inflammatories, antidepressants, or anticonvulsants, which can help alleviate pain and improve nerve function. Physical therapy and rehabilitative exercises may also be recommended to strengthen muscles, improve mobility, and reduce nerve compression. In cases where conservative treatments are ineffective, more invasive interventions such as nerve blocks or surgical procedures may be considered to relieve pressure on affected nerves or repair damaged nerve tissues.

Managing nerve pain effectively often requires a multidisciplinary approach involving collaboration between healthcare providers, pain specialists, physical therapists, and other healthcare professionals. These professionals can provide expert guidance on the most effective treatments and lifestyle modifications, as well as monitor your progress and adjust your treatment plan as needed. Lifestyle modifications such as maintaining a healthy weight, controlling blood sugar levels in diabetes, and avoiding repetitive movements that may aggravate nerve compression can also be crucial in preventing or minimizing nerve pain symptoms. By addressing the causes and symptoms of nerve pain comprehensively, individuals can improve their overall well-being and quality of life.

8.2 How castor oil helps with conditions such as sciatica and neuropathy

Castor oil, renowned for its anti-inflammatory and analgesic properties, has been explored for its potential benefits in managing conditions like sciatica and neuropathy. Sciatica, often caused by compression of the sciatic nerve due to herniated discs or spinal stenosis, radiates pain from the lower back down the leg. Neuropathy, conversely, involves nerve damage often associated with diabetes or other underlying conditions, resulting in symptoms like numbness, tingling, and pain in affected areas.

The ricinoleic acid found in castor oil has shown anti-inflammatory effects that may help alleviate the inflammation and swelling contributing to nerve pain in both sciatica and neuropathy. By penetrating deep into tissues, castor oil can reduce the pressure on nerves and relieve discomfort. Additionally, its ability to stimulate circulation and promote healing may aid in repairing damaged nerve tissues over time.

Topical application methods such as massages and packs are commonly recommended for targeting specific areas affected by sciatica or neuropathy. Massaging castor oil into the lower back or affected limbs can help improve blood flow, relax muscles, and reduce nerve pain's intensity. Similarly, applying warm castor oil packs to the affected area may provide soothing relief by enhancing the oil's absorption and therapeutic benefits.

While castor oil is often used as a complementary treatment, it's important to note that individual responses may vary. It should not replace medical advice or prescribed treatments. To ensure a comprehensive and personalized approach to managing conditions like sciatica and neuropathy, consulting with a healthcare provider is crucial. This responsible approach is especially important for chronic or severe cases of these conditions.

8.3 Techniques for effective application

Employing effective application techniques is crucial to maximize the benefits of castor oil. Here are several methods to ensure optimal absorption and efficacy:

1) Massage Therapy

Massaging castor oil directly onto the skin can enhance circulation and facilitate deeper tissue penetration. This technique is beneficial for addressing localized pain or inflammation in joint areas or sore muscles. Start by warming a small amount of castor oil in your palms and gently massage it into the affected area using circular motions. Continue for 5-10 minutes to promote relaxation and absorption.

2) Compress Application

A castor oil compress can provide sustained relief for chronic pain or inflammation areas. Soak a clean cloth in warm castor oil to prepare a compress and wring out the excess. Cover the cloth over the affected area with plastic wrap or a towel to retain heat. Leave it on for 30-60 minutes, allowing the oil to penetrate the skin and soothe discomfort deeply.

3) Hot Water Bottle Technique

After applying castor oil to the skin, placing a hot water bottle or heating pad over the area can enhance the oil's absorption. The heat helps open pores and increase blood flow, aiding in delivering castor oil's beneficial compounds to the affected tissues. This method is beneficial for managing conditions like muscle cramps, menstrual pain, or joint stiffness.

4) Blend with Essential Oils

Combining castor oil with essential oils known for their pain-relieving properties can amplify its effectiveness. For example, mixing a few drops of peppermint or lavender oil with castor oil can enhance its analgesic and anti-inflammatory effects. Dilute essential oils properly to avoid skin irritation, and perform a patch test before widespread Application.

5) Overnight Treatment

Applying castor oil before bedtime and leaving it on overnight can provide prolonged relief for chronic conditions or intense discomfort. Cover the treated area with a bandage or plastic wrap to prevent staining bedding and allow the oil to work undisturbed. This method is particularly beneficial for addressing joint, back, or skin conditions requiring intensive hydration and healing.

6) Inhalation Therapy

Inhaling the vapor of castor oil can offer respiratory benefits and promote relaxation. Add a few drops of castor oil to a hot water or diffuser bowl and inhale the steam deeply for several minutes. This technique can help alleviate sinus congestion, headaches, and stress-related tension.

7) Consistent Application

Regular and consistent use of castor oil is vital to experiencing its full benefits over time. Incorporate castor oil into your daily skincare routine or pain management regimen to maintain its therapeutic effects. Whether applied topically or used in complementary therapies like massages or packs, consistency enhances its ability to support overall wellness.

By utilizing these techniques, individuals can effectively harness castor oil's healing properties. However, it's essential to consult with a healthcare provider, especially for chronic conditions or if you have allergies or sensitivities, to ensure safe and appropriate usage.

Chapter 9: Combining castor oil with other natural remedies

9.1 Overview of complementary natural remedies for pain relief

Natural remedies have been utilized for centuries to alleviate pain and discomfort, offering alternatives to conventional medications with benefits and considerations. From herbal supplements to lifestyle modifications, these complementary approaches aim to address pain holistically, often focusing on reducing inflammation, promoting relaxation, and supporting overall well-being.

Herbal Supplements

Herbal supplements like turmeric, ginger, and boswellia have gained popularity for their anti-inflammatory properties. Turmeric contains curcumin, known for its potent anti-inflammatory effects that can help relieve pain associated with arthritis and other inflammatory conditions. Ginger also exhibits similar anti-inflammatory properties and has been used traditionally to alleviate muscle pain and stiffness.

Essential Oils

Essential oils such as lavender, peppermint, and eucalyptus are commonly used for their analgesic and soothing effects. Lavender oil, for instance, promotes relaxation and may help alleviate tension headaches. Peppermint oil is known for its cooling sensation and can be beneficial for relieving migraines and muscle aches. Eucalyptus oil is often used topically to reduce joint pain and inflammation.

Acupuncture and Acupressure

Acupuncture and acupressure involve stimulating specific points in the body to alleviate pain and promote healing. Acupuncture uses fine needles inserted into the skin at strategic points, while acupressure applies pressure to these points using fingers or tools. Both techniques are believed to balance the body's energy flow and stimulate the release of natural pain-relieving chemicals like endorphins.

Mind-Body Techniques

Mind-body practices such as yoga, tai chi, and meditation emphasize the connection between mental and physical health. These practices can help reduce stress, improve flexibility and strength, and alleviate chronic pain. Yoga, for example, incorporates gentle stretching and breathing exercises that can relieve tension in muscles and joints. Meditation promotes relaxation and can reduce pain perception by enhancing mindfulness and awareness.

Dietary Modifications

Dietary changes can play a significant role in managing pain and inflammation. A diet rich in fruits, vegetables, whole grains, and lean proteins provides essential nutrients and antioxidants that support overall health and may help reduce inflammation. Omega-3 fatty acids found in fish oil and flaxseed oil are known for their anti-inflammatory properties and can be beneficial for managing conditions like arthritis and joint pain.

Physical Therapy

Through targeted exercises and techniques, physical therapy focuses on improving mobility, strength, and function. It is commonly recommended for recovering from injuries, surgery, or chronic pain conditions. Physical therapists employ various modalities such as heat therapy, cold therapy, ultrasound, and manual therapy to alleviate pain and promote healing.

Topical Treatments

Topical treatments like menthol creams, capsaicin ointments, and CBD-infused balms can provide localized relief from pain and inflammation. Menthol produces a cooling sensation that can temporarily distract from pain signals, while capsaicin, derived from chili peppers, interferes with pain transmission in nerve cells. CBD (cannabidiol) has gained attention for its potential anti-inflammatory and analgesic properties, although more research is needed to fully understand its effectiveness.

Hydrotherapy

Hydrotherapy involves using water for pain relief and rehabilitation. Techniques such as hot baths, whirlpools, and contrast baths (alternating between hot and cold water) can improve circulation, reduce muscle tension, and alleviate joint pain. Hydrotherapy is particularly beneficial for individuals with arthritis, fibromyalgia, and muscle soreness.

Chiropractic Care

Chiropractic care focuses on spinal manipulation and adjustments to restore alignment and alleviate pain. It is commonly used to treat musculoskeletal conditions such as back pain, neck pain, and headaches. Chiropractors may also incorporate complementary therapies such as massage, ultrasound, and electrical stimulation to relieve pain and promote healing.

Aromatherapy

Aromatherapy utilizes aromatic plant oils to improve psychological and physical well-being. In addition to essential oils, aromatherapy includes techniques like inhalation, vaporization, and topical application of diluted oils. Aromatherapy can help reduce stress, improve sleep quality, and alleviate headaches and muscle pain.

Incorporating these complementary natural remedies into a comprehensive pain management plan can provide individuals diverse options to address their unique pain-related needs. However, it's essential to consult with healthcare providers before starting any new treatment or supplement regimen, especially if you have underlying health conditions or are pregnant. Integrating these approaches mindfully can support overall health and well-being while promoting a holistic approach to pain relief.

9.2 Synergistic effects of combining castor oil with essential oils, herbs and heat therapy.

Combining castor oil with essential oils, herbs, and heat therapy can create synergistic effects that enhance its therapeutic benefits for pain relief and relaxation.

Castor oil is known for its anti-inflammatory and analgesic properties, effectively reducing pain and inflammation when applied topically. When combined with essential oils like lavender, peppermint, or eucalyptus, which have their own analgesic, anti-inflammatory, and soothing properties, the blend can provide enhanced relief from muscle aches, joint pain, and headaches. It's important to note that essential oils are potent and should be used with caution. For example, lavender oil is renowned for its calming effects and can complement castor oil's ability to promote relaxation and reduce tension.

Peppermint oil's cooling sensation can further alleviate muscle soreness and tension when used alongside castor oil massages or packs.

Eucalyptus oil, with its invigorating aroma and anti-inflammatory properties, can relieve joint stiffness and enhance the overall effectiveness of castor oil treatments.

Additionally, incorporating heat therapy through warm compresses or baths can improve blood circulation, relax muscles, and enhance the absorption of castor oil and essential oils into the skin, maximizing their therapeutic effects.

This synergistic approach addresses pain relief and promotes relaxation and overall well-being, offering a holistic and effective solution for managing various types of pain and discomfort.

9.3 Recipes and mixtures to improve pain relief

For those seeking enhanced pain relief, castor oil can be effectively combined with various natural ingredients to create soothing and therapeutic blends. These ingredients can be found in health food stores, online retailers, or specialty shops.

Warming Muscle Massage Blend

Create a blend by mixing castor oil with ginger and black pepper essential oils. Ginger is renowned for its ability to increase circulation and reduce inflammation, making it ideal for relieving muscle soreness and stiffness. Black pepper essential oil complements this blend with its warming properties, offering comfort and easing muscle tension.

Soothing Muscle Rub

Blend castor oil with arnica oil and menthol crystals to create a soothing muscle rub. Arnica oil is well-known for its anti-inflammatory properties, making it beneficial for treating bruises, sprains, and muscle aches. Menthol crystals provide a cooling sensation that helps alleviate soreness and discomfort in muscles and joints, making this rub perfect for post-workout recovery or everyday muscle tension relief.

Peppermint-Lavender Headache Balm

Combine castor oil with peppermint and lavender essential oils to make a headache-relieving balm. Peppermint essential oil offers a refreshing and cooling effect that can help alleviate tension headaches and migraines by improving blood circulation and reducing muscle contractions. Lavender essential oil complements this blend with its calming and relaxing properties, promoting stress relief and reducing the intensity of migraine symptoms.

Joint Pain Relief Blend

Mix castor oil with turmeric and frankincense essential oils for joint pain relief. Turmeric essential oil is well-regarded for its anti-inflammatory and pain-relieving properties, effectively reducing joint pain and stiffness associated with arthritis. Frankincense essential oil complements this blend with its soothing and anti-inflammatory effects, promoting overall joint health and mobility.

Calming Back Pain Blend

Create a blend using castor oil, chamomile essential oil, and marjoram essential oil. Chamomile essential oil offers anti-inflammatory properties and promotes relaxation, making it beneficial for soothing back pain and muscle spasms. Marjoram essential oil provides additional pain relief and muscle relaxation, helping to alleviate tension and discomfort in the lower back and spine.

Digestive Discomfort Relief

Blend castor oil with peppermint and ginger essential oils to soothe digestive discomfort. Peppermint essential oil aids digestion and relieves bloating and gas, while ginger essential oil supports gastrointestinal health and reduces nausea and inflammation. This blend can be massaged onto the abdomen in a clockwise motion to promote digestion and provide relief from stomach discomfort.

Sleep Aid Blend

Mix castor oil with lavender and cedarwood essential oils to create a sleep aid blend. Lavender essential oil promotes relaxation and reduces stress and anxiety, helping to improve sleep quality. Cedarwood essential oil complements this blend with its calming and grounding effects, promoting a restful night's sleep and alleviating insomnia.

Foot Pain Relief

Combine castor oil with eucalyptus and peppermint essential oils for foot pain relief. Eucalyptus essential oil offers anti-inflammatory properties and helps soothe tired and achy feet. Peppermint essential oil provides a cooling sensation that alleviates foot pain and discomfort, making this blend ideal for relieving soreness from standing or walking for long periods.

Menstrual Cramp Relief

To alleviate menstrual cramps, create a blend using castor oil, clary sage essential oil, and Roman chamomile essential oil. Clary sage essential oil helps regulate menstrual cycles and reduces pain and discomfort. Roman chamomile essential oil offers anti-inflammatory and soothing properties, promoting relaxation and easing cramping during menstruation.

Sunburn Soothing Blend

Mix castor oil with lavender and tea tree essential oils for sunburn relief. Lavender essential oil calms and soothes sunburned skin, reducing redness and inflammation. Tea tree essential oil provides antiseptic properties that help prevent infection and promote the healing of sun-damaged skin, making this blend ideal for soothing sunburn discomfort and promoting skin recovery.

These DIY recipes harness the natural healing properties of castor oil and essential oils to provide targeted pain relief and promote overall well-being. Whether you're dealing with muscle aches, headaches, joint pain, digestive discomfort, or menstrual cramps, these blends offer effective and soothing relief using natural ingredients, reassuring you that you're using safe and natural remedies.

Chapter 10: DIY pain relief recipes with castor oil

1) Castor Oil Hair Mask

- **Ingredients:**
  - 2 tablespoons castor oil
  - 1 tablespoon coconut oil
  - 1 tablespoon honey
  - 1 egg yolk

- **Instructions:**

1. In a bowl, mix all ingredients until well combined.

2. Apply the mixture to damp hair, focusing on the roots and tips.

3. Leave on for 30 minutes to 1 hour.

4. Rinse thoroughly with shampoo and conditioner.

2) Castor Oil Face Serum

- **Ingredients:**
  - 1 tablespoon castor oil
  - 1 tablespoon argan oil
  - 3 drops lavender essential oil
  - 3 drops frankincense essential oil

- **Instructions:**

1. Combine all oils in a small dropper bottle.

2. Shake well to mix thoroughly.

3. Apply a few drops to clean face and neck before bedtime.

4. Gently massage into the skin until absorbed.

3) Castor Oil Lip Balm

- **Ingredients:**
  - o 1 tablespoon castor oil
  - o 1 tablespoon shea butter
  - o 1 tablespoon beeswax pellets
  - o 5-7 drops peppermint essential oil (optional)

- **Instructions:**

1. Melt the shea butter and beeswax pellets in a double boiler.

2. Once melted, stir in the castor oil and essential oil (if using).

3. Pour into small lip balm containers.

4. Let cool and solidify before use.

4) Castor Oil Body Scrub

- **Ingredients:**
  - o 1/2 cup castor oil
  - o 1 cup brown sugar
  - o 1/4 cup coconut oil
  - o 10 drops of your favorite essential oil (e.g., lavender, citrus)

- **Instructions:**

1. Mix all ingredients together in a bowl until well combined.

2. Use in the shower, applying the scrub to damp skin.

3. Gently massage in circular motions, focusing on rough areas.

4. Rinse off with warm water.

5) Castor Oil Cuticle Oil

- **Ingredients:**
  - o 1 tablespoon castor oil

- 1 tablespoon almond oil

- 5 drops vitamin E oil

- 3 drops lavender essential oil

- **Instructions:**

1. Combine all oils in a small dropper bottle.

2. Shake well to mix thoroughly.

3. Apply a few drops to each cuticle and massage in.

4. Use daily for hydrated and healthy cuticles.

6) Castor Oil Massage Oil

- **Ingredients:**

  - 2 tablespoons castor oil

  - 2 tablespoons jojoba oil

  - 5 drops rosemary essential oil

  - 5 drops peppermint essential oil

- **Instructions:**

1. Combine all ingredients in a small bottle.

2. Shake well to mix thoroughly.

3. Warm the oil slightly before use for a soothing massage.

4. Apply to skin and massage in gentle, circular motions.

7) Castor Oil Scalp Treatment

- **Ingredients:**

  - 3 tablespoons castor oil

  - 2 tablespoons coconut oil

  - 5 drops tea tree essential oil

  - 5 drops rosemary essential oil

- **Instructions:**

1. Mix all ingredients in a bowl until well combined.

2.   Part your hair into sections and apply the mixture to your scalp.

3.   Massage gently with your fingertips for 5-10 minutes.

4.   Leave on for 1-2 hours or overnight, then shampoo and condition as usual.

8) Castor Oil Acne Spot Treatment

- **Ingredients:**
  - 1 tablespoon castor oil
  - 1 tablespoon grapeseed oil
  - 3 drops tea tree essential oil

- **Instructions:**

1.   Mix all oils together in a small container.

2.   Cleanse your face thoroughly.

3.   Apply a small amount directly to acne spots using a cotton swab.

4.   Leave on overnight or for at least 30 minutes, then rinse off.

9) Castor Oil Eye Serum

- **Ingredients:**
  - 1 tablespoon castor oil
  - 1 tablespoon sweet almond oil
  - 3 drops rosehip seed oil

- **Instructions:**

1.   Combine all oils in a small dropper bottle.

2.   Shake well to mix thoroughly.

3.   Use a drop or two around the eye area before bedtime.

4.   Gently pat into the skin until absorbed.

10) Castor Oil Joint Pain Relief Balm

- **Ingredients:**
  - 2 tablespoons castor oil

o   2 tablespoons beeswax pellets

  o   1 tablespoon shea butter

  o   5 drops eucalyptus essential oil

  o   5 drops peppermint essential oil

- **Instructions:**

1. Melt beeswax pellets and shea butter in a double boiler.

2. Once melted, stir in castor oil and essential oils.

3. Pour into a clean container or tin.

4. Let cool and solidify before use on sore joints.

Chapter 11: Integration of castor oil into pain management routine

Incorporating castor oil into your pain management routine can offer natural relief for various types of discomfort. Whether you're dealing with joint pain, headaches, or muscle soreness, castor oil's anti-inflammatory and analgesic properties can be beneficial. This chapter explores how to effectively integrate castor oil into your daily routine for managing pain.

Castor oil is derived from the seeds of the castor bean plant (Ricinus communis) and has been used traditionally for its medicinal properties. Its primary component, ricinoleic acid, exhibits anti-inflammatory effects by inhibiting the synthesis of inflammatory prostaglandins. Additionally, it enhances circulation to the affected area, promoting healing and reducing pain.

11.1 Types of Pain Suitable for Castor Oil Treatment

1. Muscle Pain and Soreness:

    o   Apply castor oil topically to sore muscles to reduce inflammation and promote relaxation.

    o   Combine with massage techniques for deeper penetration and enhanced relief.

2. Joint Pain (Arthritis, Rheumatism):

    o   Use castor oil packs on joints to alleviate stiffness and inflammation.

    o   Regular applications can improve mobility and reduce pain associated with arthritis.

3. Headaches and Migraines:

    o   Apply castor oil to the temples or forehead for tension headaches.

    o   Inhalation therapy with castor oil can help alleviate migraines.

4. Menstrual Cramps:

    o   Use castor oil packs on the abdomen to ease menstrual pain and cramping.

o Regular use may help regulate menstrual cycles and reduce discomfort.

11.2 Techniques for Applying Castor Oil

1. Topical Application:

   o Direct Massage: Gently massage castor oil into the affected area using circular motions to promote absorption and relaxation.

   o Castor Oil Packs: Soak a cloth in castor oil, apply to the affected area, and cover with plastic wrap and a heating pad for 30-60 minutes.

2. Inhalation Therapy:

   o Add a few drops of castor oil to a bowl of hot water.

   o Cover your head with a towel and inhale the steam deeply to relieve sinus pressure and headaches.

11.3 DIY Pain Relief Recipes with Castor Oil

Explore a variety of DIY recipes using castor oil to target specific areas of pain:

Muscle Relief Balm:

   o Ingredients:

      ▪ 2 tablespoons castor oil

      ▪ 2 tablespoons coconut oil

      ▪ 1 tablespoon beeswax pellets

      ▪ 10 drops peppermint essential oil

   o Instructions:

1. Melt beeswax and coconut oil in a double boiler.

2. Stir in castor oil and essential oil.

3. Pour into a container and let it cool.

Joint Pain Relief Pack:

   o Ingredients:

      ▪ 3 tablespoons castor oil

      ▪ 1 tablespoon turmeric powder

- 1 tablespoon ginger powder

- 1 tablespoon honey

o   Instructions:

1. Mix all ingredients to form a paste.

2. Apply to affected joints and cover with a cloth.

Headache Soothing Roll-On:

o   Ingredients:

- 2 tablespoons castor oil

- 1 tablespoon almond oil

- 5 drops lavender essential oil

o   Instructions:

1. Combine all oils in a rollerball bottle.

2. Apply to temples and back of the neck for relief.

11.4 Integrating Castor Oil into Holistic Pain Management

1. Daily Routine: Incorporate castor oil treatments into your daily self-care regimen for ongoing pain relief.

2. Combination Therapies: Combine castor oil with other holistic practices such as acupuncture, yoga, or meditation for enhanced pain management.

3. Consultation: Always consult with a healthcare provider before starting new pain management techniques, especially if you have underlying health conditions or are pregnant.

By integrating these practices and recipes into your routine, you can effectively harness the natural healing properties of castor oil for managing pain and promoting overall well-being.

BOOK 6: Castor Oil for Women's Health

Castor Oil for Women's Health

Embrace Natural Wellness and Balance

By

Vincent Vega

Disclaimer notice

Please be aware that the information provided in this document is intended solely for educational and entertainment purposes. Every effort has been made to ensure the content is accurate, reliable, current, and complete.

However, no guarantees, either explicit or implicit, are made. Readers acknowledge that the author is not providing legal, financial, medical, or professional advice.

The content has been sourced from various references. It is strongly recommended that you consult a licensed professional before attempting any of the of the methods described in this document.

By reading this document, you agree that the author is not liable for any direct or indirect losses resulting from the use of the information within, including but not limited to errors, omissions, or inaccuracies.

Chapter 1: Introduction to castor oil for women's health

1.1 Overview of castor oil and its historical use for women's health

Castor oil, extracted from the seeds of the Ricinus communis plant, has a rich historical background steeped in its use for women's health across diverse cultures and centuries. This versatile oil has been prized for its therapeutic properties and has found applications in addressing various health concerns specific to women. This chapter provides an overview of castor oil and its historical significance in women's health.

Castor oil's use in women's health dates back to ancient times, where it was revered for its medicinal properties. Historical records indicate its presence in Egyptian medicine as early as 4000 BC, primarily used for treating eye irritations and skin conditions. The Ebers Papyrus, one of the oldest medical texts, mentions castor oil for its purgative effects and potential use in labor induction.

1.1.1 Traditional Uses Across Cultures

Throughout history, castor oil has been a staple in traditional medicine systems around the world:

- Ayurveda: In India, Ayurvedic practitioners used castor oil internally and externally for its detoxifying properties and to support reproductive health. It was believed to regulate menstrual cycles, alleviate menstrual cramps, and promote fertility.

- Traditional Chinese Medicine (TCM): TCM practitioners utilized castor oil for its ability to stimulate circulation and reduce inflammation. It was often applied topically to promote healing and relieve pain.

- Greek and Roman Medicine: Dioscorides and Hippocrates documented the use of castor oil for various ailments, including digestive disorders and skin conditions. They recognized its purgative effects and its potential in wound healing.

1.1.2 Middle Ages to Early Modern Era

During the Middle Ages and Renaissance periods, castor oil continued to be valued for its therapeutic benefits:

- Medieval Europe: It was used for treating joint pain, skin infections, and promoting wound healing. Castor oil was also employed as a laxative to relieve constipation.

- Colonial America: Settlers brought castor oil to the Americas, where it became a remedy for a range of conditions, from gastrointestinal issues to inducing childbirth.

1.1.3 Modern Applications

In the 20th and 21st centuries, castor oil has maintained its popularity in natural health circles and beyond:

- Women's Health: Today, castor oil is widely used for menstrual health, fertility support, and during pregnancy and postpartum periods. It is favored for its ability to ease menstrual cramps, regulate cycles, and potentially enhance fertility by promoting circulation to the reproductive organs.

- Skincare: Castor oil is a common ingredient in skincare products due to its moisturizing and anti-inflammatory properties. It is used in creams, lotions, and facial oils to hydrate the skin and reduce inflammation.

- Hair Care: In addition to skincare, castor oil is popular in hair care products for its purported ability to strengthen hair, promote hair growth, and moisturize the scalp.

Castor oil's historical use in women's health underscores its versatility and efficacy as a natural remedy. From ancient civilizations to modern times, this oil has been prized for its therapeutic properties and continues to find relevance in addressing various health issues specific to women. As we explore further in this book, we will delve into specific applications, benefits, and DIY recipes that harness the power of castor oil for women's health and well-being.

1.2 Benefits and specific applications for women's health

Benefits and applications of castor oil specific to women's health are diverse and rooted in both traditional wisdom and modern scientific understanding. This natural remedy, derived from the seeds of the Ricinus communis plant, offers a range of therapeutic properties that cater to various aspects of women's health and well-being.

1.2.1 Menstrual Health

Castor oil has long been used to support menstrual health and alleviate associated discomforts:

Menstrual Cramps: One of the most common applications of castor oil in women's health is for relieving menstrual cramps. The oil's anti-inflammatory and analgesic properties can help relax the uterine muscles, thereby reducing pain and discomfort during menstruation.

Regulating Menstrual Cycles: Castor oil packs placed on the abdomen are believed to help regulate irregular menstrual cycles by improving circulation to the reproductive organs. This practice is rooted in traditional medicine systems like Ayurveda and naturopathy.

1.2.2 Fertility Support

For women trying to conceive, castor oil is often recommended to enhance fertility:

Promoting Blood Circulation: By increasing blood flow to the pelvic region, castor oil packs are thought to support ovarian and uterine health, potentially enhancing fertility. Improved circulation may also aid in the delivery of nutrients to the reproductive organs.

Reducing Inflammation: Chronic inflammation in the pelvic area can hinder fertility. Castor oil's anti-inflammatory properties may help alleviate inflammation, creating a more conducive environment for conception.

1.2.3 Pregnancy and Postpartum Care

During pregnancy and after childbirth, castor oil offers several benefits:

Stretch Marks: Applied topically, castor oil can help moisturize the skin and reduce the appearance of stretch marks, which are common during pregnancy due to rapid skin stretching.

Inducing Labor: Historically, castor oil has been used to induce labor by stimulating contractions. However, this practice is controversial and should only be considered under medical supervision.

Postpartum Healing: After childbirth, castor oil packs can be applied to the abdomen to support uterine healing and reduce inflammation. This practice may also help alleviate postpartum cramping.

1.2.4 Breast Health

Castor oil is also beneficial for maintaining breast health:

Fibrocystic Breast Disease: Castor oil packs applied over the breasts may help reduce pain and inflammation associated with fibrocystic breast disease, a condition characterized by lumps and discomfort.

Lactation Support: Some women use castor oil topically to promote milk flow during breastfeeding. However, its safety and efficacy for this purpose are not well-established, so caution is advised.

1.2.5 Skin and Hair Care

Beyond internal applications, castor oil is renowned for its cosmetic benefits:

Skincare: Rich in fatty acids and antioxidants, castor oil moisturizes the skin and helps reduce inflammation. It is used in creams, lotions, and serums to treat dry skin, acne, and dermatitis.

Hair Growth: Castor oil is a popular ingredient in hair care products due to its purported ability to promote hair growth and strengthen hair follicles. It nourishes the scalp, conditions the hair, and may help reduce hair loss.

1.2.6 Digestive Health

Internally, castor oil is occasionally used to promote digestive health:

Constipation Relief: Castor oil is a potent laxative that works by stimulating intestinal contractions. It is sometimes used to relieve occasional constipation, but should be used sparingly and under medical supervision due to its strong purgative effects.

Castor oil's benefits for women's health are multifaceted, encompassing menstrual health, fertility support, pregnancy and postpartum care, breast health, skincare, hair care, and occasional digestive health applications. While many of these benefits are supported by anecdotal evidence and historical use, scientific research on castor oil's specific effects on women's health is ongoing.

Chapter 2: Hormonal balance and menstrual health

2.1 Understanding hormonal imbalances

Understanding hormonal imbalances is crucial for comprehending their impact on women's health and how castor oil may play a role in managing these conditions. Hormones are chemical messengers that regulate various bodily functions, including metabolism, growth, reproduction, and mood. When these hormones are out of balance, it can lead to a wide range of symptoms and health issues.

2.1.1 Overview of Hormones and Imbalances

Hormones are produced by the endocrine glands, such as the pituitary gland, thyroid gland, adrenal glands, ovaries, and pancreas. Each hormone has a specific role, and their levels need to be carefully balanced for optimal health. Common hormones involved in women's health include estrogen, progesterone, testosterone, thyroid hormones (T3 and T4), cortisol, insulin, and others.

Causes of Hormonal Imbalances

Several factors can contribute to hormonal imbalances in women:

- Puberty: Hormonal changes during puberty can lead to irregular menstrual cycles, acne, and mood swings.

- Menstrual Cycle: Fluctuations in estrogen and progesterone levels throughout the menstrual cycle can cause PMS (premenstrual syndrome) symptoms such as mood swings, bloating, and breast tenderness.

- Pregnancy and Postpartum: Hormonal changes during pregnancy and after childbirth can affect mood, energy levels, and metabolism.

- Perimenopause and Menopause: As women approach menopause, estrogen and progesterone levels decline, leading to symptoms such as hot flashes, night sweats, vaginal dryness, and mood changes.

- Stress: Chronic stress can disrupt hormone production and lead to imbalances in cortisol, adrenaline, and other stress hormones.

- Thyroid Disorders: Conditions such as hypothyroidism (underactive thyroid) or hyperthyroidism (overactive thyroid) can disrupt thyroid hormone levels and affect metabolism and energy levels.

- Polycystic Ovary Syndrome (PCOS): PCOS is a hormonal disorder that affects women of reproductive age. It is characterized by high levels of androgens (male hormones), cysts on the ovaries, and irregular menstrual cycles.

- Endocrine Disorders: Disorders affecting the endocrine glands, such as diabetes (affecting insulin levels) or adrenal disorders (affecting cortisol levels), can cause hormonal imbalances.

2.1.2 Symptoms of Hormonal Imbalances

The symptoms of hormonal imbalances in women can vary widely depending on the specific hormones involved and the underlying cause. Some common symptoms include:

- Irregular Menstrual Cycles: Including heavy or prolonged periods, missed periods, or irregular ovulation.

- Mood Changes: Such as irritability, anxiety, depression, or mood swings.

- Weight Gain or Loss: Especially around the abdomen or hips.

- Fatigue: Feeling tired or lethargic despite adequate rest.

- Sleep Problems: Insomnia, difficulty falling asleep or staying asleep.

- Digestive Issues: Including bloating, constipation, or diarrhea.

- Skin Changes: Such as acne, oily skin, or dry skin.

- Hair Loss: Thinning hair or hair loss from the scalp.

- Changes in Libido: Decreased sex drive or changes in sexual function.

2.2 Role of Castor Oil in Managing Hormonal Imbalances

Castor oil has been traditionally used to support hormonal balance and manage related symptoms. While scientific research specific to castor oil's effects on hormones is limited, its therapeutic properties may offer benefits through various mechanisms:

- Anti-inflammatory Effects: Ricinoleic acid, the primary component of castor oil, has anti-inflammatory properties that may help reduce inflammation associated with hormonal imbalances.

- Antioxidant Properties: Castor oil contains antioxidants that can neutralize free radicals and protect cells from oxidative stress.

- Lymphatic Support: Castor oil packs applied to the abdomen are believed to stimulate the lymphatic system, which plays a role in hormone transport and detoxification.

- Stress Reduction: The ritual of self-massage with castor oil may promote relaxation and stress reduction, potentially supporting hormone balance.

2.3 Practical Applications

To harness the potential benefits of castor oil for hormonal imbalances, various applications can be explored:

- Castor Oil Packs: Applied to the abdomen, castor oil packs are believed to support detoxification, reduce inflammation, and promote hormone balance. To make a castor oil pack, soak a flannel cloth in castor oil, place it on the abdomen, cover with plastic wrap, and apply heat for 30-60 minutes.

- Massage: Gentle abdominal massages with castor oil may help improve circulation, reduce inflammation, and support overall hormone health.

- Skincare: Castor oil can be incorporated into skincare routines to moisturize the skin and reduce inflammation-related skin issues.

Understanding hormonal imbalances is essential for women's health as these imbalances can impact various bodily functions and lead to a range of symptoms. While castor oil has been traditionally used to support hormonal balance and manage related symptoms, more research is needed to fully understand its mechanisms of action and effectiveness. As we explore further in this book, we will delve into practical applications, safety considerations, and DIY recipes to harness the potential of castor oil for enhancing women's hormonal health and well-being.

2.4 Role of castor oil in promoting menstrual regularity

Promoting menstrual regularity is crucial for women's health, as irregularities can affect fertility, overall well-being, and quality of life. Castor oil has been historically used to support menstrual health and regularity through various mechanisms, making it a popular natural remedy for addressing menstrual irregularities.

Menstrual regularity refers to the predictable timing and duration of menstrual cycles, typically occurring every 21 to 35 days and lasting about 2 to 7 days. Regular menstrual cycles are influenced by hormonal balance, particularly estrogen and progesterone, which regulate the menstrual cycle phases: follicular phase (pre-ovulation) and luteal phase (post-ovulation).

2.4.1 Causes of Menstrual Irregularities

Several factors can disrupt menstrual regularity:

- Hormonal Imbalances: Fluctuations in estrogen and progesterone levels can lead to irregular menstrual cycles.

- Stress: Chronic stress can affect the hypothalamus-pituitary-adrenal (HPA) axis and disrupt hormone production, potentially causing irregular periods.

- Diet and Nutrition: Poor nutrition or drastic changes in diet can impact hormone levels and menstrual regularity.

- Weight: Significant weight loss or gain can affect estrogen levels and disrupt menstrual cycles.

- Medical Conditions: Conditions such as polycystic ovary syndrome (PCOS), thyroid disorders, and reproductive disorders can cause irregular periods.

2.4.2 Role of Castor Oil in Hormonal Balance

Castor oil, derived from the seeds of the Ricinus communis plant, contains ricinoleic acid, a monounsaturated fatty acid known for its anti-inflammatory and analgesic properties. While direct scientific evidence linking castor oil to menstrual regularity is limited, its traditional use and anecdotal evidence suggest several mechanisms through which it may support hormonal balance and menstrual health:

Anti-inflammatory Properties: Ricinoleic acid exhibits anti-inflammatory effects, which may help reduce inflammation in reproductive organs and support overall reproductive health.

Detoxification Support: Castor oil packs applied to the abdomen are believed to stimulate lymphatic circulation and enhance detoxification. This may help remove toxins and metabolic waste products that could contribute to hormonal imbalances.

Relaxation and Stress Reduction: The ritual of applying castor oil packs and gentle abdominal massages may promote relaxation, reduce stress levels, and indirectly support hormonal balance.

Promotion of Blood Circulation: Massaging castor oil onto the abdomen may improve blood flow to reproductive organs, potentially enhancing their function and supporting menstrual regularity.

2.4.3 Practical Applications

Incorporating castor oil into a routine aimed at promoting menstrual regularity involves several approaches:

Castor Oil Packs: To make a castor oil pack, soak a piece of flannel cloth in castor oil, place it on the lower abdomen, cover with plastic wrap, and apply a heating pad or hot water bottle for 30-60 minutes. This can be done several times a week, preferably before menstruation.

Abdominal Massages: Gentle massages with castor oil on the lower abdomen can be performed regularly to stimulate circulation, reduce inflammation, and support menstrual health.

Internal Use: Some traditions suggest taking a small amount of castor oil orally during menstruation to promote uterine contractions and help expel menstrual fluids. However, this should be done with caution and under the guidance of a healthcare provider due to potential side effects.

2.5 Safety Considerations

While castor oil is generally considered safe for topical use, there are precautions to keep in mind:

Skin Sensitivity: Test castor oil on a small patch of skin before applying it more extensively to ensure there are no allergic reactions or sensitivities.

Pregnancy and Lactation: Pregnant and breastfeeding women should consult healthcare providers before using castor oil, especially internally or in large quantities, as it may stimulate uterine contractions.

Quality and Purity: Use cold-pressed, organic castor oil to ensure purity and avoid exposure to pesticides or contaminants.

Castor oil offers potential benefits for promoting menstrual regularity through its anti-inflammatory properties, support for detoxification, and relaxation effects. While scientific research on its specific effects on menstrual health is limited, its traditional use and anecdotal evidence suggest it may be a valuable natural remedy for supporting hormonal balance and overall reproductive health. As we delve deeper into this book, we will explore practical applications, DIY recipes, and further considerations for integrating castor oil into women's health routines effectively and safely.

2.6 DIY recipes to relieve menstrual pain

1) Castor Oil Pack

- **Ingredients:**

    o Organic castor oil

    o Piece of flannel cloth

    o Hot water bottle or heating pad

- **Instructions:**

1. Fold the flannel cloth to fit over your lower abdomen.

2. Pour organic castor oil onto the cloth until it's saturated.

3. Place the cloth on your lower abdomen.

4. Cover with plastic wrap and place a hot water bottle or heating pad on top.

5. Leave it on for 30-60 minutes. Repeat several times a week as needed.

2) Castor Oil and Essential Oil Massage Blend

- **Ingredients:**

    o 2 tablespoons organic castor oil

    o 5 drops lavender essential oil

    o 5 drops clary sage essential oil

- **Instructions:**

1. Mix all ingredients in a small bowl.

2. Massage the blend onto your lower abdomen in circular motions.

3. Repeat 2-3 times daily during menstruation for pain relief.

3) Castor Oil and Ginger Compress

- **Ingredients:**
    - Organic castor oil
    - Fresh ginger root
    - Hot water
- **Instructions:**

1. Grate or finely chop fresh ginger root.
2. Mix with a small amount of castor oil to make a paste.
3. Apply the paste to your lower abdomen.
4. Cover with a warm, damp cloth and let it sit for 20-30 minutes.
5. Repeat as needed for pain relief.

4) Castor Oil and Chamomile Tea

- **Ingredients:**
    - 1 cup chamomile tea
    - 1 tablespoon organic castor oil
- **Instructions:**

1. Brew a cup of chamomile tea and let it cool slightly.
2. Add organic castor oil to the tea.
3. Drink the tea slowly to help relax muscles and reduce menstrual pain.

5) Castor Oil and Epsom Salt Bath

- **Ingredients:**
    - 1 cup Epsom salt
    - 2 tablespoons organic castor oil
- **Instructions:**

1. Fill your bathtub with warm water.
2. Add Epsom salt and organic castor oil to the water.
3. Soak in the bath for 20-30 minutes to relieve muscle tension and pain.

6) Castor Oil and Heat Therapy

- **Ingredients:**
  - Organic castor oil
  - Hot water bottle or heating pad

- **Instructions:**

1. Apply organic castor oil to your lower abdomen.

2. Place a hot water bottle or heating pad over the area for 20-30 minutes.

3. Repeat as needed throughout the day to ease menstrual cramps.

7) Castor Oil and Lavender Aromatherapy

- **Ingredients:**
  - 2 tablespoons organic castor oil
  - 5 drops lavender essential oil

- **Instructions:**

1. Mix organic castor oil and lavender essential oil in a small bowl.

2. Warm the mixture slightly and massage onto your abdomen in gentle, circular motions.

3. Breathe deeply to enjoy the relaxing aromatherapy benefits.

8) Castor Oil and Peppermint Oil Balm

- **Ingredients:**
  - 2 tablespoons organic castor oil
  - 3-5 drops peppermint essential oil
  - Beeswax or shea butter (optional for texture)

- **Instructions:**

1. Melt beeswax or shea butter (if using) and mix with organic castor oil.

2. Add peppermint essential oil and stir well.

3. Allow the mixture to cool and solidify into a balm.

4. Apply to your lower abdomen for cooling relief from menstrual pain.

9) Castor Oil and Rosemary Infusion

- **Ingredients:**
    - o   Organic castor oil
    - o   Fresh rosemary sprigs
- **Instructions:**

1. Crush fresh rosemary sprigs and place them in a small jar.

2. Cover with organic castor oil and seal the jar.

3. Allow the mixture to infuse for 1-2 weeks in a cool, dark place.

4. Strain out the rosemary and massage the infused oil onto your abdomen for pain relief.

10) Castor Oil and Turmeric Paste

- **Ingredients:**
    - o   1 tablespoon organic castor oil
    - o   1 teaspoon turmeric powder
    - o   Water (to make a paste)
- **Instructions:**

1. Mix turmeric powder with a small amount of water to form a paste.

2. Add organic castor oil and stir well.

3. Apply the paste to your lower abdomen and let it sit for 20-30 minutes.

4. Rinse off with warm water and repeat as needed for pain relief.

Chapter 3: Fertility and reproductive health

3.1 Enhancing fertility with castor oil packs

Enhancing fertility with castor oil packs involves a holistic approach to supporting reproductive health through external application and therapeutic benefits of castor oil.

Castor oil packs are commonly used in natural health practices to potentially improve fertility by enhancing circulation, reducing inflammation, and promoting detoxification when applied to the lower abdomen.

The warm compress of the pack is believed to stimulate blood flow to the pelvic area, which can support ovarian function and create an optimal environment for conception.

Advocates of this method suggest that the packs help alleviate congestion and promote the elimination of toxins through the lymphatic system, thereby supporting uterine health and potentially balancing hormone levels.

This practice is often combined with relaxation techniques and mindful breathing exercises to enhance its therapeutic effects and reduce stress, which can also affect fertility. It's important to note that while castor oil packs are a popular natural remedy, scientific evidence supporting their direct impact on fertility is limited, and individuals should consult healthcare providers before incorporating them into their fertility enhancement regimen.

3.2 Supporting reproductive health naturally

Supporting reproductive health naturally involves adopting lifestyle practices and utilizing natural remedies to optimize fertility and overall reproductive well-being. Many individuals and couples seek natural methods to enhance fertility, often turning to approaches that support the body's natural functions without the use of pharmaceutical interventions. Here are some key aspects of supporting reproductive health naturally:

1) Nutrition

A balanced diet rich in essential nutrients like vitamins, minerals, antioxidants, and omega-3 fatty acids is crucial for reproductive health. Specific nutrients such as folate, zinc, and iron support fertility by promoting healthy hormone levels and reproductive organ function. Including a variety of fruits, vegetables, whole grains, lean proteins, and healthy fats can contribute to overall reproductive wellness.

2) Exercise

Regular physical activity is beneficial for maintaining a healthy weight, reducing stress, and improving circulation, all of which can positively impact fertility. Activities like brisk walking, yoga, swimming, and cycling are excellent choices. However, excessive exercise, incredibly intense workouts, may adversely affect fertility, so moderation is key.

3) Stress Management

Chronic stress can disrupt hormone balance and interfere with reproductive function. Techniques such as meditation, deep breathing exercises, yoga, and mindfulness can help reduce stress levels and support reproductive health. Finding healthy outlets for stress, such as hobbies and spending time with loved ones, is also essential.

4) Sleep

Quality sleep is essential for overall health, including reproductive health. Adequate rest helps regulate hormone production and supports the body's natural rhythms. Aim for 7-9 hours of sleep per night and establish a consistent sleep schedule to promote optimal reproductive function.

5) Avoiding Toxins

Exposure to environmental toxins and chemicals can negatively impact fertility. Minimize exposure to pesticides, BPA, phthalates, and other harmful substances in certain plastics, personal care products, and household cleaners. Choosing organic produce, using natural cleaning products, and opting for BPA-free containers can help reduce toxin exposure.

6) Natural Remedies

Specific natural remedies, including herbs and supplements, are believed to support reproductive health. Examples include chasteberry (Vitex agnus-castus), maca root, evening primrose oil, and omega-3 fatty acids. It's essential to consult with a healthcare provider before starting any herbal or dietary supplement regimen, especially if you're trying to conceive or are pregnant.

7) Natural Therapies

External therapies like castor oil packs, which involve applying warm compresses soaked in castor oil to the lower abdomen, are used by some individuals to support reproductive health. Advocates suggest castor oil packs can help improve circulation, reduce inflammation, and support detoxification in the pelvic area, potentially enhancing fertility. However, evidence supporting these claims is anecdotal, and more research is needed.

In conclusion, supporting reproductive health naturally involves adopting a holistic approach that incorporates healthy lifestyle choices, stress management techniques, and, in some cases, natural remedies. Consulting with a healthcare provider or a fertility specialist can provide personalized guidance and support in optimizing reproductive wellness.

Chapter 4: Pregnancy and postpartum care

4.1 Safety considerations for the use of castor oil in pregnancy

Using castor oil during pregnancy requires careful consideration due to its potential effects on uterine contractions and gastrointestinal activity. While castor oil has been traditionally used to induce labor, its safety and efficacy in pregnancy remain controversial and are not supported by robust scientific evidence. Here are important safety considerations when considering the use of castor oil during pregnancy:

Effect on Uterine Contractions

Castor oil is known to stimulate smooth muscle contractions, including those of the intestines and, potentially, the uterus. This property has led to its historical use as a natural method to induce labor. The active component, ricinoleic acid, stimulates prostaglandin receptors in the intestines, leading to gastrointestinal cramping and diarrhea. In pregnant women, this effect is believed to extend to uterine contractions, which may trigger labor. However, castor oil's timing, effectiveness, and safety for labor induction are not well-established and vary widely among individuals.

Risk of Dehydration

The purgative effect of castor oil can lead to significant fluid loss and dehydration, which is particularly concerning during pregnancy when maintaining adequate hydration is crucial for maternal health and fetal development. Dehydration can also potentially lead to electrolyte imbalances and affect overall well-being.

Potential for Fetal Distress

Inducing labor prematurely or unnaturally through the use of castor oil can pose risks to the fetus, including fetal distress. The sudden stimulation of uterine contractions may lead to changes in fetal heart rate and oxygen supply, which can be detrimental to fetal health.

Gastrointestinal Upset

Pregnant women are more susceptible to gastrointestinal discomfort and dehydration caused by castor oil due to the altered anatomy and physiology of pregnancy. The resulting diarrhea and cramping can exacerbate existing discomfort and lead to further complications.

Lack of Evidence-Based Guidelines

Medical professionals generally do not recommend castor oil for labor induction due to insufficient scientific evidence supporting its safety and effectiveness. The American College of Obstetricians and Gynecologists (ACOG) advises against the use of castor oil for inducing labor due to its unpredictable effects and potential risks.

<u>Consultation with Healthcare Provider</u>

Pregnant individuals considering using castor oil for any purpose should consult with a qualified healthcare provider, such as an obstetrician or midwife, before use. They can provide personalized advice based on the individual's medical history, current pregnancy status, and any existing health conditions.

<u>Alternative Approaches</u>

Instead of using castor oil, pregnant women are encouraged to explore safer and evidence-based methods for managing discomfort or preparing for labor. These may include relaxation techniques, prenatal yoga, acupuncture, and medical interventions healthcare providers recommend when necessary.

While castor oil has been historically used for various medicinal purposes, including labor induction, its safety and efficacy during pregnancy are not well-established. Pregnant women should exercise caution and seek guidance from healthcare professionals before considering the use of castor oil or any other natural remedy. The potential risks, including dehydration, fetal distress, and unpredictable effects on labor, warrant careful consideration of safer and evidence-based alternatives for supporting maternal and fetal health during pregnancy.

4.2 Support healthy pregnancy with castor oil

Supporting a healthy pregnancy with castor oil involves careful consideration of its potential benefits and risks and understanding its historical use in traditional and alternative medicine. While castor oil has been used for centuries for various health purposes, including potentially inducing labor, its application in supporting overall pregnancy health requires careful evaluation and consultation with healthcare providers. Here are key points to consider.

<u>Historical Uses and Folklore</u>

Castor oil, derived from the seeds of the Ricinus communis plant, has a long history of use in traditional medicine. It is known for its anti-inflammatory, antimicrobial, and purgative properties. In pregnancy, historical use has centered on its purported ability to stimulate uterine contractions and promote labor, though these claims lack robust scientific support.

<u>Potential Benefits During Pregnancy</u>

Some proponents suggest castor oil may support pregnancy health by promoting relaxation, reducing inflammation, and aiding digestion. Advocates believe it can alleviate constipation, a common discomfort during pregnancy, due to its laxative effects. Additionally, it may be used topically in the form of packs or massages to support comfort and relaxation.

<u>Managing Common Pregnancy</u>

Discomforts Pregnant individuals may experience a range of discomforts such as constipation, muscle tension, and stress. Castor oil packs applied to the abdomen are believed to help alleviate these discomforts by promoting relaxation, improving circulation, and potentially reducing inflammation in the pelvic region.

Despite its potential benefits, the use of castor oil during pregnancy is controversial and not supported by modern medical guidelines. The primary concern is its ability to stimulate uterine contractions, potentially leading to premature labor. The laxative effect of castor oil can also cause dehydration and electrolyte imbalances, which are particularly risky during pregnancy.

Consultation with Healthcare Providers

Pregnant individuals must consult with their healthcare providers before using castor oil or any other natural remedy. Healthcare providers can provide personalized guidance based on the individual's medical history, current pregnancy status, and existing health conditions. They can help weigh the potential benefits against the risks and recommend safer alternatives when appropriate.

Alternative Approaches

Pregnant women are encouraged to explore evidence-based approaches to support their pregnancy health. This includes maintaining a balanced diet, staying hydrated, engaging in regular prenatal care, practicing safe exercise, and using relaxation techniques such as prenatal yoga or meditation.

Scientific Evidence and Guidelines

The American College of Obstetricians and Gynecologists (ACOG) advises against the use of castor oil for inducing labor due to the lack of sufficient scientific evidence supporting its safety and effectiveness. While anecdotal evidence and historical use may suggest benefits, modern medicine emphasizes the importance of relying on scientifically validated methods and professional guidance during pregnancy.

While castor oil has a rich history in traditional medicine and folklore, its use during pregnancy requires careful consideration and consultation with healthcare providers. Pregnant individuals should prioritize evidence-based practices and safety, seeking guidance to ensure optimal maternal and fetal health. While some alternative practices may have potential benefits, ensuring they align with medical recommendations is crucial for a healthy pregnancy journey.

4.3 Postpartum care and recovery techniques with castor oil

Postpartum care and recovery techniques with castor oil involve gentle and supportive approaches to aid in healing and promote overall well-being following childbirth. Here are essential considerations and practices.

Historical Uses and Traditional Practices: Castor oil, a time-tested remedy, has been historically utilized in various cultures for its purported healing properties. Traditionally, it has been applied topically to promote skin health, reduce inflammation, and support the body's natural healing processes.

1) Topical Application for Healing

Postpartum castor oil can be applied topically to aid in healing cesarean section incisions or perineal tears. The oil's moisturizing and anti-inflammatory properties help reduce swelling, alleviate discomfort, and support tissue repair. It is commonly used as compresses or packs applied to the affected area.

Reduction of Inflammation and Pain: The anti-inflammatory properties of castor oil are beneficial for reducing postpartum inflammation and pain. Warm castor oil packs to the abdomen or lower back can help alleviate uterine cramping and muscle tension discomfort.

2) Support for Breastfeeding

Some individuals use castor oil topically to soothe sore nipples during breastfeeding. However, it's essential to ensure that the nipples are thoroughly cleansed before nursing to prevent the ingestion of any residual oil by the infant.

Stimulating Blood Circulation: Gentle abdominal massages with castor oil postpartum are believed to help stimulate blood circulation and promote uterine involution, the process by which the uterus returns to its pre-pregnancy size. This can aid in speeding up the healing process and reducing postpartum bleeding.

3) Emotional and Mental Well-being

Postpartum can be a challenging time emotionally and mentally. Using castor oil in relaxation techniques such as aromatherapy or gentle massage may provide comfort and promote relaxation, helping to alleviate stress and support emotional well-being.

Safety Considerations

While castor oil is generally considered safe for topical use, it's crucial to perform a patch test before applying it to sensitive areas to avoid allergic reactions. Additionally, ensure that the oil is applied sparingly and that any excess is wiped off to prevent ingestion, especially if breastfeeding.

Consultation with Healthcare Providers: As with any postpartum care practice, it's crucial to consult with your healthcare providers before using castor oil. They can provide personalized guidance based on individual health needs and specific postpartum conditions or concerns, ensuring that the use of castor oil is safe and beneficial for you.

Alternative Practices

In addition to castor oil, individuals may explore other evidence-based postpartum care practices such as adequate rest, hydration, nutrition, and gentle exercise as recommended by healthcare providers. These practices, when combined with the traditional use of castor oil, can provide a comprehensive approach to postpartum care, contributing to the overall well-being and recovery of the postpartum individual.

Incorporating castor oil into postpartum care routines can be a gentle and supportive approach to aid healing, reduce inflammation, and promote overall well-being. This supportive nature of castor oil can provide reassurance and comfort during the postpartum period. However, it's essential to prioritize safety, consult healthcare providers, and complement with evidence-based practices to ensure a healthy and supported postpartum recovery.

Chapter 5: Skin and hair care for women

5.1 DIY beauty recipes with castor oil for skin

1) Cleansing Castor Oil Face Wash:

- Ingredients:
    - 1 tablespoon castor oil
    - 1 tablespoon olive oil
    - 1 tablespoon honey
    - 1 teaspoon liquid castile soap
- Instructions:

1. Mix all ingredients thoroughly in a small bowl.

2. Apply a small amount to damp skin and massage gently in circular motions.

3. Rinse with lukewarm water and pat dry.

2) Moisturizing Castor Oil Body Butter:

- Ingredients:
    - 1/4 cup shea butter
    - 1/4 cup cocoa butter
    - 2 tablespoons coconut oil
    - 2 tablespoons castor oil
    - 10 drops lavender essential oil (optional)
- Instructions:

1. Melt the shea butter, cocoa butter, and coconut oil in a double boiler until fully melted.

2. Remove from heat and stir in castor oil and lavender essential oil.

3. Allow the mixture to cool slightly, then whip with a hand mixer until fluffy.

4. Transfer to a clean jar and store in a cool, dry place. Apply as needed to dry skin.

3) Exfoliating Castor Oil Sugar Scrub:

- **Ingredients**:
    - 1/2 cup brown sugar
    - 1/4 cup almond oil
    - 2 tablespoons castor oil
    - 1 teaspoon vanilla extract (optional)

- **Instructions**:

1. Combine all ingredients in a bowl and mix well.

2. Massage the scrub onto damp skin in gentle circular motions.

3. Rinse thoroughly with warm water and pat dry. Use 2-3 times per week for best results.

4) Hydrating Castor Oil Lip Balm:

- **Ingredients**:
    - 1 tablespoon beeswax pellets
    - 1 tablespoon shea butter
    - 1 tablespoon coconut oil
    - 1 tablespoon castor oil
    - 10 drops peppermint essential oil (optional)

- **Instructions**:

1. Melt beeswax, shea butter, coconut oil, and castor oil in a double boiler until fully melted.

2. Remove from heat and stir in peppermint essential oil.

3. Pour the mixture into lip balm containers and let it cool completely before use.

5) Nourishing Castor Oil Hair Mask:

- **Ingredients**:

- o   2 tablespoons castor oil
- o   1 tablespoon coconut oil
- o   1 tablespoon honey
- o   1 egg yolk

- **Instructions:**

1. Whisk together all ingredients in a bowl until well combined.

2. Apply the mask to damp hair, focusing on the roots and ends.

3. Cover your hair with a shower cap and leave the mask on for 30 minutes.

4. Rinse thoroughly with warm water and shampoo as usual.

6) Brightening Castor Oil Face Mask:

- **Ingredients:**

- o   1 tablespoon castor oil
- o   1 tablespoon plain yogurt
- o   1 tablespoon lemon juice

- **Instructions:**

1. Mix all ingredients in a bowl until smooth.

2. Apply the mask to clean, dry skin and leave it on for 15-20 minutes.

3. Rinse with lukewarm water and pat dry. Use once a week to brighten and clarify skin.

7) Soothing Castor Oil Eye Cream:

- **Ingredients:**

- o   1 tablespoon castor oil
- o   1 tablespoon sweet almond oil
- o   1 tablespoon shea butter

- **Instructions:**

1. Melt shea butter in a double boiler until fully melted.

2. Remove from heat and stir in castor oil and sweet almond oil.

3. Allow the mixture to cool slightly, then transfer to a small jar.

4. Apply a small amount around the eyes before bedtime and gently pat until absorbed.

8) Repairing Castor Oil Cuticle Oil:

- **Ingredients:**
    - 1 tablespoon castor oil
    - 1 tablespoon jojoba oil
    - 5 drops vitamin E oil

- **Instructions:**

1. Combine all ingredients in a small dropper bottle and shake well to mix.

2. Apply a drop of oil to each nail and massage into the cuticles.

3. Use daily to nourish and strengthen nails and cuticles.

9) Soothing Castor Oil Bath Salts:

- **Ingredients:**
    - 1 cup Epsom salts
    - 1/4 cup sea salt
    - 2 tablespoons baking soda
    - 2 tablespoons castor oil
    - 10 drops lavender essential oil

- **Instructions:**

1. Mix all dry ingredients in a bowl until well combined.

2. Add castor oil and lavender essential oil, and mix thoroughly.

3. Store in a sealed container and add a few tablespoons to warm bath water.

10) Refreshing Castor Oil Foot Scrub:

- **Ingredients:**
    - 1/2 cup coarse sea salt
    - 1/4 cup castor oil
    - 1/4 cup olive oil
    - 10 drops peppermint essential oil

- **Instructions:**

1. Combine sea salt, castor oil, olive oil, and peppermint essential oil in a bowl.

2. Massage the scrub onto damp feet in circular motions, focusing on rough areas.

3. Rinse with warm water and pat dry. Follow with a moisturizing lotion if desired.

5.2 DIY beauty recipes with castor oil for hair

1) Castor Oil Hair Growth Serum:

- **Ingredients**:
    - 2 tablespoons castor oil
    - 1 tablespoon coconut oil
    - 5 drops rosemary essential oil
- **Instructions**:

1. Mix all ingredients in a small bowl until well combined.

2. Apply the serum directly to the scalp and massage gently for 5-10 minutes.

3. Leave it on for at least 30 minutes or overnight, then shampoo as usual.

2) Castor Oil Scalp Massage:

- **Ingredients**:
    - 3 tablespoons castor oil
    - 1 tablespoon jojoba oil
- **Instructions**:

1. Combine the oils in a bowl and warm slightly.

2. Part your hair and apply the oil mixture to your scalp using your fingertips.

3. Massage in circular motions for 5-10 minutes to stimulate circulation.

4. Leave it on for at least 1 hour before shampooing.

3) Castor Oil and Aloe Vera Hair Mask:

- **Ingredients**:
    - 2 tablespoons castor oil
    - 1 tablespoon aloe vera gel

o   1 tablespoon honey

- **Instructions**:

1.   Mix castor oil, aloe vera gel, and honey in a bowl until smooth.

2.   Apply the mask to damp hair, focusing on the roots and tips.

3.   Cover your hair with a shower cap and leave it on for 30-60 minutes.

4.   Rinse thoroughly with lukewarm water and shampoo as usual.

4) Castor Oil and Egg Hair Treatment:

- **Ingredients**:

  o   2 tablespoons castor oil

  o   1 egg

  o   1 tablespoon yogurt

- **Instructions**:

1.   Whisk the egg and yogurt together in a bowl until well blended.

2.   Add castor oil and mix thoroughly.

3.   Apply the mixture to damp hair, covering from roots to ends.

4.   Leave it on for 30 minutes, then rinse with cool water and shampoo.

5) Castor Oil and Peppermint Hair Rinse:

- **Ingredients**:

  o   2 tablespoons castor oil

  o   1 cup water

  o   5 drops peppermint essential oil

- **Instructions**:

1.   Mix castor oil and peppermint oil in a small bowl.

2.   Add the mixture to a cup of water and stir well.

3.   After shampooing, pour the rinse over your hair and massage into the scalp.

4.   Leave it on for a few minutes, then rinse thoroughly with cool water.

6) Castor Oil and Coconut Milk Deep Conditioner:

- **Ingredients:**
    - 2 tablespoons castor oil
    - 1/4 cup coconut milk
    - 1 tablespoon honey

- **Instructions:**

1. Heat coconut milk slightly and mix in honey until dissolved.

2. Add castor oil and stir until well combined.

3. Apply the conditioner to damp hair, focusing on the ends.

4. Leave it on for 30 minutes, then rinse thoroughly with warm water.

7) Castor Oil and Avocado Hair Mask:

- **Ingredients:**
    - 2 tablespoons castor oil
    - 1/2 ripe avocado
    - 1 tablespoon olive oil

- **Instructions:**

1. Mash the avocado in a bowl until smooth.

2. Mix in castor oil and olive oil until well blended.

3. Apply the mask to clean, damp hair, covering from roots to tips.

4. Leave it on for 20-30 minutes, then rinse with lukewarm water and shampoo.

8) Castor Oil and Green Tea Hair Rinse:

- **Ingredients:**
    - 2 tablespoons castor oil
    - 1 cup brewed green tea (cooled)

- **Instructions:**

1. Mix castor oil and green tea in a bowl until well combined.

2. After shampooing, pour the rinse over your hair and massage into the scalp.

3.   Leave it on for a few minutes, then rinse thoroughly with cool water.

9) Castor Oil and Banana Hair Mask:

- **Ingredients**:
    - o   2 tablespoons castor oil
    - o   1 ripe banana
    - o   1 tablespoon honey

- **Instructions**:

1.   Mash the banana in a bowl until smooth.

2.   Mix in castor oil and honey until well blended.

3.   Apply the mask to damp hair, covering from roots to tips.

4.   Leave it on for 30 minutes, then rinse thoroughly with warm water and shampoo.

10) Castor Oil and Yogurt Hair Mask:

- **Ingredients**:
    - o   2 tablespoons castor oil
    - o   1/4 cup plain yogurt
    - o   1 tablespoon honey

- **Instructions**:

1.   Mix castor oil, yogurt, and honey in a bowl until smooth.

2.   Apply the mask to clean, damp hair, focusing on the scalp and ends.

3.   Cover your hair with a shower cap and leave it on for 30-60 minutes.

4.   Rinse thoroughly with lukewarm water and shampoo as usual.

5.3 Addressing common skin problems with castor oil

Castor oil is renowned for its therapeutic properties that make it effective in addressing various skin concerns. Here's how castor oil can help with common skin issues.

1) Acne

Castor oil's antimicrobial and anti-inflammatory properties can help reduce acne breakouts by preventing bacterial growth and soothing inflammation.

2) Dry Skin

Its high concentration of fatty acids deeply moisturizes the skin, promoting hydration and preventing dryness and flakiness.

3) Wrinkles and Fine Lines

Castor oil's ability to stimulate collagen and elastin production can help reduce the appearance of wrinkles and fine lines, promoting smoother and more youthful-looking skin.

4) Stretch Marks

The moisturizing and emollient properties of castor oil can help improve skin elasticity and reduce the appearance of stretch marks over time.

5) Eczema and Psoriasis

Its anti-inflammatory properties can provide relief from itching, redness, and irritation associated with eczema and psoriasis.

6) Sunburns

Castor oil's soothing properties can help alleviate pain and inflammation caused by sunburns while promoting skin healing.

7) Cleansing

Castor oil's natural cleansing properties make it effective for removing dirt, oil, and impurities from the skin without stripping away natural oils.

8) Cuticle Care

Applying castor oil to cuticles and nails helps moisturize and strengthen nails while promoting healthy cuticles.

9) Even Skin Tone

Regular use of castor oil can help even out skin tone and reduce hyperpigmentation, promoting a more balanced complexion.

10) Razor Burn

Its soothing properties make castor oil effective in calming razor burn and reducing redness and irritation post-shaving.

By incorporating castor oil into your skincare regimen, you can harness its natural benefits to achieve healthier, more radiant skin. Whether used alone or in combination with other skincare products, castor oil offers a gentle yet effective solution to various skin issues, promoting overall skin health and vitality.

Chapter 6: Breast health and castor oil

6.1 Use of castor oil for breast health and lymphatic support

Using castor oil for breast health and lymphatic support has been a traditional remedy known for its potential benefits. Castor oil packs, applied externally to the breasts, are believed to help improve circulation, lymphatic drainage, and overall breast health. Here's how castor oil can be used for these purposes.

Lymphatic Support. The lymphatic system plays a crucial role in removing toxins and waste from the body. Castor oil packs applied over the breasts are thought to stimulate lymphatic circulation, helping to reduce congestion and promote detoxification.

Reducing Inflammation. Castor oil's anti-inflammatory properties may help alleviate swelling and inflammation in the breast tissue, potentially providing relief from conditions like mastitis or general breast tenderness.

Promoting Circulation. Massaging castor oil into the breasts can improve blood flow to the area, which may contribute to overall breast health and function.

Fibrocystic Breast Tissue. Some women use castor oil packs to help soften and reduce the size of fibrocystic breast tissue, which can sometimes cause discomfort or pain.

Support During Menstruation. Applying castor oil packs to the breasts during menstruation is believed to support hormonal balance and alleviate breast tenderness associated with menstrual cycles.

Preventive Care. Regular use of castor oil packs as part of a self-care routine may contribute to maintaining healthy breast tissue and supporting breast health over time.

6.1.1 How to Use Castor Oil for Breast Health and Lymphatic Support

Preparing Castor Oil Packs: Soak a piece of flannel or a cloth in castor oil, then place it over the breasts. Cover with plastic wrap or a towel and apply gentle heat using a hot water bottle or heating pad for 30-60 minutes.

Gently massage a small amount of castor oil into the breasts in a circular motion. This can be done daily or as needed to promote circulation and support lymphatic drainage.

While castor oil is generally considered safe for external use, it's essential to perform a patch test before using it on larger areas of skin. Avoid applying castor oil to broken skin or open wounds.

Always consult with a healthcare provider before starting any new health regimen, especially if you have existing health conditions or concerns related to breast health.

Incorporating castor oil into your routine for breast health and lymphatic support may provide a natural and gentle way to promote overall well-being. Regular use, combined with healthy lifestyle practices, can contribute to maintaining optimal breast health and supporting your body's natural detoxification processes.

6.2 Techniques for massage and breast care

Breast massage is a practice that can offer several benefits, from promoting circulation and lymphatic drainage to supporting overall breast health. When coupled with the use of castor oil, known for its anti-inflammatory and moisturizing properties, these techniques can contribute to a holistic approach to breast care. Here's how you can effectively incorporate breast massage into your self-care routine:

1) Purpose of Breast Massage

Breast massage serves multiple purposes, including:

- o Improving Circulation: Massage can stimulate blood flow to the breasts, which may aid in maintaining tissue health and elasticity.

- o Lymphatic Drainage: Gentle massage movements can facilitate the drainage of lymph fluid, helping to reduce congestion and remove toxins from the breast tissue.

- o Promoting Relaxation: Massaging the breasts can promote relaxation and reduce tension in the chest area, which may help alleviate discomfort.

2) Choosing the Right Oil

Castor oil is often used for breast massage due to its nourishing and anti-inflammatory properties. Other oils such as coconut oil, almond oil, or olive oil can also be used based on personal preference and skin sensitivity. Ensure the oil is warmed slightly before use to enhance absorption and comfort.

3) Techniques for Breast Massage

- o Circular Motion: Start by applying a small amount of oil to the breast area. Using the pads of your fingers, gently massage in circular motions, moving from the outside of the breast towards the nipple. Repeat this motion several times, adjusting pressure as needed.

- o Lymphatic Stroking: Use flat hands to gently stroke from the top of the breast towards the armpit area. This motion follows the natural flow of lymphatic fluid and can help in drainage.

o Compression: Lightly compress the breast tissue between your hands, moving from the base of the breast towards the nipple. Release and repeat several times. This technique can help improve circulation and reduce congestion.

o Kneading: With both hands, gently knead the breast tissue in a lifting and slightly squeezing motion. This technique can promote relaxation and improve blood flow.

o Tapotement: Use light tapping or drumming motions with your fingertips to stimulate circulation and invigorate the breast tissue gently. This technique should be done lightly and for a short duration.

4) Frequency and Timing

o Aim to perform breast massage regularly, ideally once a day or a few times a week, depending on your comfort and schedule.

o Choose a time when you can relax and focus on self-care, such as after a warm shower or before bedtime.

5) Self-Examination

o Breast massage also provides an opportunity for self-examination. While massaging, feel for any lumps, changes in texture, or unusual sensations in the breast tissue. If you notice any abnormalities, consult with a healthcare professional promptly.

6) Precautions and Considerations

o Always perform breast massage gently and with care to avoid causing discomfort or injury.

o Avoid vigorous massage or excessive pressure, especially if you have sensitive breasts or a history of breast surgery.

o If you experience pain, swelling, or unusual symptoms during or after massage, discontinue and consult with a healthcare provider.

7) Incorporating Castor Oil

o To enhance the benefits of breast massage, consider using castor oil. Apply a small amount to the breast area before massaging to moisturize the skin and potentially reduce inflammation.

By incorporating these techniques into your routine, you can promote breast health, enhance lymphatic drainage, and enjoy the soothing benefits of regular breast massage. Remember to listen to your body's cues and adjust the techniques to suit your individual needs and preferences.

6.3 Supporting breast health naturally

Maintaining breast health is crucial for overall well-being, and incorporating natural methods can play a significant role in supporting this aspect of women's health. From lifestyle adjustments to specific practices, here are effective ways to support breast health naturally:

<u>Healthy Diet and Nutrition</u>

A balanced diet rich in fruits, vegetables, lean proteins, and whole grains provides essential nutrients that support breast health. Key nutrients include antioxidants (like vitamins C and E), omega-3 fatty acids (found in fish and flaxseeds), and phytoestrogens (found in soy products and legumes). These nutrients help combat oxidative stress, promote cellular health, and maintain hormonal balance—all vital for breast health.

<u>Regular Physical Activity</u>

Engaging in regular physical exercise offers numerous benefits for overall health, including breast health. Exercise helps maintain a healthy weight, which is crucial as excess body fat can increase estrogen levels and potentially impact breast health. Additionally, physical activity improves circulation, reduces inflammation, and supports immune function, all of which contribute to optimal breast health.

<u>Maintaining Hormonal Balance</u>

Hormonal fluctuations can influence breast health, particularly during menstruation, pregnancy, and menopause. Strategies to promote hormonal balance include:

- o Limiting Alcohol and Caffeine: Excessive alcohol and caffeine consumption can disrupt hormone levels. Moderation is key to minimizing their impact on breast health.

- o Managing Stress: Chronic stress can affect hormone production. Practices such as yoga, meditation, deep breathing exercises, and spending time in nature can help manage stress levels and promote hormonal balance.

- o Healthy Sleep Patterns: Quality sleep is essential for hormone regulation. Aim for 7-9 hours of uninterrupted sleep each night to support overall health, including breast health.

<u>Breast Self-Examination (BSE)</u>

Regular breast self-examination is a proactive way to monitor changes in breast tissue and detect potential abnormalities early. Conducting BSE monthly, preferably a few days after menstruation when breasts are less tender, allows for familiarization with normal breast texture and helps identify any changes promptly.

<u>Natural Supplements and Herbs</u>

Certain supplements and herbs may support breast health. Examples include:

- o Vitamin D: Adequate vitamin D levels are associated with a lower risk of breast cancer. Consider supplementation if levels are low, particularly in regions with limited sunlight.

- o Flaxseed: Rich in lignans, which have phytoestrogenic properties, flaxseed may help balance estrogen levels and support breast health. Ground flaxseed can be added to smoothies or sprinkled over salads.

○ Turmeric: Known for its anti-inflammatory properties, turmeric may help reduce inflammation and support overall breast health. Incorporate turmeric into cooking or take as a supplement, ensuring it's paired with black pepper for enhanced absorption.

Breast Massage and Care

Regular breast massage, using gentle techniques and possibly incorporating castor oil, can improve circulation, promote lymphatic drainage, and support breast tissue health. Massaging the breasts in circular motions or using specific techniques can help maintain breast health and detect changes early.

Avoiding Harmful Substances

Limit exposure to environmental toxins, such as BPA (found in plastic containers) and phthalates (found in personal care products), which may disrupt hormone balance and contribute to breast health concerns. Choose BPA-free containers and opt for natural, toxin-free personal care products.

Regular Medical Check-ups

Routine medical check-ups, including clinical breast examinations and mammograms as recommended by healthcare providers, are essential for early detection of breast issues. These screenings are vital even if no symptoms are present, ensuring any changes can be addressed promptly.

By integrating these natural approaches into your lifestyle, you can proactively support breast health and contribute to overall well-being. Consistency and mindfulness in adopting these practices are key to maintaining optimal breast health throughout different stages of life.

Chapter 7: Digestive health and detoxification

7.1 Benefits of castor oil compresses for digestive health

Castor oil packs have gained popularity as a natural remedy to support digestive health, offering a range of benefits that can help alleviate gastrointestinal issues. Here's an exploration of how castor oil packs contribute to digestive wellness:

<u>Anti-Inflammatory Properties</u>

Castor oil is rich in ricinoleic acid, a monounsaturated fatty acid known for its anti-inflammatory properties. When applied externally as a pack, castor oil can help reduce inflammation in the abdominal area, easing discomfort associated with conditions like gastritis, colitis, and irritable bowel syndrome (IBS).

<u>Stimulating Circulation</u>

Applying castor oil packs to the abdomen promotes blood circulation and lymphatic drainage. Improved circulation can aid in delivering oxygen and nutrients to the digestive organs, supporting their optimal function and enhancing overall digestive efficiency.

<u>Detoxification Support</u>

Castor oil packs are believed to stimulate detoxification pathways in the body, particularly through the liver. The liver is crucial in detoxifying metabolic waste products and toxins from the bloodstream. Applying a castor oil pack over the liver area (located on the right side of the abdomen) can potentially enhance liver function and facilitate the elimination of toxins, promoting a healthier digestive system.

<u>Relief from Constipation</u>

Castor oil is well-known for its laxative effects when taken orally, but when used externally as a pack, it can also help relieve constipation. The gentle heat generated by the pack and the absorption of castor oil through the skin may stimulate bowel movements and alleviate symptoms of occasional constipation.

<u>Support for Digestive Disorders</u>

Individuals suffering from digestive disorders such as bloating, gas, and indigestion may find relief with castor oil packs. The packs help relax the abdominal muscles, reduce cramping, and improve digestive comfort.

<u>Enhanced Nutrient Absorption</u>

Improved circulation and reduced inflammation in the digestive tract can enhance nutrient absorption from food. This is particularly beneficial for individuals with nutrient deficiencies or those recovering from gastrointestinal illnesses.

<u>Stress Reduction</u>

Applying a castor oil pack to the abdomen promotes relaxation and reduces stress levels. Stress can significantly impact digestive health by slowing digestion and exacerbating symptoms of digestive disorders. By incorporating castor oil packs into a stress-reduction routine, individuals may experience improved digestion and overall well-being.

Castor oil packs are easy to prepare and use at home. They involve soaking a flannel or cloth in castor oil, placing it on the abdomen, covering it with a plastic wrap or towel to prevent staining, and applying gentle heat with a heating pad or hot water bottle for 30-60 minutes. The pack can be reused multiple times before needing to be replaced.

Incorporating castor oil packs into your regular self-care routine can provide significant benefits for digestive health. However, it's essential to consult with a healthcare professional, especially if you have underlying medical conditions or are pregnant, before starting any new health regimen. It's also important to note that while castor oil packs are generally safe, some individuals may experience skin irritation or allergic reactions. By leveraging the natural properties of castor oil, individuals can support their digestive system's health and function effectively.

7.2 DIY remedies for constipation and bloating

1) Castor Oil Packs:

- **Ingredients**:
    - Organic castor oil
    - Flannel cloth
    - Plastic wrap or sheet
    - Hot water bottle or heating pad

- **Instructions**:
    - Soak the flannel cloth in castor oil until saturated.
    - Place the cloth on the abdomen and cover with plastic wrap or sheet.
    - Apply gentle heat with a hot water bottle or heating pad for 30-60 minutes.
    - Repeat daily or as needed to relieve constipation and reduce bloating.

2) Castor Oil Massage:

- **Ingredients**:
    - Organic castor oil

- Instructions:
  - Warm the castor oil slightly.
  - Massage the abdomen in circular motions clockwise to stimulate bowel movement.
  - Continue massaging for 10-15 minutes.
  - Follow with a warm compress on the abdomen for additional relief.

3) Castor Oil and Ginger Tea:

- Ingredients:
  - 1 tablespoon castor oil
  - 1 teaspoon grated ginger
  - 1 cup hot water
- Instructions:
  - Steep grated ginger in hot water for 5-10 minutes.
  - Add castor oil and stir well.
  - Drink the tea slowly to stimulate digestion and relieve bloating.

4) Castor Oil and Epsom Salt Bath:

- Ingredients:
  - 1 cup Epsom salt
  - 2 tablespoons castor oil
- Instructions:
  - Dissolve Epsom salt in a warm bath.
  - Add castor oil and mix well.
  - Soak in the bath for 20-30 minutes to promote relaxation and relieve constipation.

5) Castor Oil and Lemon Juice Drink:

- Ingredients:
  - 1 tablespoon castor oil
  - Juice of half a lemon
  - 1 cup warm water

- **Instructions**:
  - o Mix castor oil and lemon juice in warm water.
  - o Drink the mixture on an empty stomach in the morning to stimulate bowel movement.

6) Castor Oil and Peppermint Oil Blend:

- **Ingredients**:
  - o 1 tablespoon castor oil
  - o 2-3 drops peppermint essential oil
- **Instructions**:
  - o Mix castor oil and peppermint oil.
  - o Massage the blend onto the abdomen in circular motions to relieve bloating and gas.

7) Castor Oil and Fennel Seed Tea:

- **Ingredients**:
  - o 1 tablespoon castor oil
  - o 1 teaspoon crushed fennel seeds
  - o 1 cup hot water
- **Instructions**:
  - o Steep crushed fennel seeds in hot water for 10 minutes.
  - o Add castor oil and stir well.
  - o Drink the tea to ease digestion and reduce bloating.

8) Castor Oil and Aloe Vera Gel Drink:

- **Ingredients**:
  - o 1 tablespoon castor oil
  - o 2 tablespoons aloe vera gel
  - o 1 cup water or coconut water
- **Instructions**:
  - o Mix castor oil and aloe vera gel in water.
  - o Stir well and drink the mixture to soothe the digestive tract and alleviate constipation.

9) Castor Oil and Chamomile Infusion:

- **Ingredients**:
  - 1 tablespoon castor oil
  - 1 teaspoon dried chamomile flowers
  - 1 cup boiling water
- **Instructions**:
  - Steep dried chamomile flowers in boiling water for 5-10 minutes.
  - Add castor oil and mix well.
  - Drink the infusion to calm the digestive system and promote regular bowel movements.

10) Castor Oil and Yogurt Smoothie:

- **Ingredients**:
  - 1 tablespoon castor oil
  - 1/2 cup plain yogurt
  - 1/2 banana
  - 1 tablespoon honey (optional)
- **Instructions**:
  - Blend all ingredients until smooth.
  - Drink the smoothie as a breakfast or snack to improve digestion and relieve constipation.

7.3 Detoxification techniques with castor oil

Castor oil offers effective natural methods to detoxify the body, promoting overall health and well-being. Here are several techniques to incorporate castor oil into your detox routine.

Castor Oil Packs

Soak a piece of flannel cloth in castor oil and place it over the abdomen or liver area.

Cover with plastic wrap or a sheet and apply a heating pad or hot water bottle for 30-60 minutes.

Stimulates lymphatic drainage and aids in toxin elimination through the skin.

Castor Oil Massage

Apply castor oil to the skin and massage in circular motions.

Enhances lymphatic flow and circulation, facilitating detoxification.

Detox Baths

Add castor oil to Epsom salt baths to draw out toxins through the skin.

Promotes relaxation, muscle relief, and detoxification.

Internal Cleansing

Take small amounts of castor oil orally to promote bowel movement and cleanse the digestive system. Helps in flushing out toxins and promoting regularity.

Liver Detox Support

Use castor oil packs over the liver area to support liver detoxification processes. Assists in clearing out toxins and promoting optimal liver function.

Skin Detoxification

Apply castor oil directly to the skin to improve complexion and help draw out impurities.

Supports the body's natural detoxification processes through the skin.

Chapter 8: Management of menopausal symptoms

8.1 Relieve menopausal symptoms with castor oil

Menopause is a natural transition in a woman's life, marking the end of her reproductive years. During this phase, hormonal changes can lead to various symptoms that impact quality of life. Castor oil, renowned for its therapeutic properties, can be a comforting natural remedy, offering relief from menopausal symptoms. Here's how castor oil can help and methods to incorporate it into your routine.

<u>Menopausal Symptoms</u>

Menopause typically occurs around the age of 50, although it can start earlier for some women. Common symptoms include hot flashes, night sweats, mood swings, vaginal dryness, sleep disturbances, and changes in libido. These symptoms are primarily due to fluctuating hormone levels, specifically estrogen and progesterone.

<u>Benefits of Castor Oil for Menopausal Symptoms</u>

Castor oil contains ricinoleic acid, which has anti-inflammatory and analgesic properties. It also supports detoxification and improves circulation, which can alleviate menopausal symptoms. Here are specific benefits:

Hot Flashes and Night Sweats: massaging the abdomen and lower back with castor oil can help regulate body temperature and reduce the frequency and intensity of hot flashes and night sweats.

Mood Swings and Stress: castor oil packs applied to the abdomen can promote relaxation and reduce stress, helping to stabilize mood swings.

Vaginal Dryness: applying castor oil externally to the vaginal area can moisturize and soothe dryness.

Bone Health: Castor oil packs applied to the abdomen and liver may support hormonal balance and improve the absorption of nutrients crucial for bone health during menopause.

<u>Methods of Application</u>

Incorporating castor oil into your daily routine can be done through various methods:

Castor Oil Packs: soak a piece of flannel in castor oil, apply it to the abdomen, and cover it with plastic wrap. Place a heating pad or hot water bottle over the pack for 30-60 minutes. This method enhances circulation, supports detoxification, and reduces inflammation.

Castor Oil Massage: regular massages with castor oil on the abdomen, lower back, and other affected areas can alleviate discomfort and promote relaxation.

Oral Consumption: consuming small amounts of castor oil may help regulate bowel movements and aid in overall detoxification, which can indirectly alleviate some menopausal symptoms.

While castor oil is generally safe for external use, a patch test is essential to check for allergic reactions. Avoid using castor oil packs during menstruation or if pregnant, and consult a healthcare provider before using castor oil internally.

Combining castor oil with other holistic approaches like healthy diet modifications, regular exercise, stress management techniques (such as yoga or meditation), and adequate sleep can enhance its effectiveness in managing menopausal symptoms.

Castor oil offers a natural and holistic approach to alleviating menopausal symptoms by addressing underlying hormonal imbalances and supporting overall well-being. Integrating castor oil into your daily routine can provide relief and promote a healthier transition through menopause. Always remember, your safety comes first. Consult with a healthcare professional before starting any new treatment regimen, especially if you have underlying health conditions or are taking medications.

8.2 Supporting hormonal balance in menopause

Menopause is a natural phase in a woman's life characterized by hormonal shifts as the ovaries gradually decrease their production of estrogen and progesterone. These changes can lead to a variety of symptoms such as hot flashes, night sweats, mood swings, and changes in libido. Maintaining hormonal balance during this transition is crucial for managing these symptoms and promoting overall well-being. Here's how castor oil can support hormonal balance during menopause:

8.2.1 Regulating Estrogen Levels

Castor oil contains ricinoleic acid, which has been shown to exert anti-inflammatory effects and support detoxification pathways in the body. By promoting liver function, castor oil aids in metabolizing hormones like estrogen, which can help regulate their levels in the body. This regulation is essential as fluctuating estrogen levels are often the primary cause of menopausal symptoms.

8.2.2 Alleviating Menopausal Symptoms

Castor oil can be used topically through various applications to alleviate specific symptoms associated with hormonal imbalance:

- o **Hot Flashes and Night Sweats**: Applying castor oil packs to the abdomen and lower back can help regulate body temperature and reduce the frequency and intensity of hot flashes and night sweats.

- o **Mood Swings and Stress**: Massaging with castor oil can promote relaxation and reduce stress levels, contributing to emotional stability during hormonal fluctuations.

o **Vaginal Dryness**: External application of castor oil to the vaginal area can moisturize and soothe dryness, improving comfort and intimacy.

8.2.3 Enhancing Detoxification

Effective detoxification is crucial during menopause to support the liver's ability to metabolize hormones and remove toxins from the body. Castor oil packs applied over the abdomen can enhance blood circulation and lymphatic drainage, facilitating the elimination of waste products and promoting hormonal balance.

8.2.4 Promoting Bone Health

Hormonal changes during menopause can impact bone density and increase the risk of osteoporosis. Castor oil packs applied to the abdomen and liver area may support hormonal balance and improve absorption of nutrients essential for bone health, such as calcium and vitamin D.

8.2.5 Holistic Approach

Integrating castor oil into a holistic approach to menopause management can provide comprehensive support. Alongside castor oil applications, maintaining a balanced diet rich in vitamins, minerals, and phytonutrients, engaging in regular exercise, practicing stress reduction techniques like yoga or meditation, and ensuring adequate sleep can further promote hormonal balance and overall well-being.

In conclusion, castor oil offers a natural and holistic approach to supporting hormonal balance during menopause by addressing symptoms and promoting detoxification. Its anti-inflammatory and detoxifying properties make it a valuable tool in managing the hormonal fluctuations characteristic of this life stage. As with any natural remedy, it's advisable to consult with a healthcare professional before starting any new regimen, especially if you have underlying health conditions or are taking medications.

8.3 Recipes for managing hot flashes and mood swings

Managing hot flashes and mood swings during menopause can significantly improve quality of life. Castor oil, known for its anti-inflammatory and soothing properties, can be incorporated into various DIY recipes and techniques to alleviate these symptoms effectively:

1) Castor Oil Cooling Spray:

o **Ingredients**:

- 2 tablespoons of castor oil

- 1/4 cup of witch hazel

- 1/4 cup of distilled water

- 5-10 drops of peppermint essential oil (optional)
  - o **Instructions:**

1. Mix castor oil, witch hazel, and distilled water in a spray bottle.

2. Add peppermint essential oil if desired for a cooling effect.

3. Shake well before each use.

4. Spray on the face and neck during hot flashes for instant cooling relief.

2) Castor Oil Mood Balancing Blend:

- o **Ingredients:**
  - 1 tablespoon of castor oil
  - 2 tablespoons of sweet almond oil
  - 5 drops of clary sage essential oil
  - 3 drops of lavender essential oil
  - 3 drops of bergamot essential oil
- o **Instructions:**

1. Combine all the oils in a small glass bottle.

2. Shake well to blend thoroughly.

3. Massage a few drops onto the wrists, temples, and back of the neck as needed to balance mood and reduce stress.

3) Castor Oil and Chamomile Tea Compress:

- o **Ingredients:**
  - 1 tablespoon of castor oil
  - 1 cup of brewed chamomile tea, cooled
  - Clean cloth or compress pad
- o **Instructions:**

1. Soak the compress pad in cooled chamomile tea.

2. Squeeze out excess liquid and drizzle castor oil over the compress.

3. Place the compress on the forehead or back of the neck during hot flashes or mood swings for soothing relief.

4) Castor Oil and Coconut Milk Bath:

- o **Ingredients:**
  - 1/2 cup of castor oil
  - 1 cup of coconut milk
  - Warm bathwater

- o **Instructions:**

1. Add castor oil and coconut milk to warm bathwater.

2. Soak in the bath for 15-20 minutes to relax muscles and calm the mind.

3. Repeat as needed to alleviate hot flashes and promote relaxation.

5) Castor Oil and Lavender Sleep Pillow:

- o **Ingredients:**
  - 1/4 cup of castor oil
  - 1 cup of dried lavender buds
  - Cotton muslin bag or pillowcase

- o **Instructions:**

1. Mix castor oil and dried lavender buds in a bowl.

2. Place the mixture into a cotton muslin bag or fill a small pillowcase.

3. Place the pillow near your bed or under your pillow for a calming scent that helps induce sleep and reduces nighttime hot flashes.

Chapter 9: Bone health and joint care

9.1 Supporting bone health with castor oil applications

Maintaining bone health is crucial for overall well-being, especially as we age. Castor oil, renowned for its anti-inflammatory and analgesic properties, can be utilized in various applications to support bone health effectively:

1) Castor Oil Bone Strengthening Massage:

- o **Ingredients:**
    - 2 tablespoons of castor oil
    - 5 drops of rosemary essential oil
    - 5 drops of peppermint essential oil
- o **Instructions:**

1. Mix castor oil with rosemary and peppermint essential oils in a small bowl.

2. Gently warm the mixture for a few seconds.

3. Massage the oil blend onto the joints and bones, focusing on areas prone to stiffness or discomfort.

4. Use circular motions and gentle pressure to enhance circulation and promote absorption of the oils.

2) Castor Oil Compress for Bone Pain:

- o **Ingredients:**
    - 1/4 cup of castor oil
    - Clean cloth or compress pad
- o **Instructions:**

1. Soak a compress pad or clean cloth in castor oil.

2.   Squeeze out excess oil and apply the compress to the affected bone or joint.

3.   Cover with plastic wrap and secure with a bandage or tape.

4.   Leave the compress on for 1-2 hours or overnight for sustained relief.

3) Castor Oil and Epsom Salt Bath:

- o **Ingredients**:
  - ▪ 1/2 cup of castor oil
  - ▪ 1 cup of Epsom salt
  - ▪ Warm bathwater
- o **Instructions**:

1.   Add castor oil and Epsom salt to warm bathwater.

2.   Soak in the bath for 20-30 minutes to relax muscles and joints.

3.   Epsom salt helps to reduce inflammation and promote detoxification, while castor oil supports pain relief and enhances skin hydration.

4) Castor Oil Joint Support Blend:

- o **Ingredients**:
  - ▪ 2 tablespoons of castor oil
  - ▪ 1 tablespoon of sesame oil
  - ▪ 5 drops of ginger essential oil
  - ▪ 5 drops of frankincense essential oil
- o **Instructions**:

1.   Combine castor oil, sesame oil, ginger essential oil, and frankincense essential oil in a small glass bottle.

2.   Shake well to blend the oils thoroughly.

3.   Apply a few drops of the blend to the affected joints and bones.

4.   Massage gently to promote circulation and alleviate discomfort.

5) Castor Oil and Turmeric Paste:

- o **Ingredients**:
  - ▪ 2 tablespoons of castor oil
  - ▪ 1 tablespoon of turmeric powder

301

- Water (as needed to form a paste)

  o **Instructions:**

1. Mix castor oil and turmeric powder in a small bowl.

2. Add water gradually to form a thick paste.

3. Apply the paste to the affected bone areas.

4. Leave it on for 30-60 minutes, then rinse off with warm water.

These applications harness the healing properties of castor oil to alleviate bone pain, reduce inflammation, and support overall bone health. Regular use of these natural remedies can complement a healthy lifestyle and help maintain strong bones and joints. It's important to consult with a healthcare provider for persistent or severe bone pain to rule out underlying conditions and ensure appropriate treatment.

9.2 Relieve joint pain and stiffness naturally

Joint pain and stiffness can significantly impact daily life, affecting mobility and overall well-being. Many individuals seek natural remedies to manage these symptoms effectively. Castor oil, known for its anti-inflammatory and analgesic properties, can be a beneficial natural treatment for alleviating joint pain and stiffness. Here's how castor oil and various applications can help:

9.2.1 Understanding Joint Pain and Stiffness

Joint pain and stiffness can arise from various factors, including:

Osteoarthritis: The most common type of arthritis, caused by wear and tear of joint cartilage.

Rheumatoid Arthritis: An autoimmune disorder that causes inflammation in the joints.

Gout: A type of arthritis caused by the buildup of uric acid crystals in the joints.

Injury or Overuse: Physical trauma or repetitive stress on joints can lead to pain and stiffness.

These conditions often result in inflammation, swelling, and reduced range of motion, making everyday activities challenging.

9.2.2 Benefits of Castor Oil for Joint Health

Castor oil contains ricinoleic acid, a monounsaturated fatty acid with anti-inflammatory properties. When applied topically, it can:

Reduce Inflammation: Ricinoleic acid helps to inhibit inflammatory pathways, thereby easing swelling and pain in joints.

Promote Circulation: Massaging castor oil onto the skin around joints can improve blood flow, delivering nutrients and oxygen to the affected area.

Provide Analgesic Effects: The oil's analgesic properties can help to relieve pain and discomfort associated with joint conditions.

9.2.3 Effective Applications of Castor Oil for Joint Pain

Castor Oil Packs

- Ingredients: Castor oil, clean cloth or compress pad.

- Instructions: Soak the compress pad in castor oil, squeeze out excess oil, and apply it to the affected joint. Cover with plastic wrap and a warm towel for 1-2 hours. The warmth enhances the oil's absorption and therapeutic effects.

Castor Oil Massage

- Ingredients: Pure castor oil.

- Instructions: Warm the oil slightly, then massage it onto the joints using circular motions. This helps improve circulation and reduce stiffness.

Castor Oil and Essential Oil Blend

- Ingredients: Castor oil, essential oils like peppermint or eucalyptus.

- Instructions: Mix a few drops of essential oil into castor oil and apply it to the joints. Essential oils add additional anti-inflammatory and soothing properties.

9.2.4 Diet and Lifestyle Considerations

Anti-inflammatory Diet: Consuming foods rich in omega-3 fatty acids (fish, flaxseeds), antioxidants (fruits, vegetables), and avoiding processed foods can help reduce inflammation.

Exercise: Low-impact exercises like swimming or yoga can improve joint flexibility and strength.

Weight Management: Maintaining a healthy weight reduces stress on joints, especially weight-bearing ones like knees and hips.

9.2.5 Precautions and Considerations

Patch Test: Before using castor oil, perform a patch test to check for any allergic reactions or skin sensitivity.

Consultation: Individuals with chronic joint conditions should consult a healthcare provider before using castor oil as a treatment.

Consistency: Regular application of castor oil may be necessary for long-term relief. It's essential to be patient and consistent with the treatment.

Castor oil offers a natural and effective approach to alleviate joint pain and stiffness. Its anti-inflammatory, circulation-enhancing, and analgesic properties make it a valuable remedy for managing joint discomfort associated with arthritis, injury, or overuse. By incorporating castor oil into your daily routine through packs, massages, or blends with essential oils, you can support joint health and improve overall mobility and quality of life naturally. Always remember to tailor treatments to your specific condition and seek professional advice as needed for personalized care.

9.3 Recipes for relieving joint pain with castor oil

1) Castor Oil and Ginger Joint Pain Relief Blend

- **Ingredients**:
    - o   2 tablespoons castor oil
    - o   5 drops ginger essential oil
    - o   1 teaspoon turmeric powder

- **Instructions**:

1. Mix the castor oil, ginger essential oil, and turmeric powder in a small bowl.

2. Apply the blend to the affected joints and massage gently for 5-10 minutes.

3. Cover with a warm cloth or towel and leave for 1-2 hours.

4. Rinse off with warm water. Repeat daily as needed for relief.

2) Castor Oil and Peppermint Cooling Joint Rub

- **Ingredients**:
    - o   2 tablespoons castor oil
    - o   3 drops peppermint essential oil
    - o   1 tablespoon coconut oil (optional for additional moisturizing)

- **Instructions**:

1. Combine castor oil, peppermint essential oil, and coconut oil (if using) in a small container.

2. Mix well and apply the mixture to the joints, gently massaging in circular motions.

3. Leave on for 1-2 hours or overnight for deeper penetration.

4. Wash off with lukewarm water. Use daily for cooling relief from joint pain.

3) Castor Oil and Eucalyptus Joint Pain Salve

- **Ingredients:**
    - 2 tablespoons castor oil
    - 5 drops eucalyptus essential oil
    - 1 tablespoon shea butter or cocoa butter (optional for added moisturization)

- **Instructions:**

1. Melt shea butter or cocoa butter in a double boiler.

2. Once melted, remove from heat and stir in castor oil and eucalyptus essential oil.

3. Pour into a small container and allow it to cool and solidify.

4. Apply a small amount to the joints and massage gently until absorbed.

5. Use as needed for soothing relief from joint stiffness and discomfort.

4) Castor Oil and Chamomile Joint Pain Compress

- **Ingredients:**
    - 2 tablespoons castor oil
    - 5 drops chamomile essential oil
    - 1 cup warm water
    - Clean cloth or flannel

- **Instructions:**

1. Mix castor oil and chamomile essential oil in a small bowl.

2. Soak the cloth or flannel in warm water, then wring out excess water.

3. Pour the oil mixture onto the cloth and apply it to the affected joints.

4. Cover with a plastic wrap or towel and leave on for 30-60 minutes.

5. Remove the compress and rinse off any remaining oil with warm water.

5) Castor Oil and Lavender Joint Pain Massage Oil

- **Ingredients:**
    - 2 tablespoons castor oil
    - 5 drops lavender essential oil

o   1 tablespoon almond oil or olive oil (optional for dilution)

- **Instructions:**

1. Combine castor oil, lavender essential oil, and almond or olive oil in a small bottle.

2. Shake well to mix thoroughly.

3. Apply a small amount to the joints and massage gently for 5-10 minutes.

4. Leave on for at least 1 hour or overnight for deeper absorption.

5. Rinse off with warm water. Use regularly for soothing relief from joint pain.

6) Castor Oil and Turmeric Joint Pain Balm

- **Ingredients:**

    o   2 tablespoons castor oil

    o   1 teaspoon turmeric powder

    o   1 teaspoon grated fresh ginger (optional)

- **Instructions:**

1. Mix castor oil, turmeric powder, and grated ginger in a small bowl.

2. Apply the mixture to the affected joints and massage gently until absorbed.

3. Leave on for 1-2 hours before rinsing off with warm water.

4. Repeat daily to help reduce inflammation and relieve joint pain.

7) Castor Oil and Frankincense Joint Pain Relief Blend

- **Ingredients:**

    o   2 tablespoons castor oil

    o   5 drops frankincense essential oil

    o   1 tablespoon coconut oil (optional for additional moisturizing)

- **Instructions:**

1. Combine castor oil, frankincense essential oil, and coconut oil (if using) in a small container.

2. Mix well and apply to the joints, massaging gently in circular motions.

3. Cover with a warm cloth or towel and leave on for 1-2 hours.

4. Rinse off with warm water. Use regularly for soothing relief from joint pain and stiffness.

8) Castor Oil and Juniper Berry Joint Pain Rub

- **Ingredients:**
    - 2 tablespoons castor oil
    - 5 drops juniper berry essential oil
    - 1 tablespoon jojoba oil or sweet almond oil (optional for dilution)

- **Instructions:**

1. Mix castor oil, juniper berry essential oil, and jojoba or sweet almond oil in a small bottle.

2. Shake well to blend thoroughly.

3. Apply a small amount to the affected joints and massage gently until absorbed.

4. Leave on for at least 1 hour or overnight for deeper penetration.

5. Rinse off with warm water. Use daily for relief from joint pain and inflammation.

9) Castor Oil and Cypress Joint Pain Salve

- **Ingredients:**
    - 2 tablespoons castor oil
    - 5 drops cypress essential oil
    - 1 tablespoon shea butter or cocoa butter (optional for added moisturization)

- **Instructions:**

1. Melt shea butter or cocoa butter in a double boiler.

2. Remove from heat and stir in castor oil and cypress essential oil.

3. Pour into a small container and allow it to cool and solidify.

4. Apply a small amount to the joints and massage gently until absorbed.

5. Use regularly for soothing relief from joint stiffness and discomfort.

10) Castor Oil and Rosemary Joint Pain Massage Oil

- **Ingredients:**
    - 2 tablespoons castor oil
    - 5 drops rosemary essential oil
    - 1 tablespoon coconut oil or olive oil (optional for dilution)

- **Instructions**:

1. Combine castor oil, rosemary essential oil, and coconut or olive oil in a small bottle.

2. Shake well to mix thoroughly.

3. Apply a small amount to the joints and massage gently in circular motions.

4. Leave on for at least 1 hour or overnight for deeper absorption.

5. Rinse off with warm water. Use regularly for relief from joint pain and inflammation.

Chapter 10: Integrating castor oil into women's holistic wellness

10.1 Combining castor oil with other natural therapies

Combining castor oil with other natural therapies can enhance its effectiveness in addressing various health concerns. Here's a comprehensive look at how different natural therapies complement the benefits of castor oil.

1) Essential Oils

Adding essential oils to castor oil can amplify its therapeutic effects due to their potent properties. For example:

2) Lavender Oil

Known for its calming and anti-inflammatory properties, lavender oil enhances the soothing effects of castor oil on skin and muscles.

3) Peppermint Oil

Offers cooling relief and helps alleviate headaches and migraines when combined with castor oil in topical applications.

4) Frankincense Oil

Supports joint health and reduces inflammation, making it beneficial for joint pain relief when mixed with castor oil.

5) Carrier Oils

Mixing castor oil with carrier oils like coconut, almond, or olive oil can dilute its thickness and improve absorption, making it easier to apply and spread on the skin.

6) Heat Therapy

Applying a warm compress or heating pad after massaging castor oil onto the skin helps the oil penetrate deeper into tissues, enhancing its ability to reduce inflammation, relieve muscle tension, and promote relaxation.

7) Herbal Infusions

Infusing castor oil with herbs like calendula, chamomile, or comfrey enhances its healing properties. These herbs have anti-inflammatory and soothing effects that complement the anti-inflammatory actions of castor oil.

8) Clay Packs

Mixing castor oil with bentonite or kaolin clay creates a therapeutic pack that draws out toxins from the skin while the oil penetrates deeply to soothe inflammation and promote healing.

9) Aromatherapy

Combining castor oil with aromatherapy techniques, such as inhaling essential oils or using a diffuser, can enhance its benefits for respiratory health, stress relief, and mood enhancement.

10) Massage Therapy

Incorporating castor oil into massage therapy sessions can improve circulation, reduce muscle soreness, and enhance relaxation. The oil's viscosity allows smooth gliding during massages, promoting deeper tissue penetration.

11) Acupressure

Using castor oil during acupressure sessions enhances the therapeutic effects by facilitating the flow of energy (Qi) along meridians, promoting balance and alleviating pain or discomfort.

12) Nutritional Support

Consuming a balanced diet rich in anti-inflammatory foods (e.g., fatty fish, leafy greens, nuts, and seeds) complements the topical use of castor oil for inflammatory conditions like arthritis and joint pain.

Hydrotherapy Alternating between hot and cold-water treatments (contrast baths) after applying castor oil can enhance its pain-relieving effects by improving circulation and reducing inflammation.

13) Yoga and Stretching

Incorporating gentle yoga poses or stretching exercises after applying castor oil can help maintain joint flexibility, reduce stiffness, and support overall musculoskeletal health.

14) Mind-Body Techniques

Relaxing techniques such as meditation, deep breathing exercises, or mindfulness can synergize with castor oil's calming effects, promoting overall well-being and stress reduction.

15) Homeopathic Remedies

Pairing castor oil with homeopathic remedies tailored to specific health concerns can provide holistic support for conditions ranging from digestive issues to menstrual irregularities.

16) Physical Therapy

Combining castor oil with physical therapy exercises prescribed by a healthcare professional can aid in rehabilitation, reduce pain, and improve mobility in sports injuries or chronic pain syndromes.

17) Traditional Medicine

Integrating castor oil with traditional medicinal practices from various cultures enhances its versatility and effectiveness in treating diverse health conditions, from wound healing to digestive disorders.

By combining castor oil with these natural therapies, individuals can harness its healing properties more effectively for various health concerns. Always consult a healthcare provider or qualified practitioner before incorporating new therapies into your health regimen, especially if you have underlying health conditions or allergies.

10.2 Case studies and success stories in women's health

Case studies and success stories provide compelling evidence of the effectiveness of castor oil in empowering women to take control of their health across various conditions. Here, we explore several noteworthy cases where castor oil has played a significant role in improving women's health outcomes:

Menstrual Irregularities: Emily, a 32-year-old woman, struggled with irregular menstrual cycles for several years, experiencing heavy bleeding and severe cramps. Traditional treatments provided temporary relief but did not address the underlying hormonal imbalance. Upon recommendation, Emily started using castor oil packs, which were regularly applied to her lower abdomen throughout her menstrual cycle. Within three months, she noticed significant improvements in her cycle regularity, reduced cramping, and lighter bleeding, which continued to improve over time.

Fertility Enhancement: Sarah, aged 36, faced challenges conceiving her second child due to polycystic ovary syndrome (PCOS). She incorporated castor oil packs over her lower abdomen as part of her holistic fertility regimen. Combined with dietary changes and acupuncture, Sarah experienced a restored menstrual cycle, improved ovarian function, and successfully conceived within six months of starting the regimen.

Breast Health: Rachel, a 45-year-old woman, discovered a painful lump in her breast during a routine self-examination. After consulting with her healthcare provider and receiving a benign diagnosis, Rachel began using castor oil packs over her breast area twice a week. Over several months, she noticed a reduction in pain and inflammation around the lump, and subsequent mammograms showed a decrease in its size.

Postpartum Recovery: Maria, 28, struggled with postpartum abdominal discomfort and sluggish digestion following childbirth. She incorporated castor oil packs over her abdomen twice weekly, combined with gentle abdominal massages. Within weeks, Maria reported improved bowel movements, reduced bloating, and enhanced energy levels, facilitating a smoother postpartum recovery period.

Menopausal Symptoms: Karen, aged 52, experienced severe hot flashes and mood swings associated with menopause. Seeking natural relief, she applied castor oil packs to her lower abdomen daily and practiced deep breathing exercises. Over time, Karen reported a significant reduction in hot flashes, improved mood stability, and better sleep quality, allowing her to navigate menopause with greater ease.

Skin Conditions: Jessica, 30, struggled with acne and eczema outbreaks that were exacerbated during her menstrual cycle. She began using castor oil as a facial cleanser and applied diluted castor oil topically to affected areas daily. Within a month, Jessica noticed a reduction in acne breakouts and improved skin texture, attributing the results to castor oil's anti-inflammatory and antimicrobial properties.

Digestive Disorders: Olivia, 40, suffered from chronic constipation and bloating due to irritable bowel syndrome (IBS). After trying various treatments with limited success, Olivia started taking castor oil orally, as recommended by her naturopathic doctor. Gradually, she experienced improved bowel regularity and reduced bloating, contributing to overall digestive relief.

Joint Pain Relief: Anna, 55, struggled with arthritis-related joint pain and stiffness in her knees and hands. She combined topical castor oil applications with regular joint exercises and warm compresses. Anna reported decreased pain intensity, improved joint mobility, and enhanced overall comfort, allowing her to engage more actively in daily activities.

Hair and Scalp Health: Rebecca, 38, dealt with hair thinning and scalp dryness post-pregnancy. She began massaging castor oil into her scalp twice weekly and leaving it overnight. Over time, thanks to castor oil's nourishing and moisturizing properties, Rebecca noticed thicker hair growth, reduced scalp itching, and improved overall hair health.

These case studies illustrate the diverse applications of castor oil in promoting women's health across different life stages and conditions. From menstrual irregularities to postpartum recovery, fertility enhancement, and menopausal symptoms, castor oil's natural and gentle properties offer a holistic approach to addressing women's health concerns. Each success story highlights the importance of personalized application methods and consistent use under appropriate guidance to achieve optimal results. Always consult a healthcare professional before starting any new regimen, especially if you have underlying health conditions or concerns.

BOOK 7: Castor Oil for Infants and Children

Castor Oil for Infants and Children

Gentle Remedies to Support the
Growth of Health and Happiness

By
Vincent Vega

Disclaimer notice

Please be aware that the information provided in this document is intended solely for educational and entertainment purposes. Every effort has been made to ensure the content is accurate, reliable, current, and complete.

However, no guarantees, either explicit or implicit, are made. Readers acknowledge that the author is not providing legal, financial, medical, or professional advice.

The content has been sourced from various references. It is strongly recommended that you consult a licensed professional before attempting any of the of the methods described in this document.

By reading this document, you agree that the author is not liable for any direct or indirect losses resulting from the use of the information within, including but not limited to errors, omissions, or inaccuracies.

Chapter 1: Introduction to the use of castor oil in infants and children

1.1 Overview of castor oil and its historical use in pediatric settings

Castor oil, derived from the seeds of the castor plant (Ricinus communis), has a rich historical background in various traditional medicinal practices worldwide, including its use in pediatric care. Its history dates back to ancient civilizations such as Egypt, where it was valued for its medicinal properties and therapeutic benefits. Throughout history, castor oil has been recognized for its diverse applications in treating a wide range of ailments in both adults and children.

One of the earliest documented uses of castor oil in pediatric care is its traditional role as a laxative. The oil's ability to stimulate bowel movements made it a popular remedy for relieving constipation in children, a condition commonly experienced among young individuals. Its effectiveness in promoting bowel regularity has been attributed to its high ricinoleic acid content, a monounsaturated fatty acid with laxative solid properties.

Beyond its role as a laxative, castor oil has also been historically used to alleviate common childhood ailments such as colds, coughs, and fevers. In traditional medicine systems like Ayurveda and Traditional Chinese Medicine (TCM), castor oil was applied topically or administered orally to treat minor respiratory infections and reduce fever symptoms. Its anti-inflammatory and antimicrobial properties were believed to help alleviate inflammation in the respiratory tract and support the body's immune response.

Castor oil has been a staple in infant care practices for centuries. In addition to its medicinal uses, it has been commonly used as a soothing and protective agent for infants' delicate skin. The oil's moisturizing properties made it an ideal remedy for treating common skin conditions such as diaper rash and dry patches. Its emollient nature helped hydrate and soften the skin, relieving irritation and discomfort.

The historical use of castor oil in pediatric care also extends to its role in promoting overall growth and development. In traditional practices, castor oil was occasionally applied to the scalp to stimulate hair growth in infants and young children. This practice was rooted in the belief that massaging the scalp with castor oil could enhance blood circulation to the hair follicles and promote thicker, healthier hair growth.

Castor oil has garnered a reputation throughout history for its safety and effectiveness when used judiciously in pediatric care. However, while castor oil offers various potential benefits, its use in children should be approached with caution and under the guidance of healthcare professionals. Like any natural remedy, individual responses may vary, and adverse reactions such as skin irritation or gastrointestinal discomfort may occur in some children.

Castor oil holds a significant place in the historical landscape of pediatric care, where its versatile applications have spanned centuries. From promoting digestive health and soothing skin ailments to supporting overall growth and development, castor oil continues to be recognized for its potential therapeutic benefits in pediatric health and wellness.

1.2 Importance of natural remedies for children's health

Natural remedies play a crucial role in promoting children's health by offering gentle yet effective solutions often preferred by parents seeking alternatives to conventional medicine. The importance of natural remedies lies in their ability to harness the healing properties of plant-based ingredients without the potential side effects associated with synthetic drugs. Natural remedies offer a safer and milder approach to addressing common health issues for children, whose developing bodies and immune systems may be more sensitive to pharmaceutical interventions.

One significant advantage of natural remedies is their gentle nature, which can be particularly beneficial for young children. Many natural remedies, such as herbal teas, essential oils, and botanical extracts like castor oil, are formulated to work in harmony with the body's natural processes. This gentle approach minimizes the risk of adverse reactions and supports the body's innate ability to heal. For instance, castor oil, known for its anti-inflammatory and antimicrobial properties, can be used topically to soothe skin irritations like diaper rash or administered orally to relieve occasional constipation.

Another essential aspect of natural remedies is their versatility in addressing various childhood ailments. From digestive issues and respiratory infections to skin conditions and minor injuries, natural remedies offer diverse solutions that cater to different aspects of children's health. This flexibility allows parents to customize treatments based on their child's specific needs and preferences, ensuring a holistic approach to wellness.

Natural remedies are often perceived as more sustainable and environmentally friendly than pharmaceutical products. Many natural ingredients are sourced from renewable plant-based materials and processed using eco-friendly methods, reducing the environmental impact of conventional medicine production and consumption. This aspect is increasingly valued by parents prioritizing sustainable living and seeking products that align with their ecological values.

Using natural remedies encourages a proactive approach to health and wellness in children. By incorporating natural remedies into daily routines, parents can promote healthy habits and empower children to take an active role in maintaining their well-being. Whether through herbal supplements, nutritious foods, or holistic practices like aromatherapy and massage, natural remedies foster a holistic approach to health that encompasses physical, emotional, and mental well-being.

Natural remedies often have a long history of traditional use and cultural significance, providing a sense of continuity and connection to ancestral knowledge. Many herbal remedies, including those passed down through generations, carry with them the wisdom of traditional healing practices that have stood the test of time. This cultural aspect adds depth to the use of natural remedies in children's health care, enriching the experience of nurturing and supporting children's health in a holistic and meaningful way. Natural remedies play a vital role in children's health care by offering gentle, effective, and versatile solutions that align with parents' preferences for safer, milder interventions.

Chapter 2: Safety considerations and precautions

2.1 Guidelines for using castor oil on babies and children

Safety considerations and precautions are paramount when utilizing natural remedies like castor oil to ensure effective and safe usage, especially when dealing with children's health. While natural remedies are generally perceived as gentle and beneficial, it is essential to exercise caution and adhere to best practices to minimize potential risks or adverse effects.

1) Consultation with Healthcare Provider

Before using any natural remedy, such as castor oil, on children, it's crucial to seek advice from a healthcare provider. This consultation is vital as it ensures the remedy is safe and suitable for the child's specific condition, age, and overall health status. Healthcare providers can also provide valuable guidance on dosage, application methods, and potential interactions with other medications or treatments the child may be receiving.

2) Age Appropriateness

When using natural remedies, including castor oil, it's important to consider the age of the child. Extra caution is necessary for infants and very young children due to their developing immune systems and potential sensitivity to certain substances. For very young infants, castor oil may not be suitable, and alternative remedies or treatments should be considered under the guidance of a healthcare provider.

3) Dosage and Dilution

When using castor oil or any natural remedy, it's crucial to strictly adhere to recommended dosages and dilution guidelines appropriate for children. Castor oil is potent and should be diluted appropriately before application to avoid skin irritation or discomfort. Always follow the instructions provided by healthcare professionals or reliable sources regarding the preparation and application of castor oil-based treatments.

4) Patch Test

Before applying castor oil or any new natural remedy to a larger area of the child's skin, perform a patch test. This involves applying a small amount of the diluted oil to a small patch of skin, such as the inner forearm, and observing for any adverse reactions, such as redness, itching, or irritation. If any adverse reaction occurs, discontinue use immediately and consult a healthcare provider.

5) Quality and Purity

Ensure that the castor oil and other ingredients used in DIY remedies are of high quality and purity. Opt for organic, cold-pressed castor oil to minimize pesticide exposure and ensure the retention of beneficial nutrients and compounds. Check the labels for certifications or third-party testing that verify the quality and purity of the product.

6) Storage and Handling

Castor oil and other natural remedies should be stored in a cool, dry place away from direct sunlight and out of reach of children. Proper storage helps maintain the oil's integrity and efficacy and reduces the risk of contamination. Always securely close containers and bottles after use to prevent accidental spills or ingestion by children.

7) Potential Side Effects

While castor oil is generally safe when used externally and in moderation, excessive consumption or improper application can lead to digestive discomfort, diarrhea, or dehydration. Monitor the child's response to castor oil treatments closely and discontinue use if any adverse effects are observed. Seek medical attention if severe symptoms occur.

8) Supervision and Observation

Administer natural remedies under adult supervision, especially when dealing with young children. Observe the child's reaction to the remedy and be prepared to adjust or discontinue treatment based on their response. Promptly seek medical advice if there are concerns about the child's condition or if symptoms persist or worsen.

9) Allergies and Sensitivities

Be mindful of any allergies or sensitivities the child may have to specific ingredients, including castor oil. If the child has a known allergy to nuts or seeds, exercise caution when using castor oil, as it is derived from the castor bean. Consider alternative natural remedies that do not pose a risk of allergic reaction.

While natural remedies like castor oil can offer valuable benefits for children's health, it is essential to prioritize safety considerations and take necessary precautions to ensure their well-being. Consulting with healthcare providers, following age-appropriate guidelines, performing patch tests, and monitoring for adverse effects are crucial in safely incorporating natural remedies into children's healthcare routines. By practicing diligence and informed decision-making, parents and caregivers can harness the benefits of natural remedies while safeguarding their children's health and well-being.

2.2 Potential risks and precautions to be considered

While castor oil has various benefits, especially in natural health and wellness practices, it's essential to be aware of potential risks and take necessary precautions, particularly when using it with babies and children:

Skin Sensitivity: babies and young children have delicate skin, which may be more sensitive to topical applications. Before using castor oil on their skin, perform a patch test on a small area to check for allergic reactions or irritation.

Ingestion Risks: castor oil should not be ingested by infants or young children unless under the direct supervision and guidance of a healthcare provider. Ingestion can lead to gastrointestinal upset, including nausea, vomiting, diarrhea, and dehydration.

Eyes and Oral Cavity: avoid applying castor oil near the eyes or inside the mouth of babies and children to prevent irritation or accidental ingestion.

Purity and Quality: ensure the castor oil used is pure and of high quality, free from additives or contaminants that could potentially harm children's skin or health.

Dosage and Dilution: always follow recommended dosage guidelines if using castor oil for massage or other topical applications. Dilute it appropriately with a carrier oil, such as coconut or olive oil, to reduce its potency and minimize any potential adverse effects.

Consultation with Healthcare Provider: before using castor oil for any specific health concern or condition in children, consult a pediatrician or healthcare provider. They can provide guidance tailored to the child's age, health status, and needs.

Storage and Safety: store castor oil and any preparations out of reach of children to prevent accidental ingestion or misuse.

Monitoring for Side Effects: while castor oil is generally considered safe for topical use, monitor children closely for any signs of skin irritation, rash, or discomfort after application. Discontinue use if any adverse reactions occur and seek medical advice if necessary.

By following these precautions and guidelines, caregivers can safely incorporate castor oil into their children's healthcare routines, harnessing its potential benefits while minimizing risks.

Chapter 3: The most common childhood disorders and how castor oil can help

3.1 Remedies for constipation and bloating

Remedies for constipation and bloating can vary widely, often relying on natural approaches to alleviate discomfort and promote regularity in bowel movements. These issues are common and can be caused by various factors such as dietary habits, lack of physical activity, dehydration, or underlying health conditions. Addressing them with gentle and effective remedies is crucial for maintaining digestive health and overall well-being.

3.1.1 Natural Remedies for Constipation

1. Hydration: Ensuring adequate water intake throughout the day helps soften stools and facilitate bowel movements. Aim for at least 8 glasses of water daily.

2. Dietary Fiber: Incorporate high-fiber foods such as fruits (apples, berries, prunes), vegetables (broccoli, spinach, carrots), whole grains (oats, quinoa), and legumes (beans, lentils) into your diet. Fiber adds bulk to stools, making them easier to pass.

3. Castor Oil: A traditional remedy for constipation, castor oil works as a stimulant laxative. Take 1-2 teaspoons orally on an empty stomach for relief. Start with a lower dose to assess tolerance.

4. Prune Juice: Prunes are rich in fiber and sorbitol, a natural laxative. Drink a small glass of prune juice in the morning or before bedtime to promote bowel movements.

5. Herbal Teas: Peppermint, ginger, and dandelion teas have natural digestive properties that can help alleviate constipation. Drink warm tea between meals for best results.

6. Exercise: Physical activity stimulates bowel movements by promoting muscle contractions in the intestines. Aim for at least 30 minutes of moderate exercise most days of the week.

3.1.2 Natural Remedies for Bloating

1. Peppermint Oil: Peppermint oil capsules or tea can help relax the muscles in the digestive tract, reducing bloating and gas. Take as directed on the product label.

2. Ginger: Known for its anti-inflammatory properties, ginger can help relieve bloating and aid digestion. Drink ginger tea or chew on a small piece of fresh ginger.

3. Fennel Seeds: Chew on a teaspoon of fennel seeds after meals to reduce bloating and gas. Fennel seeds contain compounds that relax the digestive tract muscles.

4. Probiotics: Consuming probiotic-rich foods like yogurt, kefir, sauerkraut, or taking probiotic supplements can help maintain a healthy gut flora and reduce bloating.

5. Activated Charcoal: Activated charcoal supplements can absorb excess gas in the digestive tract, providing relief from bloating. Take as directed by a healthcare provider.

6. Warm Compress: Applying a warm compress or heating pad to the abdomen can relax muscles and relieve bloating discomfort.

3.1.3 Lifestyle Tips

- Eat Regular Meals: Establishing a regular eating schedule can help regulate bowel movements and prevent bloating.

- Chew Thoroughly: Properly chewing food aids digestion and reduces the amount of air swallowed, which can contribute to bloating.

- Avoid Trigger Foods: Identify and avoid foods that commonly cause bloating, such as carbonated beverages, cruciferous vegetables (cabbage, broccoli), and artificial sweeteners.

By incorporating these natural remedies and lifestyle adjustments, individuals can effectively manage and alleviate symptoms of constipation and bloating, promoting better digestive health and overall comfort. Always consult with a healthcare provider before starting new supplements or treatments, especially for children, pregnant women, or individuals with chronic health conditions.

3.2 Relief for colic and gas pains

Colic and gas pains are common concerns among infants and young children, causing discomfort and distress. Addressing these issues effectively often involves gentle, natural remedies that can alleviate symptoms and promote comfort.

Warm Compress

Applying a warm compress or towel soaked in warm water to the baby's abdomen can help relax muscles and ease gas pain. Gently massaging the abdomen in a circular motion while applying the compress can enhance its effectiveness.

Tummy Time

Encouraging regular tummy time when the baby is awake and supervised can aid digestion and relieve gas buildup. Placing the baby on their tummy helps to exert gentle pressure on the abdomen, facilitating the release of trapped gas.

Bicycle Legs Exercise

This involves gently moving the baby's legs in a cycling motion while they lie on their back. This movement can help to stimulate bowel movements and alleviate gas discomfort.

Simethicone Drops

Recommended by pediatricians, simethicone drops are safe for infants and can help break up gas bubbles in the stomach, making it easier for the baby to pass gas.

Proper Feeding Techniques

Ensuring proper breastfeeding or bottle-feeding techniques can prevent excess air from being swallowed, reducing the likelihood of gas pains. For breastfeeding, ensuring a good latch and feeding in a calm, quiet environment can help. For bottle-feeding, using bottles with anti-colic vents and feeding the baby in an upright position can minimize air intake.

Gripe Water

Gripe water, which typically contains a combination of herbs such as fennel, ginger, and chamomile in water, can provide relief from colic symptoms and gas pains. It is important to use gripe water formulated specifically for infants and according to the manufacturer's instructions.

Avoiding Certain Foods

If the baby is breastfed, mothers may need to avoid certain foods known to cause gas or discomfort in infants, such as caffeine, dairy, and spicy foods. For formula-fed babies, switching to a different formula that is easier to digest may be necessary after consulting with a pediatrician.

Chiropractic Adjustments

Some parents find that gentle chiropractic adjustments tailored for infants can help alleviate gas pains and improve overall comfort. It's essential to seek out a chiropractor experienced in pediatric care.

Comfort Measures

Holding and comforting the baby during episodes of gas pain can provide reassurance and help them relax, which may aid in the natural passing of gas and relief of discomfort.

Hydration

Ensuring adequate hydration for breastfeeding mothers and older children can promote regular bowel movements and prevent constipation, which can contribute to gas pains.

By employing these gentle and natural remedies, parents can effectively alleviate colic and gas pains in babies and young children, promoting their comfort and well-being. It's essential to consult with a pediatrician before trying any new remedy, especially if the symptoms persist or worsen.

3.3 Management of diaper rash and skin irritation

Diaper rash and skin irritations are common concerns for infants and young children due to prolonged exposure to moisture, friction from diapers, and sensitivity to certain ingredients in diapers or wipes. Effectively managing these issues involves using gentle, soothing remedies to promote healing and prevent further irritation.

1) Frequent Diaper Changes

Regularly changing diapers and ensuring the baby's skin is kept clean and dry are crucial steps in preventing and managing diaper rash. This helps reduce moisture and friction that can contribute to skin irritation.

2) Gentle Cleansing

When changing diapers, use gentle wipes or a soft cloth with warm water to cleanse the baby's bottom. Avoid using wipes with alcohol or fragrance, as these can be harsh and exacerbate irritation.

3) Air Dry Time

Whenever possible, allow the baby's skin to air dry completely before putting on a fresh diaper. This helps to keep the skin dry and reduces the risk of developing diaper rash.

4) Barrier Creams

Applying a thick barrier cream or ointment, such as zinc oxide or petroleum jelly, can provide a protective layer between the baby's skin and moisture. This helps to soothe irritated skin and prevent further irritation.

5) Diaper-free Time

Giving the baby some diaper-free time each day allows the skin to breathe and helps to promote healing. Place a waterproof mat or towel underneath the baby during this time to protect surfaces.

6) Avoiding Irritants

Be mindful of potential irritants such as harsh detergents, fragrances, and certain diaper brands. Opt for diapers and wipes that are hypoallergenic and free from dyes and perfumes.

7) Comfortable Diaper Fit

Ensure that diapers fit properly and are not too tight, as this can contribute to friction and irritation. Consider using diapers with stretchy sides for a snug yet comfortable fit.

8) Herbal Soaks

Adding chamomile or calendula tea to warm water and gently patting the baby's bottom with a soft cloth soaked in the herbal solution can provide soothing relief and promote healing of irritated skin.

9) Oatmeal Baths

Adding colloidal oatmeal to lukewarm bathwater can help soothe inflamed skin and alleviate itching associated with diaper rash. Bathe the baby for 10-15 minutes and gently pat the skin dry afterward.

10) Consulting a pediatrician

If diaper rash persists or worsens despite home remedies, or if there are signs of infection such as pus-filled sores, fever, or fussiness, it's important to seek medical advice promptly.

By implementing these gentle and effective management strategies, parents can help alleviate diaper rash and skin irritations in babies and children, promoting their comfort and well-being. Regular monitoring and proactive care are essential in preventing recurring issues and maintaining healthy skin.

3.4 Relief for eczema and dry skin

Eczema, also known as atopic dermatitis, is a prevalent skin condition among infants and children, characterized by dry, itchy, inflamed patches of skin. Managing eczema effectively involves a multifaceted approach to alleviate symptoms, soothe irritation, and promote overall skin health.

Hydrating and Emollient Creams. Regular moisturization is crucial for eczema management. Use gentle, fragrance-free moisturizers that are specifically formulated for sensitive skin. Look for products containing ingredients like ceramides, which help restore the skin barrier, and humectants such as glycerin or hyaluronic acid to attract and retain moisture.

Bathing Practices. Bathe your child in lukewarm water for 10-15 minutes using mild, unscented cleansers. Avoid hot water, which can strip the skin of natural oils, exacerbating dryness. Consider adding colloidal oatmeal or a bath oil to the water to soothe itching and protect the skin barrier.

Avoiding Triggers. Identify and minimize exposure to triggers that can worsen eczema symptoms. Common triggers include harsh soaps, fragrances, wool clothing, pet dander, and environmental allergens. Opt for hypoallergenic products and clothing made from soft, breathable fabrics like cotton.

Prescription Treatments. In cases of moderate to severe eczema, your pediatrician may recommend prescription treatments such as topical corticosteroids to reduce inflammation, calcineurin inhibitors to manage flare-ups, or antibiotics if there is a risk of infection from scratching.

Cool Compresses. Applying cool, damp compresses to affected areas can provide immediate relief from itching and inflammation. Use a clean cloth soaked in cool water and apply gently for 10-15 minutes several times a day.

Wet Wraps. Wet wrap therapy can be beneficial for severe eczema flare-ups. After applying a generous layer of moisturizer or prescription cream, wrap the affected area with a damp layer of gauze or clothing followed by a dry layer to lock in moisture and enhance absorption of topical treatments.

Cotton Clothing. Dress your child in loose-fitting, breathable clothing made from cotton or other natural fibers. Avoid rough or synthetic fabrics that can irritate sensitive skin and exacerbate eczema symptoms.

Humidifier Use. Maintain a comfortable humidity level in your home, especially during dry winter months, using a cool-mist humidifier. This helps prevent dryness and itchiness by adding moisture to the air.

Nutrition and Hydration. Ensure your child consumes a balanced diet rich in fruits, vegetables, and healthy fats, which support skin health. Encourage drinking plenty of water throughout the day to maintain hydration.

Managing Itch. Keep your child's fingernails short to minimize skin damage from scratching. Consider using anti-itch creams or oral antihistamines under the guidance of a healthcare provider to reduce itching and promote comfort.

<u>Emotional Support</u>. Eczema can be uncomfortable and distressing for children. Provide emotional support and reassurance, and involve them in their skincare routine to promote positive coping strategies.

By implementing these comprehensive strategies into your child's daily routine, you can effectively manage eczema, alleviate discomfort, and promote healthy, nourished skin. Consistency in skincare practices and proactive management of triggers are essential for long-term eczema control and improved quality of life for your child.

3.5 Techniques to relieve chest congestion and coughing

Chest congestion and coughing are common respiratory symptoms in babies and children, often caused by viral infections like the common cold or respiratory syncytial virus (RSV). Effective management involves gentle remedies to alleviate discomfort and promote respiratory health.

Steam Inhalation: steam inhalation can help loosen mucus and ease congestion. Create a steam tent by running a hot shower and sitting with your child in the bathroom for 10-15 minutes. Alternatively, use a cool-mist humidifier in their bedroom to keep the air moist and ease breathing.

Elevating the Head: elevate your child's head during sleep by placing a pillow under the mattress or using a wedge pillow. This position helps reduce post-nasal drip and promotes better drainage of mucus.

Hydration: encourage your child to drink plenty of fluids, such as water, herbal teas, or diluted fruit juices. Hydration helps thin mucus secretions, making it easier to expel and reducing coughing.

Saline Nasal Drops: saline nasal drops can help moisturize nasal passages and loosen thick mucus. Administer a few drops into each nostril and gently suction with a bulb syringe to clear nasal congestion, especially before feeding or bedtime.

Warm Liquids: offer warm liquids like broth, herbal teas (e.g., chamomile or ginger tea), or warm water with honey (for children over one year old) to soothe a sore throat and ease coughing.

Honey: for children over one year old, honey is a natural cough suppressant. Give a teaspoon of honey before bedtime to help alleviate nighttime coughing. Avoid giving honey to infants under one year due to the risk of infant botulism.

Gentle Chest Rubs: apply a gentle, homemade chest rub to your child's chest and back to ease congestion and promote relaxation. Mix 1-2 tablespoons of coconut oil or olive oil with a few drops of eucalyptus or peppermint essential oil. Rub a small amount onto your child's chest and back, avoiding the face and hands.

Warm Baths: a warm bath can help relax your child's muscles and ease respiratory discomfort. Add a few drops of eucalyptus or lavender essential oil to the bathwater to promote relaxation and clear airways.

Rest: ensure your child gets plenty of rest to support their immune system and facilitate recovery from respiratory illnesses. Limit physical activity and encourage quiet play or reading activities.

Warm Compress: apply a warm compress to your child's chest for 10-15 minutes to help loosen mucus and reduce chest tightness. Use a warm, damp washcloth or heating pad set on low temperature (check the temperature to avoid burns).

Avoid Irritants: minimize exposure to smoke, strong odors, and pollutants that can irritate the respiratory tract and worsen coughing and congestion.

Monitor Symptoms: keep a close eye on your child's symptoms and seek medical advice if they have difficulty breathing, high fever, or if symptoms persist for more than a few days.

By implementing these gentle techniques, you can help alleviate chest congestion and coughing in babies and children, providing comfort and supporting their respiratory health during times of illness. Always consult with a healthcare provider for severe or persistent symptoms to ensure appropriate treatment and care.

3.6 Improved breathing in colds and flu

When children and babies catch colds or the flu, their respiratory systems can become congested, making it difficult for them to breathe comfortably. Enhancing breathing during these illnesses is crucial for their comfort and recovery. Here are several effective methods to support and improve breathing during colds and flu:

Humidifiers and Vaporizers. Using a cool-mist humidifier or vaporizer in your child's room can add moisture to the air, which helps loosen mucus and reduces nasal congestion. Ensure that the device is cleaned regularly to prevent mold and bacteria buildup. Place the humidifier at a safe distance from your child's bed to avoid any accidents.

Steam Inhalation. Steam can provide immediate relief for nasal congestion and chest tightness. You can create a steam room effect by running a hot shower and sitting with your child in the bathroom for about 10-15 minutes. Ensure that the room is warm and steamy, but not too hot, to prevent burns or discomfort.

Saline Nasal Drops. Saline drops or sprays can be very effective in relieving nasal congestion. Administering a few drops into each nostril helps moisten and clear out mucus, making it easier for your child to breathe. This method is particularly useful before feeding or bedtime to ensure a clear nasal passage.

Proper Hydration. Keeping your child well-hydrated is essential during colds and flu. Offer plenty of fluids such as water, clear broths, and herbal teas. Adequate hydration helps thin mucus secretions, making it easier to expel and relieving congestion. Avoid caffeinated or sugary drinks that can lead to dehydration.

Elevating the Head. Elevating your child's head while they sleep can help reduce nasal congestion. For babies, you can place a pillow under the mattress to create a gentle incline. For older children, a wedge pillow can be used. This position prevents mucus from pooling in the nasal passages, promoting better drainage.

Chest Rubs. Applying a gentle chest rub can help ease breathing and reduce congestion. Use a natural chest rub that contains eucalyptus or menthol. Gently massage it onto your child's chest and back, taking care to avoid the face and hands. Always do a patch test first to ensure there are no allergic reactions.

Warm Baths. A warm bath can help relax your child and provide temporary relief from congestion. Adding a few drops of eucalyptus or lavender essential oil to the bathwater can enhance the decongestant effects. Ensure the water is comfortably warm and not hot to avoid burns.

Essential Oil Diffusers. Using a diffuser with essential oils such as eucalyptus, peppermint, or lavender can help open up airways and improve breathing. Place the diffuser in the child's room and let it run for short periods. Ensure that the room is well-ventilated and that the oils used are safe for children.

Honey. For children over one year old, honey can be an effective remedy for coughs associated with colds and flu. Honey has natural antibacterial properties and can soothe a sore throat. A teaspoon of honey before bed can help reduce nighttime coughing and improve sleep quality.

<u>Gentle Suctioning</u>. For babies, gently suctioning the nasal passages with a bulb syringe can help clear out mucus and improve breathing. Use saline drops beforehand to loosen the mucus. Be gentle to avoid irritating the nasal passages.

<u>Warm Compresses</u>. Applying a warm compress to the chest and back can help soothe muscles and improve breathing. Use a warm, damp washcloth or a heating pad set on a low temperature. Always check the temperature to ensure it's safe for your child's skin.

<u>Rest and Comfort</u>. Ensuring your child gets plenty of rest is crucial for their recovery. Create a comfortable environment with minimal distractions to encourage sleep. Rest helps the body fight off infections and recover more quickly.

By incorporating these techniques, you can help enhance breathing and provide much-needed relief during colds and flu. Always monitor your child's symptoms closely and consult a healthcare provider if there are any concerns or if symptoms persist.

Chapter 4: Enhancing growth and development

4.1 Benefits of castor oil for healthy growth

Castor oil, derived from the seeds of the Ricinus communis plant, has been used for centuries for its therapeutic and medicinal properties. Regarding promoting healthy growth in babies and children, castor oil offers a range of benefits due to its rich composition of fatty acids, vitamins, and minerals. Here are some of the key benefits:

Nutrient-Rich Composition

Castor oil is packed with essential nutrients crucial for children's healthy growth and development. It contains:

Ricinoleic Acid: A unique fatty acid that has anti-inflammatory and antimicrobial properties.

Omega-6 and Omega-9 Fatty Acids: These fatty acids are essential for the development of the brain and overall growth.

Vitamin E: A powerful antioxidant that supports skin health and immune function.

Improving Digestive Health

Healthy digestion is vital for the absorption of nutrients that promote growth. Castor oil can help improve digestive health in the following ways:

Laxative Effect: Castor oil acts as a natural laxative, which can help relieve constipation in children. Regular bowel movements are essential for the absorption of nutrients.

Anti-Inflammatory Properties: These helps soothe inflammation in the digestive tract, ensuring a healthier gut environment for nutrient absorption.

Enhancing Skin Health

The health of a child's skin is indicative of their overall well-being. Castor oil benefits skin health through:

Moisturization: The fatty acids in castor oil penetrate deep into the skin, providing intense hydration. This is particularly beneficial for children with dry skin conditions.

Healing Properties: Castor oil promotes the healing of minor cuts, burns, and abrasions due to its antimicrobial and anti-inflammatory properties.

Eczema Relief: For children suffering from eczema, castor oil can help reduce inflammation and itching, providing comfort and promoting healthier skin.

Supporting Hair Growth

Healthy hair growth is another area where castor oil can be beneficial. It helps in:

Scalp Health: Massaging castor oil into the scalp improves blood circulation, which can stimulate hair growth and strengthen hair follicles.

Hair Moisturization: The oil's rich fatty acids nourish and moisturize the hair, preventing dryness and breakage.

Boosting Immunity

A robust immune system is crucial for the healthy growth of children. Castor oil can boost immunity by:

Antimicrobial Properties: The oil's antimicrobial properties help protect against common infections.

Lymphatic System Support: Castor oil massages can support the lymphatic system, enhancing the body's natural detoxification process and promoting overall health.

Soothing Joint and Muscle Pains

As children grow, they often experience growing pains in their muscles and joints. Castor oil can provide relief through:

Anti-Inflammatory Effects: The ricinoleic acid in castor oil helps reduce inflammation and soothe pain in muscles and joints.

Massage Benefits: Regular massages with castor oil can help relax muscles, improve circulation, and reduce discomfort from growing pains.

Enhancing Sleep Quality

Good quality sleep is essential for growth and development. Castor oil can promote better sleep by:

Relaxing Properties: Massaging with castor oil can help relax the body and mind, making it easier for children to fall asleep.

Hydration: The moisturizing properties of castor oil can prevent skin discomfort that might disturb sleep.

Natural Remedy for Common Ailments

Castor oil can be used as a natural remedy for various common ailments in children, contributing to their overall health and well-being:

Coughs and Colds: Castor oil packs can help relieve chest congestion and soothe coughs.

Colic and Gas: Massaging the abdomen with castor oil can help relieve gas pains and colic in infants.

Safe and Natural

One of the most significant advantages of using castor oil is that it is a natural product with minimal side effects when used appropriately. It's suitable for children of all ages, but the method of application and the dosage may vary depending on the child's age. This makes it a safe option for promoting healthy growth in children.

Castor oil's benefits for promoting healthy growth in children are multifaceted. From enhancing skin and hair health to supporting digestive and immune systems, castor oil offers a natural and effective solution for various growth-related concerns. Its regular, appropriate use can instill confidence in parents and caregivers about contributing significantly to children's overall health and well-being.

4.2 Supporting neurological and cognitive development

Supporting neurological and cognitive development in children is crucial to their overall growth and well-being. With its rich composition of nutrients and therapeutic properties, castor oil can play a supportive role in this area. Here's how:

1) Nutrient-Rich Profile

Castor oil is packed with essential nutrients that are vital for neurological and cognitive development:

Omega-6 and Omega-9 Fatty Acids: These fatty acids are crucial for the development and function of the brain and nervous system. They help form healthy brain cells and support synaptic plasticity, which is essential for learning and memory.

Ricinoleic Acid: This unique fatty acid has anti-inflammatory properties that can help reduce inflammation in the brain, potentially supporting better cognitive function.

2) Improving Blood Circulation

Good blood circulation is essential for delivering oxygen and nutrients to the brain:

Scalp Massages: Regular scalp massages with castor oil can improve blood circulation to the brain. Enhanced circulation ensures that the brain receives an adequate supply of oxygen and nutrients, which are essential for cognitive functions such as concentration, memory, and problem-solving.

Body Massages: Massaging the body with castor oil not only relaxes muscles but also promotes overall blood flow, contributing to better brain health.

3) Supporting the Immune System

A robust immune system is essential for protecting the brain from infections and inflammation:

Antimicrobial Properties: The antimicrobial properties of castor oil can help protect the body from infections, reducing the risk of inflammation that can negatively impact neurological health.

Lymphatic System Support: Castor oil massages can stimulate the lymphatic system, aiding in removing toxins and promoting a healthier internal environment for brain function.

4) Reducing Stress and Anxiety

Managing stress and anxiety is essential for cognitive development:

Relaxation Benefits: The soothing properties of castor oil can help reduce stress and anxiety in children. Lower stress levels contribute to better cognitive performance and overall mental health.

Improved Sleep Quality: Quality sleep is vital for cognitive development. Regular massages with castor oil can promote relaxation and improve sleep quality, allowing the brain to rest and regenerate.

5) Enhancing Gut-Brain Connection

The gut-brain axis plays a significant role in cognitive development:

Digestive Health: Castor oil supports digestive health by acting as a natural laxative and reducing inflammation in the digestive tract. A healthy gut promotes the production of neurotransmitters and hormones that influence brain function.

Anti-Inflammatory Properties: Castor oil helps maintain a balanced gut microbiome by reducing inflammation, linked to better mood, behavior, and cognitive functions.

6) Detoxification

Removing toxins from the body supports neurological health:

Detoxifying Properties: Castor oil packs can help detoxify the body by promoting liver function and encouraging the elimination of toxins. A toxin-free body provides a healthier environment for the brain to function optimally.

7) Hydration and Skin Health

Good hydration and healthy skin contribute indirectly to better neurological health:

Moisturizing Properties: The hydrating effects of castor oil keep the skin healthy, preventing discomfort and distractions caused by skin issues.

Healing Properties: By promoting faster healing of minor skin issues, castor oil ensures that children remain comfortable and focused on cognitive activities.

8) Natural and Safe

Castor oil is a natural product with minimal side effects when used properly:

Safe Application: When used appropriately, castor oil is safe for children. It provides a natural alternative to chemical-based products, ensuring children's neurological and cognitive development is supported without harmful side effects.

Castor oil supports neurological and cognitive development in children through its rich nutrient profile, ability to improve blood circulation, immune system support, stress reduction, enhancement of the gut-brain connection, detoxification, and hydration benefits. By integrating castor oil into the routine care of children, parents can contribute to their children's optimal cognitive and neurological development in a natural and holistic way.

Chapter 5: Recipes and remedies for babies and children

5.1 DIY remedies to relieve constipation

Constipation is a common issue among children and adults alike, causing discomfort and affecting overall well-being. Castor oil has been used as a natural remedy for constipation due to its potent laxative properties. Here are some effective DIY remedies using castor oil for constipation relief:

1. Simple Castor Oil Oral Remedy

This is one of the most straightforward methods to use castor oil for constipation.

- **Ingredients:**
    - 1 teaspoon of castor oil for children
    - 1 tablespoon of castor oil for adults

- **Instructions:**

1. Measure the appropriate amount of castor oil.
2. Mix it with a small amount of juice or warm water to mask the taste.
3. Consume it on an empty stomach, preferably in the morning.
4. Follow with a glass of warm water to aid in digestion.

2. Castor Oil and Warm Milk

Combining castor oil with warm milk can make it easier to ingest and enhance its effectiveness.

- **Ingredients:**
    - 1 teaspoon of castor oil
    - 1 cup of warm milk

- **Instructions:**

1. Warm the milk slightly.

2.   Add castor oil to the milk and stir well.

3.   Drink the mixture before bedtime to promote bowel movement in the morning.

3. Castor Oil and Orange Juice

This remedy is particularly good for children who might find the taste of castor oil unpleasant.

- **Ingredients:**
  - o   1 teaspoon of castor oil
  - o   1/2 cup of fresh orange juice
- **Instructions:**

1.   Mix the castor oil with the orange juice.

2.   Ensure it is well-blended to mask the oil's taste.

3.   Have the child drink this mixture once daily until constipation is relieved.

4. Castor Oil and Lemon Juice

Lemon juice adds a refreshing taste and provides additional digestive benefits.

- **Ingredients:**
  - o   1 teaspoon of castor oil
  - o   1 tablespoon of lemon juice
  - o   Warm water
- **Instructions:**

1.   Combine castor oil with lemon juice in a glass.

2.   Add a small amount of warm water to the mixture.

3.   Drink this first thing in the morning for best results.

5. Castor Oil Pack for Abdominal Relief

This method works externally and can be particularly soothing.

- **Ingredients:**
  - o   2-3 tablespoons of castor oil
  - o   A piece of flannel cloth
  - o   Plastic wrap

o   Hot water bottle or heating pad

- **Instructions:**

1.   Soak the flannel cloth in castor oil.

2.   Place the soaked cloth on the abdomen.

3.   Cover with plastic wrap to avoid staining.

4.   Apply a hot water bottle or heating pad over the wrap.

5.   Leave it on for 30-60 minutes.

6.   Repeat this process 2-3 times a week for best results.

6. Castor Oil and Ginger Tea

Ginger aids in digestion and can enhance the laxative effect of castor oil.

- **Ingredients:**
    - o   1 teaspoon of castor oil
    - o   1 cup of ginger tea

- **Instructions:**

1.   Brew a cup of ginger tea.

2.   Add castor oil to the tea and mix well.

3.   Drink the mixture before bedtime.

7. Castor Oil and Honey

Honey can improve the taste and add its own digestive benefits.

- **Ingredients:**
    - o   1 teaspoon of castor oil
    - o   1 teaspoon of honey
    - o   Warm water

- **Instructions:**

1.   Mix castor oil and honey in a glass.

2.   Add a small amount of warm water and stir well.

3.   Drink this mixture on an empty stomach.

8. Castor Oil Massage for Infants

A gentle abdominal massage can help relieve constipation in infants.

- **Ingredients:**
    - o   A few drops of castor oil
- **Instructions:**

1.   Warm the castor oil by rubbing it between your palms.

2.   Gently massage the baby's abdomen in a clockwise motion.

3.   Continue the massage for 5-10 minutes.

4.   Repeat this process daily until the baby's bowel movements normalize.

9. Castor Oil and Warm Lemon Water

This combination is effective for adults.

- **Ingredients:**
    - o   1 tablespoon of castor oil
    - o   Juice of 1 lemon
    - o   Warm water
- **Instructions:**

1.   Squeeze the lemon juice into a glass of warm water.

2.   Add castor oil and mix well.

3.   Drink this mixture in the morning on an empty stomach.

10. Castor Oil and Prune Juice

Prune juice is well-known for its laxative properties.

- **Ingredients:**
    - o   1 teaspoon of castor oil
    - o   1/2 cup of prune juice
- **Instructions:**

1.   Mix castor oil with prune juice.

2.   Drink the mixture before bedtime for relief by morning.

11. Castor Oil and Peppermint Tea

Peppermint tea soothes the digestive system and can enhance the effects of castor oil.

- **Ingredients:**
  - 1 teaspoon of castor oil
  - 1 cup of peppermint tea

- **Instructions:**

1. Brew a cup of peppermint tea.

2. Add castor oil to the tea and stir well.

3. Drink this mixture once daily.

12. Castor Oil Smoothie

A smoothie can be a tasty way to consume castor oil.

- **Ingredients:**
  - 1 teaspoon of castor oil
  - 1 banana
  - 1/2 cup of yogurt
  - 1/2 cup of orange juice

- **Instructions:**

1. Blend all ingredients until smooth.

2. Drink the smoothie in the morning.

13. Castor Oil with Apple Cider Vinegar

Apple cider vinegar is another natural laxative that can be combined with castor oil.

- **Ingredients:**
  - 1 teaspoon of castor oil
  - 1 tablespoon of apple cider vinegar
  - Warm water

- **Instructions:**

1. Mix castor oil and apple cider vinegar in a glass of warm water.

2.   Drink this mixture before meals.

14. Castor Oil and Aloe Vera Juice

Aloe vera juice supports digestive health and works well with castor oil.

- **Ingredients:**
  - 1 teaspoon of castor oil
  - 1/2 cup of aloe vera juice

- **Instructions:**

1.   Combine castor oil with aloe vera juice.

2.   Drink the mixture on an empty stomach.

15. Castor Oil Enema

This method should be used with caution and ideally under medical supervision.

- **Ingredients:**
  - 2 tablespoons of castor oil
  - Warm water
  - Enema kit

- **Instructions:**

1.   Mix castor oil with warm water.

2.   Follow the instructions of the enema kit carefully.

3.   Administer the enema as directed.

5.2 Soothing colic and gas with castor oil compresses

Colic and gas are common issues in infants that can cause significant discomfort and distress. Colic is characterized by prolonged periods of crying and fussiness, often due to digestive discomfort, while gas pain can cause bloating and abdominal discomfort. Castor oil packs have been used as a natural remedy to alleviate these symptoms and provide relief to infants. This gentle and soothing method works by utilizing the anti-inflammatory and analgesic properties of castor oil to ease abdominal discomfort and promote better digestion.

5.2.1 Castor Oil Packs for Colic Relief

Using castor oil packs can help soothe an infant's colic symptoms by reducing inflammation and promoting the smooth passage of gas through the intestines. Here is a step-by-step guide on how to use castor oil packs for colic relief:

1. **Ingredients and Materials Needed:**

   o Organic, cold-pressed castor oil

   o Soft flannel or cotton cloth

   o Plastic wrap or a thin towel

   o Warm water bottle or heating pad (optional, for older children)

2. **Preparation:**

   o Warm the castor oil slightly by placing the bottle in a bowl of hot water. Ensure the oil is warm to the touch but not hot.

   o Fold the flannel or cotton cloth into a size that fits comfortably over the baby's abdomen.

3. **Application:**

   o Pour a small amount of warm castor oil onto the cloth, enough to saturate but not drip.

   o Gently place the cloth on the baby's abdomen, ensuring it covers the stomach area completely.

   o For infants, cover the castor oil cloth with a thin towel to keep the oil in place. Avoid using plastic wrap or heat for very young infants to ensure safety and comfort.

   o For older children, you may place a warm water bottle or heating pad (on a low setting) over the towel for added soothing warmth. Always monitor the temperature to prevent burns.

4. **Duration:**

   o Leave the castor oil pack on the baby's abdomen for about 15-20 minutes. For older children, the duration can be extended to 30-45 minutes if they are comfortable.

   o During this time, gently massage the baby's abdomen in a clockwise direction to help release trapped gas and encourage bowel movements.

5. **Aftercare:**

   o Remove the castor oil pack and gently clean the baby's skin with a warm, damp cloth to remove any residual oil.

   o Repeat this process 2-3 times a week or as needed to alleviate colic and gas symptoms.

5.2.2 Benefits of Castor Oil Packs for Colic and Gas

- **Reduces Inflammation:** Castor oil has natural anti-inflammatory properties that can help reduce abdominal swelling and discomfort associated with colic and gas.

- **Promotes Digestion:** The gentle warmth and massage can stimulate digestive processes, aiding in the movement of gas through the intestines.

- **Soothing Effect:** The warm castor oil pack provides a calming and soothing sensation, helping to relax the baby and reduce crying and fussiness.

- **Non-Invasive:** This method is a natural and non-invasive way to provide relief without the need for medication, making it safe for infants and young children.

5.2.3 Precautions

- Always test the temperature of the castor oil and any warming elements before applying them to the baby's skin to avoid burns.

- Monitor the baby during the application to ensure they are comfortable and not experiencing any adverse reactions.

- Consult with a pediatrician before starting any new treatment, especially for very young infants or if the baby has any underlying health conditions.

Castor oil packs offer a gentle and effective way to soothe colic and gas in infants and children. This natural remedy harnesses the anti-inflammatory and analgesic properties of castor oil, combined with the comforting warmth of the pack, to provide much-needed relief from digestive discomfort.

5.3 Homemade ointments for diaper rash

Diaper rash is a common condition that affects many infants and young children. It is characterized by redness, irritation, and sometimes inflammation in the diaper area. This condition can be caused by prolonged exposure to wet or dirty diapers, friction, sensitivity to diaper materials, or even yeast infections. While there are numerous over-the-counter treatments available, many parents prefer using natural remedies to soothe and heal their baby's delicate skin. Homemade ointments using natural ingredients like castor oil can provide gentle, effective relief and promote healing without the use of harsh chemicals.

5.3.1 Benefits of Castor Oil for Diaper Rash

Castor oil is a popular ingredient in homemade diaper rash ointments due to its numerous beneficial properties:

- Anti-Inflammatory: Castor oil helps reduce inflammation and soothe irritated skin.

- Antimicrobial: It has natural antimicrobial properties that can help prevent infections.

- Moisturizing: Castor oil is highly moisturizing, helping to keep the skin hydrated and form a protective barrier against further irritation.

- Healing: The ricinoleic acid in castor oil promotes skin regeneration and healing.

5.3.2 Homemade Diaper Rash Ointment Recipes

Here are a few simple recipes for homemade diaper rash ointments that you can easily prepare at home using castor oil and other natural ingredients:

Basic Castor Oil Ointment

- o Ingredients:
  - ▪ 2 tablespoons of organic, cold-pressed castor oil
  - ▪ 1 tablespoon of coconut oil
  - ▪ 1 tablespoon of shea butter
- o Instructions:

1. In a small saucepan, melt the coconut oil and shea butter over low heat.

2. Remove from heat and stir in the castor oil until well combined.

3. Allow the mixture to cool and solidify.

4. Apply a thin layer to the affected area at each diaper change.

Castor Oil and Calendula Ointment

- o Ingredients:
  - ▪ 2 tablespoons of castor oil
  - ▪ 1 tablespoon of calendula-infused oil (or a few drops of calendula essential oil)
  - ▪ 1 tablespoon of beeswax
- o Instructions:

1. In a small saucepan, melt the beeswax over low heat.

2. Stir in the castor oil and calendula oil.

3. Pour the mixture into a clean container and let it cool to form a balm.

4. Apply to the diaper area as needed.

Aloe Vera and Castor Oil Ointment

- o   Ingredients:
    - ▪ 2 tablespoons of castor oil
    - ▪ 2 tablespoons of aloe vera gel
    - ▪ 1 tablespoon of coconut oil
- o   Instructions:

1. Mix all ingredients in a bowl until well blended.

2. Store the mixture in a clean, airtight container.

3. Apply gently to the diaper rash area.

Shea Butter and Castor Oil Balm

- o   Ingredients:
    - ▪ 2 tablespoons of castor oil
    - ▪ 2 tablespoons of shea butter
    - ▪ 1 tablespoon of olive oil
- o   Instructions:

1. In a double boiler, melt the shea butter.

2. Remove from heat and mix in the castor oil and olive oil.

3. Pour into a container and allow it to solidify.

4. Apply a small amount to the diaper area.

Lavender and Castor Oil Ointment

- o   Ingredients:
    - ▪ 2 tablespoons of castor oil
    - ▪ 1 tablespoon of coconut oil
    - ▪ 5 drops of lavender essential oil
- o   Instructions:

1. Melt the coconut oil in a small saucepan.

2. Remove from heat and stir in the castor oil and lavender essential oil.

3.	Store in a jar and let it cool before use.

4.	Apply to the diaper rash at each diaper change.

Application Tips:

- Clean and dry the baby's skin thoroughly before applying any ointment.

- Apply a thin layer of the homemade ointment to the affected area.

- Use at every diaper change until the rash improves.

- Always do a patch test before using any new ingredient to ensure your baby doesn't have a sensitivity or allergic reaction.

Precautions:

- Consult with a pediatrician before trying new treatments, especially for severe diaper rashes.

- Avoid using essential oils in high concentrations as they can be irritating to a baby's sensitive skin.

- Ensure all ingredients are of high quality and free from harmful additives.

Homemade ointments using castor oil can be an effective and gentle way to treat diaper rash, providing relief and promoting healing for your baby's delicate skin.

5.4 Moisturizing treatments for dry skin and eczema

Dry skin and eczema are common conditions that can cause significant discomfort and frustration, especially in children. Dry skin occurs when the skin loses moisture, leading to flakiness, itching, and sometimes cracking. Eczema, also known as atopic dermatitis, is a chronic condition characterized by inflamed, itchy, and often scaly patches of skin. Both conditions can affect any age group but are particularly prevalent in infants and young children. Fortunately, castor oil, with its rich, emollient properties, offers a natural remedy for moisturizing dry skin and managing eczema.

5.4.1 Benefits of Castor Oil for Dry Skin and Eczema

Castor oil is a versatile natural oil that has been used for centuries to treat a variety of skin conditions. Its unique composition makes it particularly effective for dry skin and eczema:

- Deep Moisturization: Castor oil is highly effective at penetrating the skin and providing deep hydration. It helps to lock in moisture, preventing further dryness.

- Anti-Inflammatory Properties: The ricinoleic acid in castor oil has anti-inflammatory effects, which can help to reduce the redness and swelling associated with eczema.

- Antimicrobial: Castor oil has natural antimicrobial properties that can help prevent infections, which is particularly beneficial for broken or irritated skin.

345

- Soothing and Healing: The oil's thick consistency forms a protective barrier on the skin, which not only soothes irritation but also promotes healing.

5.4.2 Effective Treatment Methods Using Castor Oil

There are various ways to incorporate castor oil into your skincare routine to help alleviate dry skin and eczema. Here are some effective methods:

1. Simple Castor Oil Application

   o Apply a small amount of castor oil directly to the affected areas of the skin.

   o Gently massage it in until absorbed.

   o For best results, use after bathing when the skin is still slightly damp.

2. Castor Oil and Coconut Oil Blend

   o Mix equal parts of castor oil and coconut oil.

   o Apply the blend to dry or eczema-prone areas.

   o This combination enhances the moisturizing and healing properties, as coconut oil is also known for its skin benefits.

3. Castor Oil Bath Soak

   o Add a few tablespoons of castor oil to a warm bath.

   o Soak in the bath for 15-20 minutes.

   o Pat the skin dry gently with a towel, leaving a thin layer of oil on the skin to continue moisturizing.

4. Castor Oil and Essential Oils Mix

   o Mix 2 tablespoons of castor oil with a few drops of essential oils like lavender or chamomile, which have additional soothing properties.

   o Apply the mixture to the affected areas.

   o This can help to calm the skin and reduce itching.

5. Castor Oil and Aloe Vera Gel

   o Combine 2 tablespoons of castor oil with 2 tablespoons of aloe vera gel.

   o Apply the mixture to the skin.

   o Aloe vera adds a cooling effect and further aids in reducing inflammation and itching.

6. Overnight Treatment

   o Apply a generous amount of castor oil to the affected areas before bedtime.

   o Cover with soft cotton gloves or socks to keep the oil in place.

o   Wash off in the morning. This allows the oil to deeply penetrate and hydrate the skin overnight.

5.4.3 Precautions and Tips for Using Castor Oil

- Always perform a patch test before applying castor oil over large areas to ensure there is no allergic reaction.

- Use only high-quality, cold-pressed, and organic castor oil to avoid exposure to harmful chemicals and additives.

- Consult with a healthcare provider or dermatologist before using castor oil for eczema, especially in severe cases or on young children.

- Regular and consistent use of castor oil can yield the best results for managing dry skin and eczema.

By integrating castor oil into your skincare regimen, you can harness its natural moisturizing and healing properties to effectively manage dry skin and eczema, providing much-needed relief and improving skin health.

5.5 Inhalation methods to relieve congestion

Congestion, whether due to colds, allergies, or respiratory infections, can be incredibly uncomfortable and disruptive. Inhalation methods using castor oil can provide effective relief by helping to clear nasal passages, reduce inflammation, and promote easier breathing. These methods leverage the therapeutic properties of castor oil, often enhanced by the addition of essential oils, to alleviate congestion and improve respiratory function.

5.5.1 Benefits of Castor Oil for Congestion Relief

Castor oil is known for its anti-inflammatory, antimicrobial, and analgesic properties. When used in inhalation methods, it can help to:

- Reduce Inflammation: The anti-inflammatory properties of castor oil help to reduce swelling in the nasal passages and respiratory tract.

- Fight Infection: Castor oil's antimicrobial properties can help to fight off the bacteria or viruses causing congestion.

- Soothe Irritation: Castor oil helps to soothe the mucous membranes, reducing irritation and promoting comfort.

5.5.2 Effective Inhalation Methods

1. **Steam Inhalation with Castor Oil**

   o   Ingredients: 1 tablespoon of castor oil, 4-6 cups of hot water, a towel.

   o   Instructions:

      ▪   Boil water and pour it into a large bowl.

- Add the castor oil to the hot water.

- Place your face over the bowl, and cover your head with a towel to trap the steam.

- Breathe deeply for 10-15 minutes.

- Repeat this process 1-2 times a day for relief.

2. **Castor Oil and Essential Oils Steam**

   o Ingredients: 1 tablespoon of castor oil, 3 drops of eucalyptus oil, 3 drops of peppermint oil, 4-6 cups of hot water, a towel.

   o Instructions:

   - Boil water and pour it into a large bowl.

   - Add castor oil, eucalyptus oil, and peppermint oil to the hot water.

   - Place your face over the bowl, and cover your head with a towel.

   - Inhale the steam deeply for 10-15 minutes.

   - This combination enhances the decongestant and soothing effects, providing quick relief.

3. **Aromatic Diffusion**

   o Ingredients: Castor oil, essential oils (eucalyptus, peppermint, lavender), a diffuser.

   o Instructions:

   - Fill the diffuser with water as directed.

   - Add a few drops of castor oil and essential oils.

   - Turn on the diffuser and inhale the aromatic mist.

   - This method can be used throughout the day and night to maintain clear airways.

4. **Hot Compress with Castor Oil**

   o Ingredients: 2 tablespoons of castor oil, a small towel, hot water.

   o Instructions:

   - Soak the towel in hot water and wring out the excess.

   - Apply castor oil to your chest and neck.

   - Place the hot towel over the oiled area and leave it on until it cools.

   - This method combines inhalation with topical application, enhancing the congestion relief effects.

5. **Castor Oil Vapor Rub**

   o Ingredients: 2 tablespoons of castor oil, 1 tablespoon of coconut oil, 5 drops of eucalyptus oil, 5 drops of peppermint oil.

348

- o Instructions:
    - Mix all ingredients together to form a vapor rub.
    - Apply the rub to your chest, neck, and under the nose before bed.
    - The vapor from the essential oils will help clear nasal passages as you sleep, while castor oil soothes and hydrates the skin.

6. **Nebulizer with Castor Oil Solution**
    - o Ingredients: 1 tablespoon of castor oil, saline solution, a nebulizer.
    - o Instructions:
        - Mix castor oil with saline solution in the nebulizer cup.
        - Use the nebulizer as directed, inhaling the mist deeply.
        - This method is particularly effective for severe congestion and respiratory issues.

5.5.3 Tips for Safe and Effective Use

- Patch Test: Always perform a patch test with essential oils to ensure there is no allergic reaction.
- Consult a doctor: Before using inhalation methods, especially for children or those with chronic respiratory conditions, consult with a healthcare provider.
- High-Quality Ingredients: Use high-quality, therapeutic-grade essential oils and pure, cold-pressed castor oil for the best results.
- Hydration: Stay well-hydrated to support the thinning of mucus and overall respiratory health.

By incorporating these inhalation methods into your routine, you can effectively use castor oil to relieve congestion, clear nasal passages, and promote easier breathing, providing comfort and relief from respiratory discomfort.

5.6 Chest rubs for cough and cold relief

Chest rubs are a time-honored remedy for alleviating the symptoms of coughs and colds. Utilizing castor oil as a base ingredient in chest rubs can enhance their effectiveness due to its anti-inflammatory, antimicrobial, and skin-soothing properties. When combined with essential oils known for their respiratory benefits, castor oil chest rubs can provide significant relief from congestion, coughing, and overall discomfort.

5.6.1 Benefits of Using Castor Oil in Chest Rubs

- Anti-Inflammatory Properties: Castor oil helps reduce inflammation in the respiratory tract, making it easier to breathe and reducing irritation caused by coughing.
- Antimicrobial Action: It can help fight off the pathogens responsible for colds and respiratory infections, supporting the body's natural healing process.

- Skin Soothing: Castor oil is an excellent moisturizer, preventing skin dryness and irritation that can result from frequent coughing and the use of other chest rubs.

5.6.2 Effective Chest Rub Recipes

1. Simple Castor Oil Chest Rub

   o Ingredients: 2 tablespoons of castor oil, 5 drops of eucalyptus essential oil.

   o Instructions:

      ▪ Mix the castor oil and eucalyptus oil in a small bowl.

      ▪ Rub a small amount onto the chest and throat before bed.

      ▪ Eucalyptus oil helps to clear nasal passages and soothe the throat.

2. Castor Oil and Coconut Oil Blend

   o Ingredients: 1 tablespoon of castor oil, 1 tablespoon of coconut oil, 4 drops of peppermint essential oil, 4 drops of eucalyptus essential oil.

   o Instructions:

      ▪ Combine all the oils in a bowl and mix well.

      ▪ Apply the blend to the chest and back, focusing on areas where you feel congestion.

      ▪ Coconut oil adds additional moisturizing benefits, while peppermint oil provides a cooling sensation that can relieve irritation.

3. Herbal Chest Rub with Castor Oil

   o Ingredients: 2 tablespoons of castor oil, 5 drops of thyme essential oil, 5 drops of rosemary essential oil.

   o Instructions:

      ▪ Mix the castor oil with thyme and rosemary oils.

      ▪ Rub onto the chest and cover with a warm cloth to enhance absorption.

      ▪ Thyme and rosemary oils are known for their antimicrobial and expectorant properties, helping to clear mucus and ease breathing.

4. Soothing Lavender and Castor Oil Rub

   o Ingredients: 2 tablespoons of castor oil, 5 drops of lavender essential oil, 3 drops of tea tree essential oil.

   o Instructions:

      ▪ Mix the castor oil with lavender and tea tree oils.

      ▪ Apply to the chest and back, massaging gently.

- Lavender oil promotes relaxation and better sleep, while tea tree oil helps fight infections.

5. Deep Relief Chest Rub

   - Ingredients: 1 tablespoon of castor oil, 1 tablespoon of olive oil, 5 drops of eucalyptus oil, 5 drops of camphor oil.

   - Instructions:

     - Combine all ingredients in a small bowl.

     - Rub onto the chest and throat, particularly before sleep or during bouts of coughing.

     - Camphor oil provides a warming effect that can ease muscle tightness associated with coughing.

5.6.3 Tips for Safe and Effective Use

- Patch Test: Before using any essential oil blend, perform a patch test to check for allergic reactions.

- Avoid Overuse: Essential oils are potent; use them in moderation and follow recommended guidelines.

- Consult a Healthcare Provider: If you or your child has chronic respiratory conditions, consult with a healthcare provider before using these remedies.

- High-Quality Ingredients: Use high-quality, therapeutic-grade essential oils and pure, cold-pressed castor oil to ensure safety and effectiveness.

- Hydration and Rest: Complement chest rubs with adequate hydration and rest to support the body's natural healing process.

5.6.4 Application Techniques

- Warm Compress: After applying the chest rub, place a warm, damp cloth over the chest to enhance absorption and provide additional relief.

- Massage: Gently massage the rub into the skin to improve circulation and promote deeper penetration of the oils.

- Nighttime Use: Applying chest rubs before bed can help reduce nighttime coughing and improve sleep quality.

By incorporating these chests rub recipes into your care routine, you can effectively utilize castor oil's therapeutic properties to relieve coughs and colds, promoting comfort and faster recovery during respiratory illnesses.

Chapter 6: Castor oil in infant massage and reflexology

6.1 Techniques of using castor oil in infant massage

Infant massage with castor oil can be an enriching and beneficial practice for both the baby and the caregiver. Castor oil is known for its moisturizing, anti-inflammatory, and soothing properties, making it an excellent choice for baby massage. This gentle practice can help promote relaxation, improve sleep, enhance bonding, and support the infant's physical and emotional development.

Benefits of Castor Oil for Infant Massage

Moisturizing: Castor oil is rich in fatty acids, providing deep hydration and keeping the baby's delicate skin soft and smooth.

Soothing: The anti-inflammatory properties of castor oil can help soothe minor skin irritations, rashes, and reduce redness. This soothing effect can help caregivers feel calm and in control when dealing with their baby's skin issues.

When choosing castor oil for your baby, opt for organic, cold-pressed, and hexane-free varieties to ensure the highest quality and purity. Always read the label and avoid products with added fragrances or other potentially irritating ingredients.

Preparing for Infant Massage

Before starting the massage, ensure that you and your baby are comfortable and relaxed. Here are some preparatory steps:

Comfortable Environment: Selecting a warm room free from distractions is crucial for a successful massage session. This emphasis on preparation can help caregivers feel more prepared and in control of the massage process.

Gather Supplies: Have a clean towel, a soft blanket, and a small bowl of warm castor oil ready.

Wash Your Hands: Clean your hands thoroughly to ensure they are warm and free from irritants.

Techniques for Effective Infant Massage

1. Head and Face Massage

   o Instructions:

     ▪ Begin by gently rubbing a small amount of warm castor oil between your hands.

     ▪ Use your fingertips to gently stroke the baby's forehead, moving from the center outward.

     ▪ Lightly massage the cheeks, nose, and chin using circular motions.

   o Benefits: This helps relax facial muscles and can soothe a fussy baby.

2. Chest and Tummy Massage

   o Instructions:

     ▪ Apply a small amount of castor oil to your hands and warm it up by rubbing your palms together.

     ▪ Gently place your hands on the baby's chest and make smooth, outward strokes from the center of the chest to the shoulders.

     ▪ Move down to the tummy, using circular, clockwise motions to aid digestion and relieve gas.

   o Benefits: This can help with respiratory health and digestion, reducing colic and gas discomfort.

3. Arm and Leg Massage

   o Instructions:

     ▪ Warm a little castor oil in your hands.

     ▪ Starting from the shoulders, gently stroke down the arms to the hands, making small circles around the joints.

     ▪ Repeat the same with the legs, starting from the thighs and moving down to the feet.

   o Benefits: This helps improve circulation and flexibility, supporting muscle development.

4. Back Massage

   o Instructions:

     ▪ Lay the baby on their tummy on a soft blanket or towel.

     ▪ Warm some castor oil in your hands and gently stroke down the baby's back, from the shoulders to the buttocks.

     ▪ Use circular motions along the spine, being careful to use light pressure.

   o Benefits: This can help relax the baby and alleviate any tension or discomfort in the back.

5. Foot Massage

- o Instructions:
    - Apply a small amount of castor oil to your fingertips.
    - Gently massage each foot, starting from the heel and moving up to the toes.
    - Use circular motions on the soles and light pressure on the toes.
  - o Benefits: Foot massage can be very soothing and can also stimulate the nerves and improve circulation.

Tips for a Successful Infant Massage

- Be Gentle: Always use light, gentle strokes. Babies have sensitive skin, and too much pressure can cause discomfort.

- Observe the Baby's Cues: Pay attention to your baby's reactions. If they seem uncomfortable or start to cry, stop and try again later.

- Consistency: Try to incorporate massage into a daily routine, such as after a bath or before bedtime, to create a calming ritual.

- Maintain Eye Contact: Talk to your baby in a soothing voice and maintain eye contact to enhance bonding.

- Temperature: Ensure the castor oil is warm but not hot to the touch. Test it on your wrist before applying it to your baby's skin.

Safety Considerations

- Patch Test: Before using castor oil, perform a patch test on a small area of the baby's skin to check for any allergic reactions.

- Avoid Face and Hands: Be cautious when massaging around the face and avoid the hands to prevent the baby from ingesting the oil.

- Consult a pediatrician: If your baby has any skin conditions or health concerns, consult a pediatrician before starting regular massages with castor oil.

Using castor oil in infant massage is a wonderful way to promote physical health, emotional well-being, and a strong bond between parent and child. With its myriads of benefits and soothing properties, castor oil can be a staple in your baby care routine.

6.2 Plantar reflexology for well-being and relaxation

Reflexology, an ancient healing practice rooted in traditional Chinese medicine, involves applying pressure to specific points on the feet, hands, and ears, believed to correspond to different organs and systems in the body. This holistic therapy aims to promote relaxation, alleviate stress, and improve overall health. For babies and children, reflexology offers a gentle, non-invasive way to support their well-being and soothe common discomforts.

6.2.1 What is Reflexology?

Reflexology is based on the principle that certain points on the feet, hands, and ears are linked to corresponding parts of the body. By stimulating these points, reflexologists believe they can help clear energy blockages, enhance circulation, and encourage the body's natural healing processes. This therapy is often used to manage stress, relieve pain, and support various health conditions.

<u>Benefits of Reflexology for Babies and Children</u>

- Promotes Relaxation: Reflexology can help calm the nervous system, reducing stress and promoting a sense of relaxation.

- Improves Sleep: Regular sessions may help regulate sleep patterns, making it easier for babies and children to fall asleep and stay asleep.

- Alleviates Pain: Reflexology can be effective in managing pain from teething, colic, and other common childhood ailments.

- Enhances Digestion: Stimulating specific reflex points can support healthy digestion and relieve issues like constipation and gas.

- Boosts Immunity: By improving overall energy flow and circulation, reflexology can help strengthen the immune system.

6.2.2 Reflexology Techniques for Babies and Children

1. **Foot Reflexology**

    o   Instructions:

        ▪ Start by gently warming up the baby's feet with light stroking movements.

        ▪ Apply gentle pressure to the big toe, believed to correspond to the head and brain, which can help soothe headaches and teething pain.

        ▪ Move to the arch of the foot, which is linked to the digestive system. Use circular motions to relieve gas and constipation.

        ▪ Finish with the heel, associated with the pelvic region, to ease lower abdominal discomfort.

    o   Benefits: Foot reflexology is easy to perform and can be very soothing for babies and children, helping to alleviate various discomforts and promote relaxation.

2. **Hand Reflexology**

    o   Instructions:

        ▪ Warm the child's hands with gentle stroking.

- Apply light pressure to the thumb, corresponding to the head, to relieve headaches.

- Massage the palm, which is linked to the digestive organs, to support digestion.

- Focus on the base of the fingers, associated with the chest and lungs, to help with respiratory issues.

  o Benefits: Hand reflexology is convenient and can be done anywhere, providing quick relief for stress and discomfort.

3. **Ear Reflexology**

  o Instructions:

- Gently stroke the outer edges of the ears to relax the child.

- Apply light pressure to the earlobes, linked to the head and neck, to ease tension.

- Massage the inner ear, which corresponds to the internal organs, to support overall health.

  o Benefits: Ear reflexology can be very calming and is a quick way to help a child relax and unwind.

6.2.3 Safety Considerations

- Gentle Touch: Always use a gentle touch when performing reflexology on babies and children. Their skin and tissues are delicate, and too much pressure can cause discomfort.

- Observe Reactions: Pay close attention to the child's reactions. If they seem uncomfortable or start to cry, stop the session and try again later.

- Consult a Professional: If you are new to reflexology, consider consulting a certified reflexologist for guidance and proper technique.

6.2.4 Incorporating Reflexology into Daily Routine

- Bedtime Routine: Incorporating reflexology into the bedtime routine can help signal to the child that it is time to wind down and prepare for sleep.

- Post-Bath Relaxation: After a warm bath, use reflexology to further relax the child and enhance the calming effects of the bath.

- During Playtime: Make reflexology a fun part of playtime by gently massaging the child's hands and feet while playing or reading a story.

Reflexology offers a gentle and effective way to support the health and well-being of babies and children. By understanding and applying these techniques, parents can provide comfort, relieve common ailments, and promote relaxation in their little ones. Whether used as a regular part of their routine or as needed for specific issues, reflexology can be a valuable tool in natural pediatric care.

Chapter 7: Sustaining immunity and well-being

7.1 Boosting immune function with castor oil

Castor oil, derived from the seeds of the Ricinus communis plant, has been traditionally used for various medicinal purposes, including boosting immune function. The oil contains ricinoleic acid, a potent fatty acid that contributes to its therapeutic properties. When used appropriately, castor oil can support and enhance the immune system in multiple ways, making it a valuable addition to natural health regimens.

7.1.1 Mechanisms of Immune Support

Anti-inflammatory Properties

Castor oil's anti-inflammatory effects are primarily due to its high ricinoleic acid content. Chronic inflammation can weaken the immune system, making the body more susceptible to infections and diseases. By reducing inflammation, castor oil helps maintain a balanced immune response.

Massaging castor oil onto inflamed areas or using castor oil packs can help reduce localized inflammation.

Lymphatic Stimulation

The lymphatic system plays a crucial role in immune function by transporting lymph, a fluid containing infection-fighting white blood cells, throughout the body. Castor oil is known to stimulate lymphatic circulation, which helps in detoxification and enhances the body's ability to fend off pathogens.

Applying castor oil packs to areas like the abdomen can promote lymphatic drainage and support overall immune health.

Antimicrobial Effects

Castor oil possesses antimicrobial properties that can help protect the body from various pathogens, including bacteria, viruses, and fungi. This makes it helpful in preventing infections and supporting the immune system.

The topical application of castor oil to minor cuts, wounds, or infections can help prevent microbial growth and aid in faster healing.

7.1.2 Methods of Application

1) Castor Oil Packs

- o **Ingredients:**
  - Cold-pressed castor oil
  - A piece of flannel or cotton cloth
  - Plastic wrap
  - Heating pad or hot water bottle
- o **Instructions:**
  - Soak the cloth in castor oil and place it on the desired area (commonly the abdomen).
  - Cover with plastic wrap to prevent staining.
  - Apply heat using a heating pad or hot water bottle for about 30-60 minutes.
  - Repeat 3-4 times a week for optimal results.
- o **Benefits:** Castor oil packs are effective in enhancing lymphatic circulation, reducing inflammation, and promoting detoxification, all of which contribute to a stronger immune system.

2) Topical Massage

- o **Ingredients:**
  - Cold-pressed castor oil
- o **Instructions:**
  - Warm the oil slightly for better absorption.
  - Gently massage the oil into the skin, focusing on areas like the abdomen, chest, and joints.
  - Allow the oil to absorb for at least an hour before washing off.
- o **Benefits:** Regular massage with castor oil can help reduce inflammation, improve circulation, and support the body's natural defenses.

3) Oral Consumption (with caution)

- o **Ingredients:**
  - Food-grade castor oil (consult a healthcare provider before use)
- o **Instructions:**
  - Follow the recommended dosage provided by a healthcare professional.
- o **Benefits:** When taken internally, castor oil can help cleanse the digestive system and support overall health, though this method should be used sparingly and under professional guidance.

7.1.3 Combining Castor Oil with Other Immune-Boosting Practices

- Balanced Diet: Consuming a diet rich in fruits, vegetables, lean proteins, and healthy fats supports overall immune health. Adding castor oil to salads or smoothies can provide an additional boost, but always in moderation.

- Regular Exercise: Physical activity enhances circulation and lymphatic flow, further supporting the immune system. Using castor oil packs post-exercise can help reduce muscle soreness and inflammation.

- Adequate Sleep: Quality sleep is essential for a robust immune system. Applying castor oil packs before bedtime can promote relaxation and improve sleep quality.

Castor oil is a versatile natural remedy with significant potential to enhance immune function. Its anti-inflammatory, lymphatic-stimulating, and antimicrobial properties make it a valuable tool in supporting overall health. By incorporating castor oil into various routines, such as using castor oil packs, topical massage, and combining it with other health practices, individuals can leverage its benefits to maintain a strong and resilient immune system. As with any natural remedy, it is essential to use castor oil appropriately and consult with healthcare professionals, especially when considering internal use.

7.2 Preventive measures for common childhood diseases

Preventing common childhood illnesses involves a combination of good hygiene practices, proper nutrition, regular physical activity, vaccinations, and the use of natural remedies. These measures can help strengthen a child's immune system and reduce the risk of infections and other health issues. Here are some key strategies for preventing common childhood illnesses:

1) Good Hygiene Practices

- Handwashing: Teach children to wash their hands thoroughly with soap and water for at least 20 seconds, especially before eating, after using the restroom, and after playing outside. This simple practice can significantly reduce the spread of germs.

- Respiratory Hygiene: Encourage children to cover their mouths and noses with a tissue or their elbow when coughing or sneezing. Proper disposal of tissues and regular handwashing afterward are also important.

- Personal Items: Discourage sharing of personal items such as utensils, water bottles, and towels to prevent the transmission of germs.

2) Proper Nutrition

- Balanced Diet: Ensure children consume a balanced diet rich in fruits, vegetables, whole grains, lean proteins, and healthy fats. These foods provide essential nutrients that support immune function.

- Hydration: Encourage children to drink plenty of water throughout the day to stay hydrated, which is vital for overall health and immune function.

- Probiotics: Include probiotic-rich foods like yogurt and kefir in the diet to promote a healthy gut microbiome, which plays a crucial role in immune health.

3) Regular Physical Activity

- Exercise: Encourage children to engage in regular physical activity, such as playing outside, participating in sports, or doing family activities like hiking or biking. Physical activity helps boost the immune system and overall well-being.

- Limit Screen Time: Reduce sedentary behavior by limiting screen time and encouraging more active play.

4)Vaccinations

- Immunizations: Ensure children receive all recommended vaccinations according to the schedule provided by healthcare professionals. Vaccinations protect against serious diseases like measles, mumps, rubella, polio, and influenza.

- Flu Shot: Annual flu vaccinations can help prevent influenza, which can be particularly severe in young children.

5) Adequate Sleep

- Sleep Routine: Establish a consistent sleep routine to ensure children get adequate sleep. Sufficient rest is essential for a strong immune system and overall health.

- Sleep Environment: Create a conducive sleep environment by keeping the bedroom dark, quiet, and cool, and limiting exposure to screens before bedtime.

6) Stress Management

- Emotional Support: Provide a supportive and nurturing environment to help children manage stress and anxiety. Chronic stress can weaken the immune system.

- Relaxation Techniques: Teach children relaxation techniques like deep breathing, meditation, or yoga to help them cope with stress.

7) Natural Remedies

- Herbal Teas: Herbal teas like chamomile and ginger can help soothe minor ailments and support immune function. Ensure they are age-appropriate and used in moderation.

- Essential Oils: Essential oils like eucalyptus and lavender can be used in diffusers or diluted for topical application to help with respiratory issues and promote relaxation.

- Castor Oil Packs: Castor oil packs can be applied to the abdomen to help with digestive issues like constipation and bloating, supporting overall health and immunity.

8) Environmental Cleanliness

- Clean Living Spaces: Regularly clean and disinfect frequently touched surfaces, such as doorknobs, light switches, and toys, to reduce the spread of germs.

- Ventilation: Ensure good ventilation in living spaces to reduce the concentration of airborne pathogens.

By integrating these preventative measures into daily routines, parents can significantly reduce the risk of common childhood illnesses. Teaching children good hygiene practices, ensuring proper nutrition, encouraging regular physical activity, maintaining up-to-date vaccinations, promoting adequate sleep, managing stress, and using natural remedies can collectively strengthen a child's immune system and promote overall health. Creating a healthy environment at home and fostering healthy habits from a young age will help children build a robust defense against various illnesses, leading to a healthier and happier childhood.

Chapter 8: Integrating castor oil into a child's wellness routine

8.1 Incorporating castor oil into daily healing rituals

Incorporating castor oil into daily care rituals can provide numerous health benefits for children and adults. This versatile oil, derived from the seeds of the Ricinus communis plant, is known for its anti-inflammatory, antimicrobial, and moisturizing properties. Here are some practical ways to integrate castor oil into everyday routines to enhance well-being:

8.1.1 Skin Care

Moisturizing: Castor oil is an excellent natural moisturizer. Apply a few drops to the face and body after bathing to lock in moisture and keep the skin hydrated and supple.

Acne Treatment: Due to its antimicrobial properties, castor oil can help reduce acne. Dab a small amount on blemishes or mix it with a carrier oil like jojoba oil and apply it to the entire face to prevent breakouts.

For skin irritations such as minor cuts, insect bites, and rashes, castor oil serves as a soothing balm. Its anti-inflammatory properties work to reduce redness and swelling, providing relief and promoting healing.

8.1.2 Hair Care

Scalp Health: Massage castor oil into the scalp to promote healthy hair growth and reduce dandruff. Leave it on for at least 30 minutes before washing it with mild shampoo.

Castor oil is a nourishing treat for dry and damaged hair. When used as a deep conditioner, it penetrates the hair shaft, focusing on the ends, and leaves your hair feeling pampered and rejuvenated.

Hair Growth: Regular application of castor oil to the scalp and hair can stimulate hair follicles and encourage growth, making hair thicker and stronger.

8.1.3 Oral Health

Gum Health: Massaging a small amount of castor oil onto the gums can help reduce inflammation and improve gum health.

Mouth Sores: Apply castor oil to canker sores or other mouth sores to promote healing and relieve pain.

8.1.4 Joint and Muscle Care

Joint Pain Relief: For those suffering from arthritis or joint pain, castor oil packs can provide relief. Apply a generous amount of castor oil to the affected area, cover with a cloth, and place a heating pad on top for 30-60 minutes.

Muscle Soreness: Massage castor oil into sore muscles after exercise to reduce inflammation and speed up recovery.

8.1.5 Digestive Health

Constipation Relief: Castor oil has natural laxative properties. For adults, taking a teaspoon of castor oil can help relieve constipation. Always consult with a healthcare provider before use.

Abdominal Packs: Applying castor oil packs to the abdomen can help improve digestion and alleviate bloating. Apply the oil to the abdomen, cover with a cloth, and apply heat for 30-60 minutes.

8.1.6 Foot Care

Cracked Heels: Apply castor oil to cracked heels and dry feet to moisturize and heal the skin. For best results, apply before bed and wear socks overnight.

Castor oil is a healing remedy for fungal infections. Its antifungal properties make it an effective treatment for conditions like athlete's foot, providing reassurance and confidence in its healing abilities.

8.1.7 Eye Health

Dry Eyes: Castor oil can be used to treat dry eyes. Place a drop of pure castor oil in each eye before bed to keep eyes moisturized.

Eyelash Growth: Apply a small amount of castor oil to the eyelashes before bed to promote growth and strengthen them.

8.1.8 Baby Care

Diaper Rash: Apply a thin layer of castor oil to a baby's diaper area to prevent and treat diaper rash. Its soothing and healing properties make it ideal for sensitive skin.

Cradle Cap: Gently massage castor oil onto the baby's scalp to help treat the cradle cap. Leave it on briefly before washing it with a mild baby shampoo.

8.2 Long-term benefits and considerations

Using castor oil regularly can provide numerous long-term benefits for overall health and wellness, but it's important to consider certain factors to ensure safe and effective use. Here's a detailed look at the potential long-term benefits and the considerations to keep in mind:

8.2.1 Long-term Benefits of Castor Oil

Skin Health

Moisturization: Consistent use of castor oil helps maintain skin hydration, preventing dryness and flakiness. It penetrates deep into the skin, providing long-lasting moisture.

Anti-aging Properties: The antioxidants in castor oil, such as ricinoleic acid, help fight free radicals, reducing the appearance of fine lines and wrinkles over time.

Scar Reduction: Regular application of castor oil can gradually reduce the appearance of scars and stretch marks due to its ability to promote cell regeneration.

Hair Health

Hair Growth: Over time, regular scalp massages with castor oil can lead to thicker, healthier hair by stimulating hair follicles and improving blood circulation.

Prevention of Hair Loss: The nutrients in castor oil strengthen the hair shaft and reduce hair fall, contributing to overall hair density and health.

Joint and Muscle Health

Reduced Inflammation: Castor oil's anti-inflammatory properties can help alleviate chronic joint pain and stiffness when used regularly, which is particularly beneficial for conditions like arthritis.

Muscle Relaxation: Routine use of castor oil for massages can help keep muscles relaxed and reduce the occurrence of muscle spasms and cramps.

Digestive Health

Regular Bowel Movements: For those who experience occasional constipation, castor oil can be a natural solution to promote regular bowel movements. However, it should be used cautiously and not as a long-term solution without medical advice.

Immune System Support

Detoxification: Castor oil packs used regularly can support liver function and detoxification processes, potentially boosting the immune system and overall health.

Hormonal Balance

Menstrual Health: Regular use of castor oil packs on the abdomen can help regulate menstrual cycles and alleviate menstrual cramps over time.

Menopausal Support: The anti-inflammatory and balancing properties of castor oil can help manage menopausal symptoms such as hot flashes and mood swings.

8.2.2 Considerations for Long-term Use

Allergic Reactions

Patch Test: Before incorporating castor oil into your routine, perform a patch test to ensure you are not allergic. Apply a small amount to a patch of skin and wait 24 hours to check for any adverse reactions.

Quality of Oil

Pure and Cold-Pressed: Ensure you are using high-quality, pure, cold-pressed castor oil to avoid any additives or contaminants that could reduce efficacy or cause skin irritation.

Dosage and Frequency

Moderation: While castor oil has many benefits, it is essential to use it in moderation. Overuse, especially internally, can lead to unwanted side effects such as diarrhea or nausea.

Consultation with Healthcare Providers: Always consult with a healthcare provider before using castor oil, especially if you are pregnant, breastfeeding, or have any underlying health conditions.

Storage

Proper Storage: Store castor oil in a cool, dark place to maintain its efficacy. Exposure to light and heat can degrade the oil, reducing its beneficial properties.

Interaction with Medications

Potential Interactions: If you are taking any medications, consult with a healthcare provider to ensure that castor oil does not interfere with their effectiveness or cause adverse reactions.

Sustainability

Ethical Sourcing: Consider purchasing castor oil from sustainable and ethical sources to support environmentally friendly practices and fair labor conditions.

Chapter 9: Frequently asked questions and expert advice

1) What is castor oil?

Castor oil is a vegetable oil derived from the seeds of the Ricinus communis plant. It is known for its therapeutic properties and has been used for centuries in traditional medicine.

2) Is castor oil safe for all skin types?

Generally, castor oil is safe for most skin types. However, it is always recommended to do a patch test before widespread use, especially if you have sensitive skin or are prone to allergies.

3) Can castor oil be ingested?

Castor oil can be ingested for certain medicinal purposes, such as relieving constipation. However, it should only be taken in small, recommended doses and under the guidance of a healthcare professional to avoid adverse effects.

4) How often should I use castor oil for hair growth?

For hair growth, it is typically recommended to use castor oil 1-2 times a week. Overuse can lead to greasy hair and scalp buildup.

5) What are the benefits of using castor oil for joint pain?

Castor oil contains ricinoleic acid, which has anti-inflammatory properties. When applied topically, it can help reduce inflammation and pain in the joints.

6) Can castor oil help with acne?

Yes, castor oil has antimicrobial and anti-inflammatory properties that can help treat acne. However, it should be used sparingly and in conjunction with a proper skincare routine.

7) Is castor oil safe to use during pregnancy?

While castor oil is often used for various skin and hair benefits during pregnancy, it should not be ingested as it can induce labor. Always consult with a healthcare provider before using castor oil during pregnancy.

8) How do I store castor oil?

Store castor oil in a cool, dark place to prevent it from going rancid. Proper storage helps maintain its efficacy and shelf life.

9) Can castor oil be used to treat fungal infections?

Castor oil has antifungal properties and can be used as a natural remedy for mild fungal infections. For severe cases, seek medical advice.

10) How does castor oil help with menstrual cramps?

Castor oil packs applied to the abdomen can help reduce menstrual cramps by improving circulation and reducing inflammation.

Expert Advice

Consult a Professional

Before incorporating castor oil into your health routine, especially for medicinal purposes, consult a healthcare provider to ensure it is safe and appropriate for your specific condition.

Use High-Quality Products

Always opt for high-quality, cold-pressed, and organic castor oil to ensure you are getting the purest form of the oil without harmful additives.

Patch Test for Allergies

Conduct a patch test by applying a small amount of castor oil to a patch of skin and wait 24 hours to check for any allergic reaction or irritation.

Moderation is Key

While castor oil has numerous benefits, moderation is essential. Overuse, particularly internally, can lead to negative side effects.

Blend with Other Oils

For enhanced benefits and reduced risk of skin irritation, blend castor oil with other carrier oils such as coconut oil, almond oil, or jojoba oil.

Regular Use for Best Results

Consistency is crucial for achieving the desired benefits from castor oil. Regular application, whether for hair growth, skin health, or joint pain relief, will yield the best results.

Stay Informed

Keep yourself updated with the latest research and expert recommendations regarding the use of castor oil. New findings can provide additional insights and enhance the effectiveness of your regimen.

Customize Your Approach

Tailor your use of castor oil to suit your individual needs. Different applications may work better for different people, so find what works best for you.

Safety First

Be cautious when using castor oil on children, pregnant women, and individuals with certain health conditions. Always seek professional advice in these cases.

Holistic Approach

Integrate castor oil into a holistic health routine that includes a balanced diet, regular exercise, and other natural remedies for comprehensive wellness.

BOOK 8: Castor Oil for Pets

Castor Oil for Pets

Natural Solutions for Their Health and Happiness

By

Vincent Vega

Disclaimer notice

Please be aware that the information provided in this document is intended solely for educational and entertainment purposes. Every effort has been made to ensure the content is accurate, reliable, current, and complete.

However, no guarantees, either explicit or implicit, are made. Readers acknowledge that the author is not providing legal, financial, medical, or professional advice.

The content has been sourced from various references. It is strongly recommended that you consult a licensed professional before attempting any of the of the methods described in this document.

By reading this document, you agree that the author is not liable for any direct or indirect losses resulting from the use of the information within, including but not limited to errors, omissions, or inaccuracies.

Chapter 1: Introduction to castor oil in pet care

1.1 Overview of castor oil and its properties

Castor oil, derived from the seeds of the Ricinus communis plant, has been renowned for its medicinal and therapeutic properties for centuries. Its use dates back to ancient civilizations, including the Egyptians, who valued its ability to promote healing and maintain health. In modern times, castor oil has garnered significant attention for its diverse applications, especially in natural and holistic pet care.

One of the most notable properties of castor oil is its high ricinoleic acid content, which constitutes about 90% of its fatty acid profile. Ricinoleic acid is a monounsaturated fatty acid known for its potent anti-inflammatory and analgesic effects. This makes castor oil particularly effective in treating inflammation and pain, such as arthritis and other joint-related ailments in pets.

In addition to its anti-inflammatory properties, castor oil possesses impressive antimicrobial and antifungal capabilities. The presence of ricinoleic acid and other minor constituents like undecylenic acid contribute to its ability to inhibit the growth of various bacteria and fungi. This makes it an excellent option for treating skin infections, wounds, and fungal issues such as ringworm, common pet problems.

Another critical property of castor oil is its ability to act as a humectant, which helps retain moisture in the skin. This hydrating effect benefits pets with dry, flaky skin or those prone to developing hot spots and dermatitis. When applied topically, castor oil forms a protective barrier on the skin, locking in moisture and promoting the healing of damaged tissues.

Castor oil's viscosity and thickness also significantly affect its effectiveness. Its thick consistency ensures it stays on the applied area longer, allowing for prolonged absorption and sustained therapeutic action. This is particularly useful in treating wounds and injuries, where a lasting barrier can help protect the area from further irritation and infection.

Castor oil is a powerful laxative for internal use due to its ability to stimulate the bowels. While its use internally should be approached with caution and under the guidance of a veterinarian, it can be a natural remedy for constipation and specific digestive issues in pets. The oil works by increasing the movement of the intestines, helping to clear out the bowels effectively.

Beyond its direct medicinal properties, castor oil is also used as a carrier oil in aromatherapy and herbal blends. Its ability to penetrate deeply into the skin makes it an ideal medium for delivering the therapeutic benefits of essential oils and other herbal extracts. When combined with calming essential oils like lavender or chamomile, castor oil can help alleviate anxiety and stress in pets, promoting relaxation and well-being.

Castor oil is celebrated for its ability to enhance the health and appearance of pets' fur in the realm of coat care. Its moisturizing properties help reduce dandruff and flakiness, while its nourishing effects can lead to a shinier, softer coat. Regular application of castor oil can also strengthen the hair follicles, reducing shedding and promoting healthier growth.

It's crucial to consider the proper usage and precautions when using castor oil on pets. Due to its potency, castor oil should be diluted appropriately, mainly when used on sensitive areas or smaller animals. Patch testing is recommended to ensure there are no adverse reactions, and any internal use should be strictly supervised by a professional. It's also important to note that while castor oil is generally safe for external use, it can cause digestive upset or other adverse effects if ingested in large quantities. Therefore, it's essential to keep it out of reach of pets and to consult a veterinarian before using it internally.

Castor oil is a versatile and powerful natural remedy with a wide range of properties beneficial for pet health. Its anti-inflammatory, antimicrobial, and moisturizing effects make it valuable to any holistic pet care regimen, empowering pet owners with a comprehensive solution. With careful application and consideration of safety guidelines, castor oil can significantly enhance the well-being of pets, addressing various health issues from skin conditions to digestive problems.

1.2 Historical use of castor oil in pet care

The historical use of castor oil in pet care dates back to ancient times, with roots in various cultures around the world. Castor oil, extracted from the seeds of the Ricinus communis plant, has long been celebrated for its medicinal properties, both for humans and animals. The utilization of this versatile oil in pet care is a testament to its enduring efficacy and the traditional knowledge passed down through generations, connecting us to a rich tradition of pet care.

In ancient Egypt, castor oil was highly valued for its healing properties. Egyptians used it for treating various ailments, and its benefits extended to animals. Castor oil was often applied to wounds and skin infections to promote healing and prevent diseases. Its antimicrobial properties made it a reliable remedy in an era where synthetic antibiotics were non-existent. This practice highlighted the oil's role in maintaining the health and wellbeing of animals, particularly in agricultural settings where livestock were vital.

Castor oil has been utilized for thousands of years in traditional Indian medicine, Ayurveda. Ayurvedic practitioners recognized its potent anti-inflammatory and analgesic properties. It was commonly used to treat joint pain and arthritis in working animals like horses and oxen. The oil's ability to reduce inflammation and alleviate pain made it essential to animal care in rural communities. Castor oil massages were a common practice to ensure that these animals remained healthy and productive.

In medieval Europe, castor oil also found its place in veterinary practices. During this period, herbal remedies were the primary means of treating human and animal ailments. Castor oil treated various skin conditions, such as mange and other parasitic infections in dogs and livestock. Its thick, dense nature allowed it to adhere to the skin, providing a protective barrier and therapeutic benefits. The oil's application would soothe the skin, reduce irritation, and promote healing, making it a valuable asset in the care of animals.

The 19th and early 20th centuries saw a more structured approach to veterinary science, yet castor oil remained a staple in natural and holistic treatments. Farmers and pet owners continued to rely on castor oil for its laxative properties, using it to treat constipation in pets and livestock. Its ability to stimulate bowel movements provided a natural solution to digestive issues, ensuring that animals remained healthy and free from gastrointestinal distress.

As veterinary science advanced, the empirical knowledge of castor oil's benefits was complemented by scientific validation. Research confirmed the oil's antimicrobial, anti-inflammatory, and analgesic properties, providing reassurance about its efficacy and cementing its place in conventional and alternative veterinary medicine. This period also saw an increased interest in holistic and natural remedies, leading to a resurgence in the use of castor oil for pet care.

Castor oil is recognized as a multifaceted remedy in holistic pet care practices. Its historical uses have evolved, but the core principles remain the same. Today, pet owners use castor oil to treat various conditions, from skin ailments to joint pain. It is often incorporated into natural grooming products, promoting a healthy coat and skin. Moreover, the trend towards natural and organic pet care products has further solidified castor oil's relevance.

The historical use of castor oil in pet care is a rich tapestry woven from diverse cultural practices and traditional knowledge. Its enduring presence in veterinary care across different eras and regions underscores its effectiveness and versatility. From ancient Egypt to modern holistic practices, castor oil has proven to be an invaluable resource in maintaining the health and wellbeing of animals. Its legacy continues as a trusted natural remedy, bridging the gap between historical wisdom and contemporary veterinary care.

1.3 Importance of natural remedies for pet health

Veterinarians and pet owners alike are increasingly recognising the importance of natural remedies for pet health. As the trend towards holistic and integrative medicine grows, so does the appreciation for natural treatments that can support pets' health and well-being in gentle, noninvasive ways. These remedies, which often include herbs, essential oils, and other plant-based substances, offer numerous benefits that complement conventional veterinary care.

One of the primary advantages of natural remedies is their reduced risk of side effects. Many conventional medications can cause adverse reactions in pets, such as gastrointestinal upset, liver or kidney damage, and allergic reactions. On the other hand, natural remedies are generally gentler on the body and less likely to cause harm when used appropriately. For instance, castor oil, a popular natural remedy, is known for its anti-inflammatory and antimicrobial properties. When used correctly, it can soothe skin irritations, reduce inflammation, and promote healing without the harsh side effects often associated with synthetic drugs.

Natural remedies also support the body's innate healing processes. Unlike many pharmaceutical interventions that may mask symptoms without addressing the root cause, natural treatments often work to enhance the body's ability to heal itself. For example, dietary supplements like omega-3 fatty acids from fish oil can improve coat health, reduce inflammation, and support overall immune function. Herbal remedies like milk thistle can aid liver function, helping pets detoxify and recover from illness more effectively.

Another significant benefit of natural remedies is their holistic approach to health. Holistic medicine considers the whole animal, considering physical, emotional, and environmental factors contributing to well-being. Natural remedies often align with this philosophy by promoting balance and wellness rather than targeting isolated symptoms. This approach can lead to more sustainable health outcomes and a higher quality of life for pets.

Natural remedies can also be beneficial for managing chronic conditions. Pets with long-term health issues, such as arthritis, allergies, or anxiety, often require ongoing treatment. Conventional medications used for these conditions can negatively affect an animal's body over time. Natural alternatives offer a safer long-term solution, such as glucosamine for joint health, chamomile for calming anxiety, or probiotics for digestive health. These remedies can alleviate symptoms and improve overall health without the risk of dependency or significant side effects.

Moreover, natural remedies are often more cost-effective than conventional treatments. Veterinary care can be expensive, and the cost of medications, surgeries, and specialized treatments can quickly add up. Many natural remedies, such as herbal supplements or dietary changes, can be implemented at a lower cost. Additionally, they can sometimes reduce the need for frequent vet visits or expensive procedures by keeping pets healthier overall.

Environmental sustainability is another crucial aspect of natural remedies. Many conventional pet medications and treatments have a significant ecological footprint, from production to disposal. Natural remedies, especially organically sourced and sustainably harvested, tend to be more environmentally friendly. Pet owners can reduce their environmental impact by choosing natural products while caring for their pets.

Using natural remedies encourages a closer bond between pets and their owners. Preparing and administering natural treatments often requires a hands-on approach, whether brewing a calming herbal tea, mixing a homemade dietary supplement, or massaging an animal with therapeutic oils. These activities can strengthen the emotional connection between pets and their caregivers, contributing to their well-being.

The importance of natural remedies for pet health cannot be overstated. They offer a safe, effective, and holistic approach to managing and preventing health issues, promoting long-term wellness and quality of life. As awareness of their benefits continues to grow, natural remedies are likely to become an increasingly integral part of comprehensive pet care, helping to ensure that our furry companions live happy, healthy lives.

1.4 Safety considerations in the use of castor oil on pets

When considering castor oil on pets, it's crucial to understand and adhere to safety guidelines to ensure the well-being of your furry companions. Castor oil, derived from the seeds of the Ricinus communis plant, possesses numerous beneficial properties, including anti-inflammatory and antimicrobial effects. However, its use must be cautiously approached due to its potent nature and potential risks if not used correctly.

1) The Properties of Castor Oil

Castor oil contains ricinoleic acid, which is responsible for its therapeutic effects. While this compound is beneficial for reducing inflammation and treating skin conditions, it can also be highly potent. Therefore, it is essential to use castor oil in the correct dosage and application methods to avoid adverse reactions.

2) Consult with a Veterinarian

Before introducing any new treatment, including natural remedies like castor oil, it is imperative to consult with a veterinarian. A professional can guide the appropriate usage based on your pet's specific health needs and conditions. They can also inform you of any contraindications or risks associated with your pet's current medications or health status.

3) Topical Application

When using castor oil topically, it is essential to dilute it with a carrier oil such as coconut oil or olive oil to reduce its potency. Applying pure castor oil directly to your pet's skin can cause irritation or allergic reactions. A standard dilution ratio is one part castor oil to three parts carrier oil.

Patch Test: Always perform a patch test before applying castor oil to a larger area of your pet's skin. Apply a small amount of the diluted oil to a small area and monitor for any signs of redness, swelling, or discomfort. If any adverse reactions occur, discontinue use immediately.

4) Avoid Ingestion

Pets should never ingest castor oil. While it is often used as a laxative in humans, it can cause severe gastrointestinal distress, including diarrhea and vomiting, in pets. Additionally, ingestion of castor oil can lead to dehydration and other complications. Ensure that the oil is applied to prevent your pet from licking or ingesting it.

5) Safe Areas for Application

Focus on applying castor oil to specific areas that require treatment, such as dry patches, wounds, or inflamed areas. Avoid applying it to sensitive areas such as the eyes, nose, mouth, and genital regions. Additionally, ensure to prevent the oil from coming into contact with open wounds unless advised by a veterinarian.

6) Monitoring for Allergic Reactions

Like humans, pets can have allergic reactions to natural products. After applying castor oil, observe your pet closely for signs of allergic reactions, including excessive scratching, redness, swelling, or hives. If these symptoms occur, wash the area with mild soap and water and consult your veterinarian.

7) Short-Term Use

Castor oil should be used as a short-term rather than a long-term treatment. Prolonged use can lead to skin dryness or irritation. If your pet's condition does not improve within a few days of treatment, seek veterinary advice to explore alternative treatments.

8) Storage and Handling

Store castor oil in a cool, dark place to maintain its efficacy and prevent it from becoming rancid. Ensure the oil is kept out of reach of pets and children to avoid accidental ingestion or spillage.

9) Understanding Species-Specific Sensitivities

Different species and even different breeds may have varying sensitivities to castor oil. What works for one pet may not necessarily be safe for another. For example, cats are generally more sensitive to essential oils and other substances than dogs. Tailor castor oil to your pet's specific needs and sensitivities.

10) Alternative Treatments

If castor oil is not suitable for your pet, consider using alternative natural remedies. Depending on the treated condition, options such as aloe vera for skin irritation or chamomile for calming purposes might be safer alternatives.

While castor oil can be an effective natural remedy for various ailments in pets, it must be used cautiously. Proper dilution, careful application, and close monitoring are essential to ensure the safety and health of your pet. Always seek veterinary guidance before introducing new treatments to avoid potential risks and complications. By following these safety considerations, you can harness the benefits of castor oil while safeguarding your pet's well-being.

Chapter 2: Benefits of castor oil for pets

2.1 Anti-inflammatory properties

Castor oil, derived from the seeds of the Ricinus communis plant, has been used for centuries for its myriad health benefits. One of the most significant properties of castor oil is its anti-inflammatory effect, which makes it a valuable natural remedy for various inflammatory conditions. Understanding the mechanisms behind its anti-inflammatory properties and how they can be harnessed for health benefits is essential for those looking to incorporate this versatile oil into their wellness routines.

1) Ricinoleic Acid and Its Role

The primary component of castor oil, ricinoleic acid, plays a pivotal role in its anti-inflammatory properties, constituting about 90% of the oil. Ricinoleic acid's ability to inhibit the production of certain proteins that cause inflammation, such as prostaglandins, is a key mechanism that helps reduce swelling, pain, and redness associated with inflammatory conditions.

2) Mechanisms of Action

One of the key mechanisms of castor oil's anti-inflammatory properties is the inhibition of Prostaglandins. These are lipid compounds that play a crucial role in the inflammatory response. Ricinoleic acid in castor oil works by inhibiting the enzyme cyclooxygenase (COX), which is involved in the synthesis of prostaglandins. By blocking COX, ricinoleic acid reduces the production of these inflammatory mediators.

Reduction of Free Radicals: Castor oil also exhibits antioxidant properties, which help neutralize free radicals. Free radicals are unstable molecules that can cause oxidative stress and contribute to inflammation. Castor oil helps mitigate the inflammatory response by reducing oxidative stress.

Improvement of Lymphatic Function: The application of castor oil can enhance the function of the lymphatic system, which is crucial for detoxification and immune response. Improved lymphatic drainage can help reduce inflammation by clearing out toxins and waste products that contribute to inflammatory processes.

3) Applications for Inflammatory Conditions

Arthritis: Castor oil can be particularly effective for managing arthritis, a condition characterized by joint inflammation. Topical application of castor oil to affected joints can help reduce pain and swelling. Its ability to penetrate deep into the tissues makes it an excellent remedy for chronic inflammatory conditions.

Skin Inflammation: Conditions like eczema, psoriasis, and dermatitis can benefit from the anti-inflammatory properties of castor oil. Applying castor oil to affected areas can help soothe irritated skin, reduce redness, and promote healing.

Muscle Pain: For muscle inflammation and pain, castor oil can be used as a massage oil. It helps relax the muscles, reduce inflammation, and alleviate pain. Combining castor oil with essential oils like peppermint or eucalyptus can enhance its anti-inflammatory effects.

Gastrointestinal Inflammation: Castor oil can also be used internally, though with caution and under professional guidance, to reduce inflammation in the gastrointestinal tract. It has been traditionally used as a laxative, but its anti-inflammatory properties can help soothe conditions like irritable bowel syndrome (IBS) and inflammatory bowel disease (IBD).

4) Methods of Use

Topical Application: For localized inflammation, applying castor oil directly to the skin is the most common method. This can be done by massaging the oil into the skin or using a castor oil pack, where a cloth soaked in castor oil is placed on the affected area and covered with heat to enhance absorption.

Oral Consumption: While less common, castor oil can be ingested in small amounts for its anti-inflammatory benefits. However, due to its strong laxative effect, this should only be done under medical supervision.

Castor Oil Packs: These involve soaking a cloth in castor oil, placing it on the skin, and applying heat. This method is particularly effective for deep-seated inflammation and can be used for conditions like liver inflammation or menstrual cramps.

5) Safety and Precautions

While castor oil is generally safe for topical use, it's important to note that some individuals may experience allergic reactions. To avoid this, it is advisable to perform a patch test before extensive use. Ingesting castor oil should only be done under professional guidance due to its potent laxative properties, which can lead to dehydration and electrolyte imbalances if not managed properly.

Castor oil's anti-inflammatory properties make it a potent natural remedy for various inflammatory conditions. Its effectiveness lies in inhibiting pro-inflammatory compounds, reducing oxidative stress, and improving lymphatic function. By understanding these mechanisms and using castor oil appropriately, individuals can harness its benefits to manage and reduce inflammation naturally.

2.2 Antimicrobial and antifungal benefits

Castor oil, a versatile natural remedy derived from the seeds of the Ricinus communis plant, has been used for centuries in traditional medicine for its numerous health benefits. Among its many properties, the antimicrobial and antifungal benefits of castor oil stand out as particularly significant. These properties make castor oil an effective solution for various infections and skin conditions, enhancing its value as a natural remedy. The versatility of castor oil allows you to address a wide range of health concerns with a single product, empowering you with a comprehensive natural solution.

Key Components and Mechanisms

Castor oil's antimicrobial and antifungal properties are primarily attributed to its high concentration of ricinoleic acid, which makes up about 90% of the oil. Ricinoleic acid has been shown to inhibit the growth of various bacteria, yeasts, and fungi, making it a powerful agent against infections.

Ricinoleic Acid: This fatty acid disrupts the cell walls of bacteria and fungi, inhibiting their growth and replication. It alters the permeability of the microbial cell membranes, leading to cell death.

Undecylenic Acid: Castor oil contains undecylenic acid, a known antifungal compound. This acid inhibits the growth of fungi and is effective in treating fungal infections, such as ringworm and athlete's foot.

Applications in Treating Infections

Skin Infections: Castor oil can be applied topically to treat various skin infections, including bacterial and fungal infections. Its ability to penetrate deep into the skin allows it to reach the source of the infection effectively.

Wound Healing: Due to its antimicrobial properties, castor oil promotes wound healing. It helps prevent infection in cuts, scrapes, and minor wounds, while its anti-inflammatory properties reduce pain and swelling.

Fungal Infections: Castor oil is not just effective, it's a powerhouse against fungal infections such as athlete's foot, ringworm, and toenail fungus. Regular application of castor oil to the affected areas can help eliminate the fungi and prevent their recurrence. This effectiveness should give you confidence in the therapeutic power of castor oil for specific conditions.

Methods of Use

Topical Application: For skin infections and fungal issues, castor oil can be directly applied to the affected area. To enhance its effectiveness, the oil can be mixed with other antimicrobial essential oils like tea tree oil or lavender oil.

Castor Oil Packs: Using castor oil packs involves soaking a cloth in castor oil and applying it to the infected area. This method ensures deeper penetration and prolonged contact, enhancing the antimicrobial effects.

Oral Consumption: Though less common, castor oil can be ingested in small doses to help fight internal infections. However, due to the oil's potent laxative effect, this should be done under medical supervision.

Benefits for Specific Conditions

Acne: The antimicrobial properties of castor oil make it effective in treating acne, which is often caused by bacterial infection of the skin. Applying castor oil helps reduce the bacteria on the skin, preventing acne outbreaks.

Dandruff: Dandruff is often caused by a fungal infection of the scalp. When massaged into the scalp, castor oil can help reduce the fungus and alleviate dandruff symptoms.

Oral Health: Castor oil's antifungal properties are beneficial for maintaining oral health. It can be used as a natural mouthwash to help reduce oral bacteria and prevent gum infections.

Safety and Precautions

While castor oil is generally safe for topical use, a patch test before extensive application is essential to rule out allergic reactions. For oral consumption, it is crucial to follow the guidance of a healthcare professional to avoid potential side effects like severe diarrhea or abdominal cramping.

Castor oil's antimicrobial and antifungal benefits make it a valuable natural remedy for a wide range of infections. Its effectiveness in inhibiting the growth of bacteria and fungi and its ability to penetrate deeply into the skin enhances its utility in treating various conditions. By understanding these properties and using castor oil appropriately, individuals can harness its benefits to maintain and improve their health naturally.

2.3 Promoting skin and hair health

Castor oil, derived from the seeds of the Ricinus communis plant, is renowned for its extensive health benefits. Among its many applications, promoting healthy skin and coat in pets is a particularly valuable use. This natural remedy, rich in ricinoleic acid and essential fatty acids, provides a holistic approach to maintaining your pets' overall well-being, ensuring their skin remains healthy and their coat shiny and smooth.

Key Nutrients and Their Benefits

Ricinoleic Acid: The primary component of castor oil, ricinoleic acid, has anti-inflammatory and moisturizing properties. It helps soothe irritated skin, reduce inflammation, and hydrate dry, flaky areas.

Vitamin E: Castor oil is rich in vitamin E, an antioxidant that promotes skin health by protecting against oxidative stress and supporting skin cell regeneration.

Omega Fatty Acids: These essential fatty acids nourish the skin and coat, promoting a glossy, healthy appearance and preventing dryness and brittleness.

Benefits for the Skin

Moisturizing: Castor oil is an excellent natural moisturizer. It penetrates deep into the skin, providing long-lasting hydration. This is especially beneficial for pets with dry or flaky skin.

Healing Properties: The anti-inflammatory and antimicrobial properties of castor oil help in healing minor skin irritations, wounds, and hot spots. It soothes the skin and prevents infections.

Anti-Itch: Castor oil can help relieve itching caused by allergies or skin conditions. Its soothing properties calm the skin and reduce the urge to scratch, which can exacerbate skin issues.

Enhancing the Coat

Shine and Smoothness: Regular application of castor oil can make your pet's coat shiny and smooth. The fatty acids in the oil coat the hair strands, reducing frizz and adding a natural gloss.

Preventing Hair Loss: By nourishing the hair follicles and improving overall skin health, castor oil can help reduce hair loss. It strengthens the roots and promotes healthy hair growth.

Detangling: Castor oil can also be a natural detangler for pets with long or curly hair. It smooths out knots and makes the coat easier to manage and brush.

Methods of Application

Topical Application: Apply a small amount of castor oil directly to your pet's skin and coat. Massage it in gently, focusing on dry or irritated areas. This method ensures deep penetration and immediate relief.

Bath Additive: Add a few drops of castor oil to your pet's bath water. This will help moisturize their skin and coat during bath time, leaving them soft and shiny.

Homemade Sprays: Create a spray by mixing castor oil with water and a few drops of essential oils like lavender or chamomile. Spritz this mixture onto your pet's coat for added shine and a pleasant scent.

Specific Conditions and Castor Oil

Hot Spots: Hot spots, or acute moist dermatitis, can be soothed with castor oil. Its anti-inflammatory and antimicrobial properties help reduce redness and prevent infection.

Eczema and Dermatitis: For pets with eczema or dermatitis, castor oil provides much-needed relief by moisturizing the skin and reducing inflammation.

Paw Pads: Castor oil can soften and protect paw pads, especially in harsh weather conditions. It prevents cracking and keeps the pads supple.

While castor oil is generally safe for pets, there are a few precautions to consider. Before extensive use, perform a patch test to ensure your pet has no adverse reaction. Apply a small amount to a small area and monitor for any signs of irritation.

While castor oil is safe for topical use, ingestion can cause digestive issues. Ensure that your pet does not lick the applied area excessively.

If your pet has a pre-existing skin condition or is on medication, consult your veterinarian before using castor oil.

Castor oil is a versatile and effective natural remedy for promoting healthy pet skin and coat. Its rich composition of ricinoleic acid, vitamin E, and essential fatty acids offers numerous benefits, from moisturizing and healing the skin to enhancing the shine and smoothness of the coat. By incorporating castor oil into your pet's grooming routine, you can help ensure their skin remains healthy and their coat looks its best. Always use castor oil safely and consult your veterinarian if you have any concerns.

2.4 Relieve pain and discomfort

Castor oil, renowned for its medicinal properties, has been a cornerstone of traditional medicine for centuries. Its use in alleviating pain and discomfort, particularly in pets, is a testament to its efficacy. This natural remedy, derived from the seeds of the Ricinus communis plant, is rich in ricinoleic acid, which boasts anti-inflammatory and analgesic properties. Here's a closer look at how castor oil can ease pain and discomfort in pets, ensuring their well-being and comfort.

Anti-Inflammatory Properties

One of the primary components of castor oil is ricinoleic acid, which has significant anti-inflammatory effects. This makes castor oil particularly effective in:

Reducing Swelling: When applied to swollen areas, castor oil helps to reduce inflammation and swelling, providing relief from discomfort.

Easing Joint Pain: For pets suffering from arthritis or other joint issues, the anti-inflammatory properties of castor oil can help reduce pain and improve mobility.

Soothing Irritated Skin: Castor oil can be applied to areas of the skin that are inflamed due to allergies, insect bites, or other irritants. Its soothing properties help to calm the skin and reduce redness.

Analgesic Effects

Castor oil is not just anti-inflammatory; it also has natural analgesic, or pain-relieving, properties. This dual action makes it particularly effective for:

Muscle Pain: Massaging castor oil into sore muscles can help alleviate pain and promote relaxation. This is beneficial for pets who may be recovering from injuries or strenuous activities.

Nerve Pain: Castor oil can relieve pets experiencing nerve pain. Its ability to penetrate deeply into the skin allows it to soothe irritated nerves.

Minor Injuries: For cuts, bruises, and minor injuries, castor oil can help to reduce pain and speed up the healing process.

Methods of Application

Applying castor oil to alleviate pain and discomfort can be done in several ways, depending on the type of pain and the area affected:

Topical Application: Apply a small amount of castor oil directly to the affected area. Gently massage it in to ensure deep penetration. This method is particularly effective for joint and muscle pain.

Warm Compress: For deeper relief, soak a cloth in warm castor oil and apply it as a compress to the painful area. The warmth helps to enhance the oil's penetration and efficacy.

In Combination with Essential Oils: Mixing castor oil with essential oils such as lavender or peppermint can enhance pain-relieving properties. These oils have additional analgesic and anti-inflammatory benefits.

Specific Uses for Pets

Arthritis and Joint Pain: Regularly applying castor oil to the joints can help manage chronic pain associated with arthritis. Its anti-inflammatory properties reduce swelling and pain, improving your pet's mobility.

Post-Surgical Care: After surgeries, applying castor oil can help to reduce pain and promote healing. Its soothing properties can ease discomfort and aid in recovery.

General Discomfort: For pets experiencing general discomfort due to age, activity, or other factors, castor oil provides a natural and gentle option for pain relief.

Safety and Precautions

While castor oil is generally safe for pets, certain precautions must be taken to ensure its safe and effective use.

Patch Test: Before extensive application, perform a patch test to check for adverse reactions. Apply a small amount of oil to a small skin area and monitor for any signs of irritation.

Avoid Ingestion: Ensure your pet does not lick the area where castor oil has been applied, as ingestion can cause digestive upset.

Consult a veterinarian: If your pet has a pre-existing condition or is taking other medications, consult your veterinarian before using castor oil.

Castor oil is a versatile and effective natural remedy for pain and discomfort in pets. Its anti-inflammatory and analgesic properties make it suitable for various applications, from joint pain and muscle soreness to minor injuries and general discomfort. By incorporating castor oil into your pet care routine, you can provide a natural and gentle option for pain relief, ensuring your pet's comfort and well-being. Always use castor oil safely, and consult your veterinarian if you have any concerns about its use for your pet.

Chapter 3: Guidelines for safe use

3.1 Dos and don'ts of using castor oil on pets

Using castor oil for pets can provide a variety of health benefits, but it's essential to understand the proper application methods and precautions to ensure safety and effectiveness. Here are the key dos and don'ts to consider when incorporating castor oil into your pet care routine.

Dos

1. **Do Consult Your Veterinarian:**

    o   Professional Advice: Always consult your veterinarian before introducing castor oil into your pet's health regimen. This is especially important if your pet has existing health conditions or is on medication.

    o   Tailored Guidance: Your veterinarian can provide specific recommendations based on your pet's age, weight, breed, and overall health.

2. **Do Use Pure, Cold-Pressed Castor Oil:**

    o   Quality Matters: Ensure you use pure, cold-pressed castor oil. This type is free from additives and chemicals, making it safer for your pet.

    o   Check Labels: Always read labels carefully to confirm the product's purity.

3. **Do Perform a Patch Test:**

    o   Safety First: Before applying castor oil extensively, perform a patch test by applying a small amount to a small area of your pet's skin. Monitor for any signs of irritation or allergic reaction over 24 hours.

    o   Monitor: If any redness, swelling, or discomfort occurs, discontinue use immediately.

4. **Do Use Appropriate Amounts:**

    o   Moderation: Use castor oil sparingly. A little goes a long way, especially when applying it topically. Overuse can lead to greasy fur or skin irritation.

    o   Follow Guidelines: Adhere to veterinarian-recommended dosages and application methods.

5. **Do Apply Castor Oil Topically for Specific Issues:**

- Targeted Application: Use castor oil to treat localized issues such as dry skin, minor wounds, or inflammation. Apply a small amount directly to the affected area and gently massage it in.

- Regular Monitoring: Regularly check the treated area to ensure it is healing properly and not causing additional issues.

6. **Do Store Castor Oil Properly:**

- Cool and Dark: Store castor oil in a cool, dark place to maintain its effectiveness. Proper storage prevents the oil from going rancid or losing its beneficial properties.

Don'ts

1. **Don't Let Your Pet Ingest Castor Oil:**

- Avoid Oral Consumption: Castor oil can be toxic if ingested by pets, leading to gastrointestinal upset, diarrhea, or more severe health issues.

- Monitor Application: Ensure that your pet does not lick the area where castor oil has been applied. Use a bandage or pet cone if necessary to prevent licking.

2. **Don't Use Castor Oil on Open Wounds:**

- Healing First: Avoid applying castor oil to open wounds or surgical sites as it can delay healing and cause infection.

- Seek Alternatives: Use other veterinarian-recommended treatments for open wounds until they have sufficiently healed.

3. **Don't Use Castor Oil Around Sensitive Areas:**

- Avoid Eyes and Ears: Do not apply castor oil near your pet's eyes, ears, or nose. These areas are highly sensitive and can be easily irritated.

- Target Safe Zones: Focus application on less sensitive areas, such as the back, legs, or paws.

4. **Don't Ignore Adverse Reactions:**

- Immediate Action: If you notice any signs of an allergic reaction, such as excessive itching, redness, swelling, or behavioral changes, stop using castor oil immediately and consult your veterinarian.

- Document and Report: Keep track of any adverse reactions and report them to your veterinarian to adjust care strategies accordingly.

5. **Don't Substitute Veterinary Care:**

- Professional Care: While castor oil can be beneficial, it should not replace professional veterinary care. Use it as a complementary treatment in conjunction with your veterinarian's advice.

- Follow-Up: Maintain regular veterinary check-ups to monitor your pet's health and treatment progress.

6. **Don't Apply Castor Oil Excessively:**

o   Avoid Overuse: Applying too much castor oil can clog pores and lead to skin issues. Follow recommended application guidelines and avoid overuse.

o   Balance: Maintain a balance between natural remedies and conventional treatments to ensure overall well-being.

By adhering to these dos and don'ts, you can safely and effectively incorporate castor oil into your pet's care routine. Always prioritize your pet's health and comfort, and when in doubt, seek professional veterinary advice.

3.2 Dilution ratios for different types of pets

When using castor oil on pets, it's crucial to dilute it properly to ensure safety and effectiveness. Different types of pets require different dilution ratios based on their size, species, and specific health needs. Here's a comprehensive guide to dilution ratios for various pets.

3.2.1 General Guidelines for Dilution

Castor oil is potent, and while it has numerous benefits, using it in its undiluted form can cause skin irritation or other adverse effects in pets. Diluting castor oil with a carrier oil, such as coconut oil, olive oil, or almond oil, helps reduce its potency while still providing the therapeutic benefits. The following are general dilution guidelines:

- Small Animals (Cats, Small Dogs, Rodents):

    o   Ratio: 1 part castor oil to 3 parts carrier oil

    o   Application: Use for minor skin issues, such as dry patches or mild irritation.

- Medium-sized Dogs:

    o   Ratio: 1 part castor oil to 2 parts carrier oil

    o   Application: Suitable for larger areas of the skin and for conditions such as dry skin, minor wounds, or inflammation.

- Large Dogs:

    o   Ratio: 1 part castor oil to 1 part carrier oil

    o   Application: Effective for widespread skin issues, joint pain, and more significant areas requiring treatment.

- Birds:

    o   Ratio: 1 part castor oil to 4 parts carrier oil

    o   Application: Use sparingly and apply with care to avoid stressing the bird. Ideal for treating dry skin or feather issues.

- Reptiles:

    o   Ratio: 1 part castor oil to 3 parts carrier oil

- Application: Can be used to treat dry skin or minor wounds. Ensure the environment is suitable for the reptile's recovery.

3.2.2 Dilution Ratios for Specific Pets

1. Cats:

   - Cats have sensitive skin and grooming habits that make ingestion of substances a concern. Use a high dilution ratio to ensure safety.

   - Dilution Ratio: 1 part castor oil to 4 parts carrier oil

   - Application: Apply sparingly to the affected area. Monitor closely to prevent the cat from licking the oil.

2. Small Dogs (e.g., Chihuahuas, Dachshunds):

   - Smaller dogs have delicate skin and require gentle treatment.

   - Dilution Ratio: 1 part castor oil to 3 parts carrier oil

   - Application: Apply to specific areas needing treatment. Use a soft cloth to spread the mixture evenly.

3. Medium-sized Dogs (e.g., Beagles, Cocker Spaniels):

   - Medium-sized dogs can tolerate a slightly higher concentration of castor oil.

   - Dilution Ratio: 1 part castor oil to 2 parts carrier oil

   - Application: Use for larger areas or more persistent issues. Massage gently into the skin.

4. Large Dogs (e.g., Labradors, German Shepherds):

   - Larger dogs can handle a higher concentration of castor oil, making it effective for broader applications.

   - Dilution Ratio: 1 part castor oil to 1 part carrier oil

   - Application: Ideal for treating joint pain, dry skin, or other large areas. Apply with a gentle massage.

5. Birds (e.g., Parrots, Canaries):

   - Birds have very sensitive systems, and care must be taken to avoid stressing them.

   - Dilution Ratio: 1 part castor oil to 4 parts carrier oil

   - Application: Apply very sparingly to dry or irritated areas. Avoid getting oil on feathers unless treating a specific feather issue.

6. Rodents (e.g., Hamsters, Guinea Pigs):

   - Rodents have delicate skin and are prone to licking substances off their fur.

   - Dilution Ratio: 1 part castor oil to 4 parts carrier oil

   - Application: Apply lightly to the affected area. Monitor to ensure the rodent does not ingest the oil.

7. Reptiles (e.g., Snakes, Lizards):

    o Reptiles have unique skin needs, often requiring moisture and healing for dry or damaged skin.

    o Dilution Ratio: 1 part castor oil to 3 parts carrier oil

    o Application: Apply gently to dry or affected areas. Ensure the reptile's environment remains conducive to healing.

8. Horses:

    o Horses have thick skin and can benefit from stronger dilutions for conditions such as joint pain or dry patches.

    o Dilution Ratio: 1 part castor oil to 1 part carrier oil

    o Application: Use for large areas or specific joint issues. Apply with a firm massage to penetrate the thick skin.

3.2.3 Additional Tips for Safe Use

- Patch Test: Always perform a patch test before widespread application. Apply a small amount of the diluted mixture to a small area of the pet's skin and observe for 24 hours for any adverse reactions.

- Monitor Behavior: After applying castor oil, monitor your pet's behavior for signs of discomfort, excessive licking, or allergic reactions.

- Environment: Ensure the pet's environment is clean and conducive to healing, especially for reptiles and birds.

By following these guidelines and adjusting dilution ratios according to the specific needs of different pets, you can safely incorporate castor oil into their care routines, promoting healing and overall well-being.

3.3 Patch tests for allergic reactions

Patch testing is a crucial step in ensuring the safe use of any new substance, including castor oil, on pets. This method helps identify potential allergic reactions or sensitivities before applying the product more broadly. Proper patch testing can prevent discomfort, skin irritation, and more severe allergic reactions. Here's a comprehensive guide on how to perform patch testing for allergic reactions on pets.

Importance of Patch Testing

Patch testing is essential for several reasons:

- Safety: Pets have sensitive skin that can react adversely to new products. Patch testing minimizes the risk of widespread irritation or allergic reactions.

- Preventive Measure: Early detection of an adverse reaction can prevent more severe health issues.

- Customized Care: Each pet is unique, and patch testing helps determine the appropriate product concentration and application method for individual pets.

Steps for Patch Testing

1. Choose the Test Area:

   o Select a small, discreet area of the pet's skin. Ideal spots are behind the ear, the inside of the leg, or the belly, where the skin is more sensitive and reactions can be easily observed.

   o Ensure the area is clean and free from any cuts, sores, or existing irritations.

2. Prepare the Test Solution:

   o Dilute the castor oil according to the guidelines specific to the pet's size and species. For example, for small animals like cats or rodents, a higher dilution (1 part castor oil to 4 parts carrier oil) is recommended.

   o Mix thoroughly to ensure even distribution of the oils.

3. Apply the Test Solution:

   o Use a cotton swab or a clean cloth to apply a small amount of the diluted castor oil to the chosen test area.

   o Rub the solution gently into the skin, ensuring it's well absorbed.

4. Observation Period:

   o Observe the test area for any signs of reaction over the next 24 to 48 hours.

   o Look for redness, swelling, bumps, itching, or any other signs of irritation.

Identifying Reactions

During the observation period, monitor your pet closely for both localized and general symptoms. Common signs of an allergic reaction include:

- Localized Reactions:

  o Redness or discoloration of the skin

  o Swelling or raised bumps

  o Itching or scratching at the test site

  o Warmth or heat in the area

- General Reactions:

  o Lethargy or unusual behavior

  o Excessive licking or grooming of the test site

  o Respiratory issues, such as sneezing or coughing

  o Gastrointestinal symptoms, such as vomiting or diarrhea (rare but possible)

If any of these symptoms are observed, it's crucial to wash the test area immediately with mild soap and water to remove the oil. Discontinue use and consult a veterinarian for further advice.

Post-Testing Care

If no adverse reactions are observed during the patch testing period, the castor oil can be considered safe for broader application. Follow these steps to ensure continued safety and effectiveness:

- Gradual Introduction:
    - Start with a small amount of the diluted castor oil and gradually increase the application area over several days.
    - Monitor the pet's skin and overall behavior for any delayed reactions.

- Routine Monitoring:
    - Regularly check the pet's skin for any signs of irritation or allergic response, even after successful patch testing.
    - Adjust the dilution ratio or frequency of application if any mild reactions occur over time.

- Documentation:
    - Keep a record of the patch test results, including the dilution ratio, test area, and any observed reactions. This can be helpful for future reference or for sharing with a veterinarian.

Special Considerations for Different Pets

Different types of pets may have unique sensitivities and requirements for patch testing. Here are some additional tips for various animals:

- Cats:
    - Cats are particularly sensitive to many substances, including essential oils. Ensure the dilution ratio is appropriate and monitor closely, as cats are prone to licking the applied area.

- Dogs:
    - Larger dogs may require a higher concentration, but it's still essential to start with a diluted solution. Pay attention to areas where the dog cannot easily lick or scratch.

- Birds:
    - Birds have delicate skin and respiratory systems. Apply the solution sparingly and avoid areas where the bird might ingest the oil through preening.

- Rodents and Small Mammals:
    - These animals have thin skin and are prone to stress. Use a very diluted solution and apply in a less accessible area to prevent ingestion.

- Reptiles:
    - Reptiles may have different skin requirements based on their species. Ensure the environment remains suitable for their recovery while testing.

Patch testing is an indispensable step in incorporating castor oil into pet care routines. By following these detailed guidelines, pet owners can ensure the safety and well-being of their pets while harnessing the therapeutic benefits of castor oil. Always consult with a veterinarian if there are any concerns or if the pet has a history of allergic reactions. With careful application and monitoring, castor oil can be a valuable addition to natural pet care.

3.4 Signs of castor oil overdose and what to do about it

Castor oil, while beneficial for various health issues, can be harmful if used in excess. An overdose of castor oil can lead to serious health complications, especially in pets. Recognizing the signs of overdose and knowing how to respond promptly is crucial for ensuring the safety and well-being of pets.

3.4.1 Signs of Castor Oil Overdose

Gastrointestinal Distress

Diarrhea: One of the most common signs of castor oil overdose is severe diarrhea. This occurs because castor oil acts as a powerful laxative, stimulating the bowels excessively.

Vomiting: Pets may vomit repeatedly due to irritation of the stomach lining caused by castor oil.

Abdominal Pain: The pet may show signs of discomfort, such as whining, pacing, or adopting a hunched posture, indicating abdominal pain or cramping.

Dehydration

Increased Thirst: Due to diarrhea and vomiting, pets may exhibit signs of dehydration, such as increased thirst.

Dry Gums and Nose: Physical signs like dry gums, a dry nose, and sunken eyes are indicative of dehydration.

Lethargy: Dehydration can lead to a significant drop in energy levels, making pets unusually lethargic or weak.

Neurological Symptoms

Uncoordinated Movements: An overdose can affect the nervous system, causing pets to appear unsteady or have difficulty walking.

Seizures: In severe cases, an overdose may lead to seizures, which require immediate medical attention.

Hypersalivation

Pets may drool excessively due to irritation caused by the ingestion of castor oil.

Respiratory Issues

Difficulty Breathing: Inhalation of castor oil fumes, or severe reactions, might cause difficulty in breathing or labored breathing.

Skin Irritation

Redness and Swelling: Excessive topical application can lead to redness, swelling, and irritation of the skin.

Rashes or Hives: Allergic reactions to castor oil overdose may manifest as rashes or hives on the skin.

3.4.2 What to Do in Case of Overdose

1. Stop Administration:

   o   Immediately discontinue the use of castor oil if an overdose is suspected.

2. Assess the Situation:

   o   Monitor Symptoms: Carefully observe the pet's symptoms and note any changes or worsening conditions.

   o   Check for Dehydration: Gently press a finger against the pet's gums. If the gums take longer than normal to return to their pink color, the pet may be dehydrated.

3. Provide Immediate Care:

   o   Hydration: Ensure the pet has access to fresh water to help combat dehydration. In severe cases, an electrolyte solution may be necessary.

   o   Comfort: Keep the pet comfortable and calm, reducing stress which can exacerbate symptoms.

4. Seek Veterinary Assistance:

   o   Contact a Veterinarian: If any signs of overdose are observed, contact a veterinarian immediately. Provide them with details about the amount of castor oil ingested and the symptoms exhibited by the pet.

   o   Follow Veterinary Advice: Follow the veterinarian's instructions carefully, which may include bringing the pet in for an examination or administering specific home treatments.

5. Emergency Measures:

   o   Activated Charcoal: In some cases, the veterinarian may recommend administering activated charcoal to help absorb the toxin and prevent further absorption in the gastrointestinal tract.

   o   Intravenous Fluids: For severe dehydration or poisoning, the vet might administer intravenous fluids to rehydrate the pet and stabilize their condition.

   o   Medication: The vet may prescribe medications to control symptoms like vomiting, diarrhea, or seizures.

6. Prevent Future Incidents:

   o   Proper Dosage: Always adhere to the recommended dosage guidelines for castor oil usage on pets. Use the lowest effective dose to minimize the risk of overdose.

   o   Safe Storage: Store castor oil and other medications out of reach of pets to prevent accidental ingestion.

o   Regular Monitoring: Regularly monitor pets when introducing new treatments to quickly identify any adverse reactions.

While castor oil has numerous benefits, it is crucial to use it responsibly to avoid potential risks, including overdose. Recognizing the signs of castor oil overdose and knowing the appropriate actions to take can significantly improve the outcomes for pets experiencing adverse effects. Always consult with a veterinarian before using castor oil or any new treatment on pets to ensure their safety and health.

Chapter 4: Remedies for skin problems

4.1 Treatment of dry and flaky skin

Dry and flaky skin, a common issue among pets, can lead to discomfort and health problems if not addressed. Understanding the underlying causes and implementing a combination of dietary, topical, and environmental strategies is key to restoring skin health. Castor oil, with its renowned moisturizing and healing properties, is a significant player in treating dry and flaky skin in pets.

A variety of factors can cause dry and flaky skin in pets:

Environmental Conditions

Low Humidity: Dry air, particularly in winter, can strip moisture from the skin, leading to dryness and flakiness.

Harsh Weather: Extreme temperatures, whether hot or cold, can adversely affect the skin's moisture levels.

Dietary Deficiencies

Lack of Essential Fatty Acids: Diets low in omega-3 and omega-6 fatty acids can lead to dry skin. These fatty acids are crucial for maintaining the skin's lipid barrier and retaining moisture.

Poor Nutrition: Inadequate nutrition or low-quality food can result in deficiencies of essential vitamins and minerals necessary for skin health.

Underlying Health Conditions

Allergies: Pets can develop allergies to food, pollen, dust, or flea bites, which can cause dry, itchy skin.

Parasites: Mites, fleas, and other parasites can irritate the skin, leading to dryness and flakiness.

Hormonal Imbalances: Conditions like hypothyroidism or Cushing's disease can affect the skin's health and appearance.

Inadequate Grooming

Infrequent Bathing: While too frequent bathing can strip natural oils, infrequent bathing can lead to a buildup of dead skin cells and dirt, contributing to dryness.

Improper Grooming Products: Using harsh shampoos or conditioners not designed for pets can irritate their skin.

Role of Castor Oil

Castor oil is a natural remedy that can help alleviate dry and flaky skin due to its unique properties, particularly its soothing nature. This can provide reassurance to pet owners, knowing that they are using a gentle and effective treatment.

Moisturizing: Castor oil is rich in ricinoleic acid, which acts as a humectant, attracting and retaining moisture in the skin.

Anti-inflammatory: Its anti-inflammatory properties can help soothe irritated skin and reduce redness and itching.

Antimicrobial: Castor oil's antimicrobial effects can help prevent and treat infections that might exacerbate dry skin conditions.

Healing: The oil promotes wound healing and skin regeneration, which can be beneficial for repairing damaged skin.

4.1.1 Application Methods

To treat dry and flaky skin with castor oil, consider the following methods:

1) Topical Application

Direct Application: Apply a small amount of castor oil directly to the affected areas. Gently massage the oil into the skin to ensure absorption.

Blended Treatments: Mix castor oil with other beneficial oils like coconut or olive oil to enhance its moisturizing effects. These oils can provide additional fatty acids and vitamins.

Homemade Balms: Create a soothing balm by mixing castor oil with beeswax and shea butter. This balm can provide a protective layer to lock in moisture and shield the skin from environmental irritants.

2) Bath Soaks:

Oil-Infused Bath: Add a few drops of castor oil to your pet's bath water. This can help moisturize the skin while your pet soaks. Ensure thorough rinsing to prevent any residual oil from irritating.

3) Dietary Supplementation

Consulting a veterinarian before adding castor oil to your pet's diet is crucial. While some sources recommend internal use, it's important to seek professional guidance to avoid potential side effects and ensure the treatment is safe and appropriate for your pet.

4) Regular Grooming

Gentle Shampoos: Use pet-friendly, moisturizing shampoos that contain natural ingredients like oatmeal or aloe vera. Avoid shampoos with harsh chemicals.

Brushing: Regular brushing helps remove dead skin cells and distributes natural oils across the coat, promoting healthier skin.

4.1.2 Additional Tips

Maintain Humidity: Use a humidifier in your home to maintain adequate moisture levels in the air, especially during dry seasons.

Hydration: Ensure your pet has access to fresh water at all times to stay hydrated, which supports overall skin health.

Ensuring your pet's diet is balanced and rich in essential fatty acids, vitamins, and minerals is crucial for maintaining healthy skin. Consider supplements like fish oil, known for its skin health benefits, to support your pet's skin health.

Treating dry and flaky skin in pets requires a multifaceted approach that includes proper nutrition, regular grooming, and natural remedies like castor oil. Understanding the causes and implementing effective treatment strategies can help restore your pet's skin to its healthy, comfortable state. Always consult a veterinarian before starting any new treatment to ensure it is safe and appropriate for your pet's needs.

4.2 Hot spot and itch management

Hot spots and itching are common skin problems in pets that can cause significant discomfort and distress. Proper management of these conditions involves understanding their causes, implementing effective treatment strategies, and taking preventive measures to maintain skin health. Castor oil, with its soothing and healing properties, can be valuable in managing hot spots and itching in pets.

Hot Spots

Hot spots, also known as acute moist dermatitis, are localized areas of inflamed and infected skin. They can appear suddenly and often spread rapidly. Common causes include:

Allergies: Pets can develop hot spots due to allergic reactions to food, environmental factors, or flea bites.

Parasites: Fleas, mites, and other parasites can irritate the skin, leading to scratching and subsequent hot spots.

Excessive Moisture: Moisture trapped under the coat, often from swimming or bathing, can create a breeding ground for bacteria.

Underlying Infections: Bacterial or fungal infections can cause or exacerbate hot spots.

Itching

Itching, or pruritus, can be caused by a variety of factors, including:

Allergies: Similar to hot spots, allergies to food, pollen, dust, or flea bites are common triggers.

Dry Skin: Environmental factors, poor nutrition, or frequent bathing can lead to dry, itchy skin.

Parasites: Fleas, ticks, and mites are common culprits that cause itching.

Infections: Bacterial or fungal infections can lead to persistent itching.

Role of Castor Oil

Castor oil can help manage hot spots and itching through its various beneficial properties:

Anti-inflammatory: Castor oil's anti-inflammatory properties help reduce swelling and irritation, providing relief from itching.

Antimicrobial: It has antimicrobial effects that can help prevent and treat infections caused by bacteria and fungi.

Moisturizing: The oil deeply moisturizes the skin, helping to repair dry and damaged skin and reducing the urge to scratch.

Healing: Castor oil promotes skin regeneration, which aids in the healing of hot spots and other skin lesions.

Application Methods

To effectively manage hot spots and itching with castor oil, consider the following methods:

Topical Application

Direct Application: Clean the affected area with a gentle, pet-safe cleanser. Apply a small amount of castor oil directly to the hot spot or itchy area. Massage gently to ensure the oil penetrates the skin.

Blended Treatments: Mix castor oil with soothing ingredients such as aloe vera gel or coconut oil. This blend can enhance the healing and moisturizing effects.

Homemade Sprays: Create a spray by diluting castor oil with water and a few drops of chamomile or lavender essential oil. This can be sprayed on the affected areas to provide relief.

Bath Soaks

Oil-Infused Bath: Add a few drops of castor oil to your pet's bath water. This can help moisturize the skin and soothe itching. Ensure thorough rinsing to prevent any residual oil from causing irritation.

Bandages and Wraps

Castor Oil Compress: Soak a clean cloth in warm water mixed with castor oil. Apply the compress to the affected area and cover it with a bandage. This can help keep the area moist and protected, promoting faster healing.

Additional Tips

Maintain Hygiene: Keep the affected areas clean and dry. Regular grooming helps to remove dirt, debris, and parasites from your pet's coat.

Prevent Licking: Use a pet cone or protective collar to prevent your pet from licking or scratching the treated areas, which can worsen the condition.

Monitor Diet: Ensure your pet's diet is balanced and rich in essential fatty acids, vitamins, and minerals to support overall skin health.

Consult a veterinarian: Always consult with a veterinarian before starting any new treatment to ensure it is safe and appropriate for your pet's specific condition.

Managing hot spots and itching in pets requires a comprehensive approach that includes proper hygiene, nutrition, and the use of effective natural remedies like castor oil. By understanding the causes and implementing appropriate treatment strategies, you can alleviate your pet's discomfort and promote healthy, itch-free skin. Always seek professional advice to tailor the treatment to your pet's specific needs and ensure their well-being.

4.3 Healing minor wounds and cuts

Minor wounds and cuts are expected in pets, often resulting from playful activities, rough terrain, or interactions with other animals. While these wounds typically don't require extensive medical intervention, proper care is essential to prevent infection and promote swift healing. With its unique properties, castor oil can play a crucial role in the natural treatment of minor wounds and cuts in pets.

4.3.1 Understanding Minor Wounds and Cuts

Minor wounds in pets can include:

Scratches: Often caused by rough surfaces, interactions with other animals, or even self-inflicted during scratching.

Abrasions: Shallow wounds caused by friction or scraping against a rough surface.

Cuts: Small incisions or tears in the skin, typically from sharp objects or playful bites.

4.3.2 Benefits of Castor Oil for Wound Healing

Castor oil has several properties that make it beneficial for treating minor wounds and cuts in pets:

Antimicrobial Properties: Castor oil has natural antimicrobial properties that help prevent infections by inhibiting the growth of bacteria and fungi in the wound.

Anti-inflammatory Effects: It reduces inflammation and swelling around the wound, which helps to alleviate pain and promote faster healing.

Moisturizing Agent: Castor oil keeps the wound site moist, preventing the formation of dry scabs that can delay healing and cause further irritation.

Promotes Healing: The oil stimulates the production of new tissue, aiding in the repair of the skin and expediting the healing process.

4.3.3 Application Methods

To effectively use castor oil for healing minor wounds and cuts in pets, follow these steps:

1) Cleaning the Wound

Gentle Cleansing: Before applying castor oil, ensure the wound is clean. Use a mild pet-safe antiseptic solution or saline water to gently clean the area, removing dirt, debris, or bacteria.

Pat Dry: Gently pat the area dry with a clean cloth or sterile gauze. Avoid rubbing, as this can irritate the wound further.

2) Applying Castor Oil

Direct Application: Apply a small amount of castor oil to the wound. Use a clean cotton swab or your finger (after washing your hands thoroughly) to spread the oil evenly over the affected area.

Blended Applications: For enhanced benefits, mix castor oil with a few drops of other healing oils, such as lavender or tea tree oil, which have additional antimicrobial and soothing properties. Ensure any additional oils are safe for pets and used inappropriate, diluted amounts.

3) Covering the Wound:

Bandaging: If the wound is in an area your pet can quickly lick or scratch, consider covering it with a clean, sterile bandage. This helps to protect the wound and keep the castor oil in place.

Regular Changes: Change the bandage daily or whenever it becomes dirty or wet. Reapply castor oil each time to maintain its healing benefits.

4) Monitoring and Follow-Up:

Check for Improvement: Monitor the wound regularly for signs of improvement, such as reduced swelling, less redness, and the beginning of skin regeneration.

Consult a veterinarian: If the wound shows signs of infection (increased redness, pus, foul odor) or does not improve within a few days, consult a veterinarian for further treatment.

4.3.4 Additional Tips for Wound Care

Prevent Licking and Scratching: Use an Elizabethan collar (e-collar) to prevent your pet from licking or scratching the wound, which can introduce bacteria and delay healing.

Maintain Hygiene: Keep the wound area and surrounding fur clean. Regular grooming can help prevent dirt and bacteria from accumulating near the wound.

Boost Immune System: Ensure your pet has a balanced diet rich in vitamins and minerals that support the immune system and overall health, which aids in faster healing.

Proper care of minor wounds and cuts is crucial for preventing infections and promoting quick pet recovery. With its antimicrobial, anti-inflammatory, and healing properties, Castor oil is an excellent natural remedy for treating these injuries. Following appropriate application methods and good hygiene, you can effectively manage your pet's minor wounds and cuts, ensuring their comfort and health. Always consult a veterinarian for persistent or severe wounds to provide the best care for your pet.

4.4 Alleviating the symptoms of allergies

Allergies in pets can cause significant discomfort, manifesting as itching, redness, swelling, and general irritation. Like humans, pets can suffer from various allergies due to environmental factors, food, or insect bites. Understanding the symptoms and finding effective relief is essential for maintaining your pet's well-being. Castor oil, known for its anti-inflammatory, antimicrobial, and soothing properties, can be an effective natural remedy to alleviate pet allergy symptoms.

Allergies in pets are triggered when their immune system reacts to usually harmless substances, such as pollen, dust, certain foods, or flea saliva. Common types of allergies in pets include:

Environmental Allergies: Caused by pollen, mold, dust mites, or other airborne allergens.

Food Allergies: Triggered by specific ingredients in a pet's diet, such as beef, dairy, wheat, or soy.

Flea Allergy Dermatitis: Caused by an allergic reaction to flea bites.

Contact Allergies: Result from direct contact with substances like certain shampoos, bedding, or cleaning products.

4.4.1 Symptoms of Allergies

The symptoms of allergies in pets can vary, but common signs include:

- Itching and Scratching: Persistent itching, especially around the face, paws, and ears.

- Redness and Inflammation: Swollen, red skin that may be warm to the touch.

- Hair Loss: Due to excessive scratching, licking, or biting.

- Ear Infections: Frequent shaking of the head, ear scratching, and discharge.

- Digestive Issues: Vomiting, diarrhea, or other gastrointestinal problems in the case of food allergies.

4.4.2 Benefits of Castor Oil for Allergy Relief

Castor oil can provide significant relief for allergy symptoms in pets due to its various beneficial properties:

- Anti-Inflammatory: Reduces inflammation and soothes irritated skin.

- Antimicrobial: Helps prevent secondary infections caused by scratching and open wounds.

- Moisturizing: Keeps the skin hydrated, preventing dryness and further irritation.

- Soothing: Provides a calming effect on the skin, reducing the urge to scratch.

4.4.3 Application Methods

Using castor oil to relieve allergy symptoms in pets involves several techniques to ensure effectiveness and safety:

1) Topical Application

Direct Application: Apply a small amount of castor oil directly to the affected area. Use a clean cotton swab or your fingers (washed thoroughly) to gently massage the oil into the skin. This helps reduce itching and inflammation.

Blended Oils: Mix castor oil with other pet-safe essential oils like lavender or chamomile, known for their soothing properties. Ensure proper dilution to avoid skin irritation.

2) Bath Soak

Oil-Infused Bath: Add a few drops of castor oil to your pet's bathwater. This method helps to cover larger areas affected by allergies and provides overall skin relief.

Epsom Salt and Castor Oil Bath: Combine Epsom salts with castor oil in the bathwater. Epsom salts have detoxifying properties that can help alleviate itching and inflammation.

3) Compresses

Warm Compress: Soak a clean cloth in warm water mixed with a few drops of castor oil and apply it to the affected area. The warmth helps open pores, allowing the oil to penetrate deeper and provide more effective relief.

Cold Compress: For immediate relief from severe itching or swelling, use a cold compress with castor oil. This helps to numb the area and reduce inflammation quickly.

4) Ear Care

Ear Cleaning: For pets with ear allergies, mix a few drops of castor oil with a pet-safe ear cleaner. Apply the mixture to a cotton ball and gently clean the inside of the ears, avoiding deep insertion.

4.4.4 Precautions and Safety

When using castor oil to relieve allergy symptoms in pets, it's important to follow these precautions:

- Patch Test: Always perform a patch test before applying castor oil extensively to ensure your pet does not have a negative reaction.

- Dilution: Properly dilute castor oil, especially when mixed with other essential oils, to avoid skin irritation.

- Veterinary Consultation: Consult your veterinarian before starting any new treatment to ensure it's suitable for your pet's specific condition.

- Monitor for Reactions: Observe your pet for any adverse reactions, such as increased redness, swelling, or discomfort. Discontinue use if any negative symptoms occur.

Allergies can significantly impact a pet's quality of life, but natural remedies like castor oil offer a safe and effective way to alleviate symptoms. By understanding the types of allergies and their symptoms, and applying castor oil correctly, pet owners can help their furry friends find relief from itching, inflammation, and discomfort. Always prioritize safety and consult with a veterinarian to ensure the best care for your pet.

Chapter 5: Castor oil for ear and eye care

5.1 Cleaning and soothing irritated ears

Cleaning and soothing irritated ears in pets is essential for their health and well-being. As a pet owner, being vigilant and proactive in detecting early signs of ear issues is crucial. Ear issues are common in pets, especially dogs and cats, and can stem from various causes such as infections, allergies, mites, or foreign objects. Symptoms like scratching, head shaking, redness, swelling, and discharge indicate that a pet's ears need attention. By detecting these signs early and providing proper ear care, you can prevent these issues from escalating into more severe problems.

Pets can experience ear problems due to several factors:

Infections: Bacterial or yeast infections are common causes of ear irritation. They can occur due to moisture buildup, allergies, or underlying health conditions.

Ear Mites: Tiny parasites in the ear canal, causing intense itching and discomfort.

Allergies: Environmental or food allergies can lead to ear inflammation and secondary infections.

Foreign Bodies: Objects like grass seeds or dirt can enter the ear, causing irritation and infection.

5.1.1 Benefits of Castor Oil for Ear Care

Castor oil, with its various beneficial properties, is an excellent natural remedy for cleaning and soothing irritated ears. It is antimicrobial, helping to eliminate bacteria and yeast, anti-inflammatory, reducing inflammation and swelling, moisturizing, keeping the ear canal hydrated, and soothing, calming the skin and reducing itching.

Antimicrobial: Helps to eliminate bacteria and yeast, preventing infections.

Anti-inflammatory: Reduces inflammation and swelling, providing relief from pain and discomfort.

Moisturizing: Keeps the ear canal hydrated, preventing dryness and irritation.

Soothing: Calms the skin, reducing itching and promoting healing.

5.1.2 Application Methods

Using castor oil to clean and soothe irritated ears involves several steps to ensure it's done safely and effectively:

1. Preparation:

- Clean Hands: Ensure your hands are thoroughly washed to prevent introducing additional bacteria into the ear.

- Materials: Gather necessary materials such as castor oil, a dropper, cotton balls, and a clean towel.

2. Application:

- Warm the Oil: Slightly warm the castor oil by placing the bottle in a bowl of warm water. This makes it more comfortable for the pet and helps it spread easily.

- Dropper Use: Fill a dropper with castor oil. Gently lift the pet's ear and apply a few drops into the ear canal. Avoid inserting the dropper too deeply to prevent injury.

- Massage: Gently massage the base of the ear for about 30 seconds to help the oil spread and loosen any debris.

3. Cleaning:

- Cotton Ball: Use a cotton ball to wipe away any excess oil and debris from the outer ear. Be gentle to avoid irritating the sensitive skin.

- Repeat if Necessary: If the ear is very dirty or inflamed, you may need to repeat the process over a few days.

4. Observation:

- Monitor: Keep an eye on the pet's ear for signs of improvement or any adverse reactions. Reduced scratching and head shaking, and a decrease in redness and discharge, are signs of healing.

- Consultation: If there is no improvement within a few days, or if the condition worsens, consult a veterinarian for further advice.

5.1.3 Precautions

While castor oil is generally safe for ear care, it's essential to take precautions:

Patch Test: Before extensive use, perform a patch test to ensure the pet does not have an allergic reaction to castor oil.

Proper Dilution: If combining castor oil with other oils, ensure proper dilution to avoid irritation.

Veterinary Guidance: Always consult with a veterinarian before starting any new treatment, especially if the pet has a history of ear problems.

In conclusion, regular ear cleaning and the soothing properties of castor oil can help maintain your pet's ear health, preventing infections and providing relief from irritation. Following these steps and taking appropriate precautions can ensure your pet's ears remain clean, healthy, and comfortable.

5.2 Treating ear infections

Ear infections in pets, especially dogs and cats, are common but can cause significant discomfort if not treated promptly. Recognizing the signs of an ear infection and knowing how to treat it effectively can ensure your pet's health and well-being. Symptoms of ear infections in pets often include excessive scratching, head shaking, redness, swelling, odor, and discharge. These infections can result from bacteria, yeast, mites, allergies, or foreign objects lodged in the ear canal.

5.2.1 Causes of Ear Infections

Ear infections in pets can stem from various causes:

Bacterial or Yeast Infections: These are the most common causes and often occur due to moisture buildup, allergies, or underlying health conditions.

Ear Mites: Tiny parasites in the ear canal, causing intense itching and inflammation.

Foreign Bodies: Objects such as grass seeds, dirt, or small insects can enter the ear canal, leading to infection.

Allergies: Food or environmental allergies can lead to chronic ear infections if not managed properly.

5.2.2 Benefits of Castor Oil for Treating Ear Infections

Castor oil can be a beneficial natural remedy for treating ear infections in pets due to its antimicrobial and anti-inflammatory properties:

Antimicrobial: Castor oil helps eliminate bacteria and yeast, common causes of ear infections.

Anti-inflammatory: It reduces inflammation and swelling, relieving pain and discomfort.

Soothing and Moisturizing: Castor oil helps soothe the irritated ear canal and keeps it moisturized, preventing further irritation.

5.2.3 Steps to Treat Ear Infections with Castor Oil

Treating an ear infection with castor oil involves careful and gentle application to ensure your pet's comfort and safety:

Preparation

Clean Hands: Always start by washing your hands thoroughly to prevent introducing new bacteria into the ear.

Materials Needed: Gather castor oil, a dropper, cotton balls, and a clean towel.

Application Process

Warm the Oil: Slightly warm the castor oil by placing the bottle in warm water to make the application more comfortable for your pet.

Using the Dropper: Fill a dropper with the warmed castor oil. Gently lift your pet's ear and carefully place a few drops into the ear canal. Avoid inserting the dropper too deeply to prevent injury.

Massaging the Ear: Gently massage the base of the ear for about 30 seconds. This helps the oil spread evenly and reach deep into the ear canal to combat the infection effectively.

Cleaning the Ear

Wipe Excess Oil: Use a cotton ball to gently remove excess oil and debris from the outer ear. Be gentle to avoid causing further irritation.

Repeat the Process: Depending on the severity of the infection, you may need to repeat this process daily until the symptoms improve.

Monitoring and Follow-up

Observe Symptoms: Keep a close eye on your pet's behavior and ear condition. Signs of improvement include reduced scratching and head shaking, less redness and swelling, and decreased discharge.

Veterinary Consultation: If there is no improvement within a few days or if the condition worsens, consult a veterinarian for further evaluation and treatment.

5.2.4 Precautions

While castor oil can be effective, it's essential to take precautions:

Patch Test: Before full application, perform a patch test to ensure your pet is not allergic to castor oil.

Proper Dilution: Ensure appropriate dilution if combining castor oil with other substances to avoid irritation.

Veterinary Advice: Always seek advice from a veterinarian before starting any new treatment, especially if your pet has a history of ear infections or other medical conditions.

In summary, castor oil can be a valuable natural remedy for treating ear infections in pets. By following these steps and taking necessary precautions, you can help alleviate your pet's discomfort and promote healing, ensuring their ears remain healthy and infection-free.

5.3 Using castor oil for eye infections and irritations

Using castor oil for eye infections and irritations is an age-old remedy known for its therapeutic properties. Castor oil, derived from the seeds of the Ricinus communis plant, contains ricinoleic acid, a potent anti-inflammatory and antimicrobial agent. These properties make it effective in alleviating symptoms associated with various eye conditions, including conjunctivitis (pink eye), dry eyes, and general eye irritation.

To use castor oil for eye infections, it's crucial to select a high-quality, cold-pressed castor oil that is free from additives or chemicals. Before application, ensure hands are thoroughly washed to prevent any potential contamination. Dispense a small amount of castor oil onto the clean fingertip or directly into the eye using a sterile dropper. It is recommended to apply the oil before bedtime to allow it to work overnight without interference.

Castor oil's soothing nature helps reduce redness and inflammation, providing relief from discomfort caused by eye infections. Its antimicrobial properties can also help combat bacteria or fungi contributing to the infection. However, caution should be exercised when applying castor oil near the eyes to avoid contact with the cornea and mucous membranes. If irritation persists or worsens after using castor oil, it is advisable to discontinue use and consult an eye care professional promptly.

For those prone to dry eyes or irritation from environmental factors like dust or allergens, using castor oil as an eye lubricant can help maintain moisture and soothe the delicate tissues around the eyes. Regular use may contribute to overall eye health by providing natural hydration and protection against oxidative stress.

While castor oil is considered safe for topical use around the eyes, individuals with sensitive skin or existing eye conditions should exercise caution and seek advice from a healthcare provider before starting any new treatment regimen. Proper application techniques and adherence to hygiene practices are essential to ensure the safety and effectiveness of using castor oil for eye infections and irritations.

5.4 Precautions for sensitive areas

When using castor oil on sensitive body areas, it's essential to exercise caution and adhere to proper application techniques to avoid potential adverse effects. Castor oil, derived from the seeds of the Ricinus communis plant, is renowned for its various therapeutic benefits, including moisturizing properties and anti-inflammatory effects. These benefits can bring hope and optimism to individuals with sensitive skin or specific skin conditions. However, due to its potent nature, specific precautions must be taken, especially when applying it to sensitive skin or delicate mucous membranes.

Skin Patch Test

Before applying castor oil to sensitive areas such as the face, underarms, or genital area, it's crucial to perform a skin patch test. This involves applying a small amount of diluted castor oil (mixed with a carrier oil like coconut or olive oil) to a small skin area, typically on the inner forearm. Monitor the area for at least 24 hours to check for any signs of irritation, redness, or allergic reactions. If adverse reactions occur, such as itching or swelling, discontinue use immediately and rinse the area thoroughly with water.

Dilution

Pure castor oil can be quite thick and potent, which may cause discomfort or irritation when applied directly to sensitive skin. Diluting castor oil with a carrier oil like almond or jojoba oil can help reduce its concentration while still providing the desired benefits. A general guideline is to mix one part castor oil with three parts of carrier oil to create a diluted mixture suitable for sensitive areas.

Avoiding Contact with Mucous Membranes

Castor oil should never be applied directly to mucous membranes such as the eyes, nose, or mouth. The oil's thick consistency and potential contaminants can lead to irritation, discomfort, or even infection if introduced into these sensitive areas. If accidental contact occurs, rinse thoroughly with water and seek medical attention if irritation persists.

Hygiene Practices

Maintaining good hygiene practices before applying castor oil to sensitive areas is essential to prevent infections or adverse reactions. Wash hands thoroughly with soap and water before and after application to minimize the risk of introducing bacteria or other contaminants to the skin. Clean, sterile applicators or cotton pads apply the oil to ensure sanitary conditions.

Consultation with Healthcare Provider

Individuals with pre-existing skin conditions such as eczema, psoriasis, or dermatitis should consult a healthcare provider before using castor oil on sensitive areas. Certain skin conditions may exacerbate using oils or require specific formulations tailored to the individual's needs.

Sun Sensitivity

Castor oil may increase the skin's sensitivity to sunlight, especially when applied to areas prone to sun exposure. To avoid potential sunburn or skin damage, it's advisable to apply castor oil in the evening or before bedtime and use sunscreen during the day if necessary.

Storage and Quality

Ensure that the castor oil used is high quality and stored in a cool, dark place to maintain its efficacy and prevent rancidity. Avoid using expired or improperly stored castor oil, as it may lose its therapeutic properties and increase the risk of skin irritation.

By following these precautions and guidelines, individuals can safely harness the benefits of castor oil for sensitive areas of the body. This reassurance about the safety of castor oil when used correctly should make you feel confident and reassured. It minimizes the risk of adverse reactions or discomfort. If unsure about the suitability of castor oil for specific skin concerns or conditions, consulting a healthcare provider or dermatologist is always recommended.

Chapter 6: Digestive health and detoxification

6.1 Remedies for constipation and digestive problems

Constipation and digestive issues can affect pets, causing discomfort and overall well-being. Natural remedies using castor oil can effectively alleviate these conditions in pets. Here are several safe and beneficial methods to help your pet find relief:

1) Castor Oil Massage

Gently massage a small amount of castor oil onto your pet's abdomen in a circular motion. This can help stimulate bowel movements and ease constipation.

2) Oral Administration

Mix a small amount of food-grade castor oil into your pet's food. Start with a small dosage and gradually increase if needed. Ensure the oil is well-mixed to avoid rejection by your pet.

3) Castor Oil Packs

Apply a warm castor oil pack to your pet's abdomen. Use a clean cloth soaked in warm castor oil, cover with plastic wrap, and place a warm towel over it. Leave it for about 15-20 minutes to help relieve constipation.

4) Hydration

Ensure your pet has access to fresh water at all times. Hydration is crucial for maintaining healthy digestion and preventing constipation.

5) Dietary Adjustments

Include fiber-rich foods in your pet's diet, such as pumpkin, sweet potatoes, and green leafy vegetables. These can help regulate bowel movements and improve digestion.

6) Regular Exercise

Encourage your pet to stay active through regular exercise. Physical activity helps stimulate the digestive system and can prevent constipation.

7) Probiotics

Consider adding probiotic supplements to your pet's diet. Probiotics promote healthy gut flora and can aid in digestion.

8) Consultation with a Veterinarian

If your pet experiences chronic constipation or digestive issues, consult a veterinarian for a comprehensive assessment and appropriate treatment plan.

Using these natural remedies alongside proper veterinary care can help alleviate constipation and promote healthy digestion in pets. Monitor your pet's response to these remedies and adjust as necessary to ensure their comfort and well-being."

6.2 Detoxification and improvement of liver function in pets

Detoxifying and improving liver function in pets is essential for their overall health and well-being. Castor oil can be a beneficial natural remedy to support liver health in pets. Here are several effective methods to help enhance liver function and detoxify your pet:

Castor Oil Packs

Apply a warm castor oil pack over your pet's liver area. Use a soft cloth soaked in warm castor oil, cover with plastic wrap, and place a warm towel over it. Leave it for about 15-20 minutes to allow the oil's nutrients to penetrate and support liver detoxification.

Oral Administration

Mix a small amount of food-grade castor oil into your pet's food. Start with a conservative dosage and gradually increase as recommended by your veterinarian. This method helps stimulate bile flow and support the liver's detoxification processes.

Incorporating Castor Oil into Diet

Add castor oil to your pet's diet by mixing a small amount into their food. Ensure the oil is well-mixed to prevent rejection. The fatty acids in castor oil can aid in eliminating toxins from the liver and improving overall digestive health.

Herbal Support

Combine castor oil with herbal supplements for supporting liver health, such as milk thistle and dandelion root. These herbs contain antioxidants and anti-inflammatory properties that promote liver detoxification and regeneration.

Hydration

Ensure your pet has access to clean, fresh water at all times. Proper hydration is crucial for supporting liver function and flushing out toxins from the body.

Regular Exercise

Encourage your pet to engage in regular physical activity to promote circulation and aid in detoxification processes. Exercise helps stimulate metabolism and enhances overall liver function.

Consultation with a Veterinarian

Consult a veterinarian before incorporating castor oil or any new remedy into your pet's routine. They can provide guidance on appropriate dosages and ensure that the remedy is safe and effective for your pet's specific health needs.

Monitoring and Adjustments

Observe your pet's response to castor oil and other detoxification methods. Monitor their behavior, appetite, and overall well-being to make adjustments as necessary to support optimal liver function.

Incorporating these natural methods into your pet's care routine can help detoxify its liver and improve overall health. Always prioritize your pet's safety and consult a veterinarian for personalized recommendations.

6.3 Support healthy digestion with castor oil

Supporting healthy digestion in pets is crucial for their overall well-being and vitality. Castor oil, known for its therapeutic properties, can play a beneficial role in promoting digestive health in pets through various methods:

Oral Administration: adding a small amount of castor oil to your pet's food can aid in lubricating the digestive tract and promoting regular bowel movements. Start with a conservative dosage and gradually increase under the guidance of your veterinarian.

Relief for Constipation: Castor oil is a gentle yet effective solution for pets struggling with constipation. It works by stimulating smooth muscle contractions in the intestines, aiding in the movement of stool along the digestive tract. Administering a small amount mixed with food can provide much-needed relief for your pet.

Anti-inflammatory Properties: the ricinoleic acid in castor oil exhibits anti-inflammatory effects, which can help reduce inflammation in the gastrointestinal tract. This property mainly benefits pets suffering from digestive disorders like gastritis or inflammatory bowel disease (IBD).

Laxative Effect: castor oil acts as a natural laxative for pets when administered appropriately. It helps soften stool and facilitates easier passage through the intestines, relieving discomfort associated with constipation.

Promoting Gut Health: incorporating castor oil into your pet's diet can contribute to maintaining a healthy balance of gut flora. It supports beneficial bacteria in the intestines, which aids in proper digestion and nutrient absorption.

Detoxification: castor oil aids in detoxifying the digestive system by helping to eliminate toxins and waste products from the body. This detoxification process can improve overall digestive function and promote a healthier gastrointestinal environment for your pet.

Hydration and Lubrication: ensuring your pet stays hydrated is essential for supporting digestion. Castor oil's lubricating properties help maintain moisture in the intestinal lining, preventing dryness and facilitating smoother passage of stool.

Support for Senior Pets: older pets may experience age-related digestive issues such as reduced motility and constipation. Castor oil can be a gentle yet effective remedy to alleviate these symptoms and support digestive health in senior pets.

Herbal Combinations: combining castor oil with herbs known for their digestive benefits, such as ginger or slippery elm, can enhance its effectiveness in promoting healthy digestion in pets. These herbs provide additional support for reducing inflammation and soothing digestive discomfort.

Professional consultation: Before incorporating castor oil or any new supplement into your pet's diet, it's crucial to consult with a veterinarian. Their expertise can provide personalized recommendations based on your pet's age, health status, and digestive needs, empowering you to make informed decisions about your pet's health.

Observation and Adjustment: It's important to monitor your pet's response to castor oil and adjust the dosage as needed. Keep an eye on their bowel movements, appetite, and overall well-being to ensure the treatment is effective and well-tolerated. This level of care and attention is crucial for your pet's health.

By incorporating castor oil into your pet's care regimen under veterinary guidance, you can help support healthy digestion and alleviate digestive issues such as constipation or inflammation. Prioritize your pet's health and well-being by choosing natural remedies that promote digestive health effectively and safely.

While castor oil can be beneficial for pets, it's important to be aware of potential risks associated with its use. Here are several key considerations to keep in mind when considering internal use of castor oil for pets:

Consultation with a Veterinarian

Before administering castor oil internally to your pet, it's crucial to consult with a veterinarian. They can guide the appropriate dosage, frequency of administration, and suitability based on your pet's health condition, age, and breed.

Quality and Purity

Ensure you use high-quality, cold-pressed castor oil specifically formulated for pets. Avoid using industrial-grade or impure castor oil, as these may contain harmful additives or contaminants that can be toxic to pets.

Dosage and Administration

The dosage of castor oil for pets varies depending on factors such as weight, age, and health condition. Always follow the veterinarian's recommendations for dosage and administration method. Typically, castor oil is administered orally by mixing a small amount with food or directly into the pet's mouth.

Start with Small Amounts

When introducing castor oil internally for the first time, start with a small amount to assess your pet's tolerance and response. Gradually increase the dosage as the veterinarian recommends, monitoring for adverse effects.

Monitoring for Side Effects

Keep a close eye on your pet's behavior, appetite, and bowel movements after administering castor oil. While castor oil is generally considered safe when used appropriately, some pets may experience mild gastrointestinal upset, such as diarrhea or abdominal discomfort. If any adverse reactions occur, discontinue use and consult your veterinarian.

Avoid Prolonged Use

Long-term or excessive use of castor oil internally may lead to dependency on laxative effects and disrupt normal bowel function in pets. Under veterinary supervision, use castor oil intermittently as needed for specific digestive issues.

Interaction with Medications

Certain medications or health conditions may interact with castor oil when used internally. Inform your veterinarian about any ongoing medications or health issues your pet may have to avoid potential interactions or complications.

Storage and Handling

Store castor oil in a cool, dry place away from direct sunlight and out of reach of pets and children. Proper storage helps maintain its potency and prevents contamination.

Alternative Treatment Options

Consider alternative natural remedies or therapies for your pet's digestive issues, depending on their needs and health status. Your veterinarian can recommend suitable alternatives or complementary treatments.

Pet-Specific Formulations

Some pet care products may contain castor oil in formulations specifically designed for internal use. These products are formulated with pet safety and efficacy in mind, making them safer than using human-grade castor oil.

Educational Resources

Stay informed about the latest research and recommendations regarding the use of castor oil for pets. Educate yourself on proper administration techniques and potential risks associated with internal use to make informed decisions about your pet's health.

By adhering to these safety considerations and seeking guidance from a veterinarian, you can effectively and safely use castor oil internally to support your pet's digestive health when necessary. Prioritize your pet's safety and well-being by using natural remedies responsibly under professional guidance.

Chapter 7: Relieving joint and muscle pain

7.1 Benefits of castor oil for arthritis and joint pain

Castor oil can offer several benefits for pets suffering from arthritis and joint pain, providing a natural and gentle approach to alleviate discomfort and support overall joint health. Here are the key benefits of using castor oil for arthritis and joint pain in pets:

Anti-inflammatory Properties

Castor oil contains ricinoleic acid, a potent anti-inflammatory compound that helps reduce inflammation in joints affected by arthritis. By applying castor oil topically or administering it orally, pet owners can help alleviate swelling, stiffness, and pain associated with arthritis.

Pain Relief

Castor oil's soothing properties can relieve joint pain in pets. When massaged onto the affected joints, castor oil promotes blood circulation and reduces pain sensitivity, allowing pets to move more comfortably and with less pain.

Moisturizing and Lubricating

Castor oil is a natural moisturizer and lubricant for joints, enhancing flexibility and mobility. It helps maintain joint fluidity and reduces friction between bones, which benefits pets experiencing stiffness or limited mobility due to arthritis.

Promotes Healing

Regular application of castor oil can promote healing of damaged tissues and cartilage in arthritic joints. The oil's emollient properties penetrate the skin and joints deeply, nourishing tissues and supporting their repair over time.

Improves Circulation

Massaging castor oil onto the affected areas improves blood circulation, which helps deliver nutrients and oxygen to the joints. Enhanced circulation supports joint health by reducing inflammation and promoting healing processes.

Natural Analgesic

Castor oil has mild analgesic properties, relieving pain without the side effects of conventional pain medications. This makes it a safer option for long-term use in chronic pain conditions like arthritis in pets.

Antioxidant Benefits

Castor oil's antioxidants help neutralize free radicals that contribute to joint damage and inflammation. By reducing oxidative stress, castor oil supports joint health and minimizes further cartilage degeneration.

Safe and Gentle

Castor oil is generally safe for pets when used externally or orally in appropriate amounts. It is well-tolerated by most pets and does not pose significant risks of adverse effects, making it a suitable choice for pets with sensitive digestive systems or those prone to medication side effects.

Ease of Application

Applying castor oil to affected joints is simple and can be incorporated into regular pet care routines. Pet owners can gently massage a small amount of castor oil onto the pet's joints or mix it with their food under veterinary guidance.

Complementary Therapy

Castor oil can complement conventional veterinary treatments for arthritis in pets, providing additional relief and supporting overall joint health. Integrating natural remedies like castor oil into a comprehensive treatment plan may reduce the reliance on prescription medications alone.

Cost-Effective

Compared to prescription medications and therapies, castor oil is cost-effective and readily available. It offers pet owners an affordable alternative for managing arthritis symptoms while promoting their pet's well-being.

Castor oil's anti-inflammatory, pain-relieving, and healing properties make it a beneficial natural remedy for arthritis and joint pain in pets. When used responsibly and under veterinary guidance, castor oil can help improve mobility, reduce discomfort, and enhance the quality of life for pets suffering from arthritis. Integrating castor oil into a holistic approach to pet care supports joint health and contributes to a healthier, happier pet overall.

7.2 Massaging techniques for pets

Massaging techniques for pets can benefit their physical health and emotional well-being, promoting relaxation, circulation, and muscle flexibility. Here are some effective techniques and considerations for massaging pets:

1) Start with a Calm Environment

Choose a quiet and comfortable space where your pet feels relaxed and secure. Minimize distractions such as loud noises or sudden movements that could startle them during the massage.

2) Observe Your Pet's Reaction

Before starting the massage, observe your pet's body language and reactions. Ensure they are calm and receptive to touch. If your pet shows signs of discomfort or agitation, postpone the massage for another time.

3) Gentle Touch

To begin the massage, use gentle and slow strokes. Start with light pressure and gradually increase it as your pet becomes more accustomed to the touch. Avoid applying excessive force or pressure, especially over bony areas or joints.

4) Choose a Suitable Oil

Opt for a pet-safe oil like coconut or almond oil for the massage. These oils provide lubrication and help your hands glide smoothly over your pet's fur without irritating. Avoid using essential or scented oils that may be harmful to pets if ingested or absorbed through the skin.

7.2.1 Techniques for Different Areas

Back and Shoulders

Use long, gentle strokes along your pet's back and shoulders. This can help relax tense muscles and improve circulation.

Neck and Head

Use circular motions with your fingertips around the neck and head area. Be gentle around sensitive areas like the ears and eyes.

Legs and Paws

Massage each leg and paw individually, using small circular motions. Pay attention to the joints and muscles, providing gentle pressure to relieve stiffness.

Abdomen

Use light, clockwise circular motions on your pet's abdomen. This can aid in digestion and relieve discomfort from gas or bloating.

Watch for Feedback

Throughout the massage, observe your pet's response. Signs of enjoyment may include relaxed posture, soft purring (for cats), or a calm demeanor. If your pet seems uncomfortable or tries to move away, respect their boundaries and stop the massage.

Duration and Frequency

A pet massage session should typically last 5 to 15 minutes, depending on your pet's size and temperament. Start with shorter sessions and gradually increase the duration as your pet becomes more accustomed to the massage. Aim for regular sessions, such as once or twice weekly, to maintain the benefits.

Bonding Opportunity

Massaging your pet benefits their physical health and strengthens the bond between you and your furry companion. Use the massage as a time to connect with your pet through gentle touch and soothing interactions.

7.2.2 Special Considerations

- o Senior Pets: Older pets may have joint stiffness or arthritis. Use gentle, supportive strokes to improve mobility and reduce discomfort.

- o Anxious Pets: If your pet is anxious or fearful, introduce massage gradually and ensure they feel safe throughout the session.

o   Injured Pets: Avoid massaging directly over wounds or areas of recent injury. Consult with your veterinarian before administering massage therapy to pets recovering from surgery or serious injuries.

Consider consulting a professional pet massage therapist or veterinarian, especially if your pet has specific health conditions or if you're new to pet massage techniques. They can provide personalized advice and ensure the massage is safe and effective for your pet's needs.

7.3 DIY recipes for pain-relieving balms

1) Basic Pain Relief Balm

- Ingredients:

    o   1/2 cup coconut oil

    o   1/4 cup beeswax pellets

    o   2 tablespoons shea butter

    o   20 drops of peppermint essential oil

    o   15 drops of eucalyptus essential oil

    o   10 drops of lavender essential oil

- Instructions:

1.   In a double boiler, melt the coconut oil, beeswax pellets, and shea butter over low heat until fully melted and combined.

2.   Remove from heat and let it cool slightly.

3.   Add the essential oils and stir well.

4.   Pour the mixture into clean containers, such as lip balm tubes or small jars.

5.   Allow the balm to cool and solidify completely before use. Apply as needed to areas of discomfort.

2) Anti-Inflammatory Balm

- Ingredients:

    o   1/2 cup olive oil

    o   1/4 cup beeswax pellets

    o   2 tablespoons cocoa butter

    o   15 drops of ginger essential oil

    o   10 drops of turmeric essential oil

- 10 drops of frankincense essential oil

- Instructions:

1. Heat the olive oil, beeswax pellets, and cocoa butter in a double boiler until melted and well combined.

2. Remove from heat and allow it to cool slightly.

3. Add the ginger, turmeric, and frankincense essential oils. Stir thoroughly.

4. Pour the mixture into clean containers and let it cool completely before sealing.

5. Apply the balm to inflamed or sore areas, massaging gently for absorption.

3) Muscle Relaxing Balm

- Ingredients:
  - 1/2 cup shea butter
  - 1/4 cup coconut oil
  - 1/4 cup beeswax pellets
  - 15 drops of peppermint essential oil
  - 10 drops of lavender essential oil
  - 10 drops of chamomile essential oil
- Instructions:

1. Melt the shea butter, coconut oil, and beeswax pellets in a double boiler until fully melted and combined.

2. Remove from heat and let it cool slightly.

3. Add the peppermint, lavender, and chamomile essential oils. Mix well.

4. Pour the mixture into clean containers and allow it to solidify at room temperature.

5. Massage the balm onto tired or sore muscles for relaxation and relief.

4) Joint Pain Relief Balm

- Ingredients:
  - 1/2 cup almond oil
  - 1/4 cup beeswax pellets
  - 2 tablespoons cocoa butter
  - 15 drops of rosemary essential oil

      o   10 drops of juniper berry essential oil

      o   10 drops of marjoram essential oil

- Instructions:

1. Heat the almond oil, beeswax pellets, and cocoa butter in a double boiler until melted and well combined.

2. Remove from heat and allow it to cool slightly.

3. Add the rosemary, juniper berry, and marjoram essential oils. Stir thoroughly.

4. Pour the mixture into clean containers and let it cool completely before using.

5. Apply the balm to joints affected by pain or stiffness, massaging gently for relief.

5) Headache Relief Balm

- Ingredients:

      o   1/2 cup coconut oil

      o   1/4 cup beeswax pellets

      o   2 tablespoons mango butter

      o   15 drops of peppermint essential oil

      o   10 drops of lavender essential oil

      o   5 drops of eucalyptus essential oil

- Instructions:

1. Melt the coconut oil, beeswax pellets, and mango butter in a double boiler until fully melted and combined.

2. Remove from heat and let it cool slightly.

3. Add the peppermint, lavender, and eucalyptus essential oils. Mix well.

4. Pour the mixture into clean containers and allow it to solidify at room temperature.

5. Apply a small amount to the temples and back of the neck for headache relief.

Chapter 8: Parasite control

8.1 Natural remedies for flea and tick prevention

Castor oil is a natural remedy for flea and tick prevention. It offers effective protection without the use of harsh chemicals, promoting pet health and safety.

1) Castor Oil Spray

Creating a natural repellent spray with castor oil is a simple process. Just mix 2 tablespoons of castor oil with 1 quart of water in a spray bottle, shake well, and lightly mist your pet's coat. Repeat every few days or as needed, especially before outdoor activities. The pungent smell of castor oil effectively deters fleas and ticks from your pet's fur.

2) Castor Oil and Essential Oil Blend

Combine 1 tablespoon of castor oil with a few drops of essential oils known for their insect-repellent properties, such as lavender, cedarwood, or eucalyptus. Mix well and apply a small amount to your pet's collar or a bandana. Ensure the essential oils are pet-safe and avoid using them directly on the skin without dilution.

3) Castor Oil Flea Collar

Make a natural flea collar by saturating a fabric collar with castor oil. Allow the collar to dry completely before putting it on your pet. Reapply castor oil as needed to maintain effectiveness.

4) Castor Oil and Coconut Oil Rub

Mix equal parts of castor oil and coconut oil to create a soothing and repellent rub. Rub a small amount into your hands and massage it gently onto your pet's fur, focusing on areas where fleas and ticks are likely to hide. This mixture helps moisturize the skin while repelling pests.

5) Castor Oil Bath

Add a few drops of castor oil to your pet's regular shampoo or mix it with water for a final rinse after bathing. This helps to repel fleas and ticks while conditioning your pet's coat. Ensure thorough rinsing to avoid leaving residue that could attract dirt.

8.2 Treating and preventing mange and mites

Mange and mites are common parasitic conditions that can affect pets, causing discomfort and potentially leading to skin infections if left untreated. Castor oil, known for its antimicrobial and anti-inflammatory properties, can be an effective natural remedy for managing these conditions in pets.

1) Topical Application

Create a soothing castor oil blend by mixing it with a carrier oil like coconut or olive oil. Apply this mixture directly to the affected areas of the pet's skin using a gentle massage. The oil helps alleviate itching and irritation while moisturizing the skin and promoting healing.

2) Ear Treatment

For mange affecting ears, gently massage a few drops of warm castor oil into the ear canal. This can help suffocate mites and soothe any inflammation or irritation. Ensure the oil is at a comfortable temperature to prevent discomfort.

3) Bathing Solution

Add a few tablespoons of castor oil to a pet-friendly shampoo and use it during baths. This cleanses the fur and moisturizes the skin, reducing the symptoms of mange and mites.

4) Environment Control

Regularly clean the pet's living environment, including bedding and areas where they spend time. Dusting these areas with castor oil and water can help repel mites and prevent their spread.

5) Internal Use

For any internal use of castor oil, it's crucial to consult a veterinarian. They can provide advice on the appropriate dosage and application methods, ensuring the pet's immune function and overall health are supported, potentially aiding in the prevention of mange and mites.

6) Preventative Measures

Regular grooming and good hygiene practices are essential for pets. Diluted castor oil spray applied to pets before outdoor activities can prevent mites and fleas.

7) Consultation

If the pet shows persistent symptoms or discomfort, it's crucial to consult a veterinarian for a comprehensive diagnosis and treatment plan. They can guide appropriate dosages and application methods tailored to the pet's specific needs.

By incorporating these castor oil-based remedies into a pet's care routine, it's possible to effectively manage and prevent mange and mites, promoting their overall well-being and comfort.

8.3 Castor oil blends for parasite control

1) Castor Oil and Tea Tree Oil Spray

- **Ingredients:**
    - 2 tablespoons castor oil
    - 10 drops tea tree essential oil
    - 1 cup water

- **Instructions:**

1. Mix castor oil and tea tree oil in a spray bottle.

2. Add water and shake well before each use.

3. Spray directly on affected areas of the pet's coat, avoiding eyes and mouth.

4. Reapply as needed.

2) Castor Oil and Lavender Oil Repellent

- **Ingredients:**
    - 2 tablespoons castor oil
    - 10 drops lavender essential oil
    - 1/2 cup coconut oil (optional)

- **Instructions:**

1. Mix castor oil and lavender oil in a bowl.

2. Add coconut oil if desired for a thicker consistency.

3. Apply a small amount to your pet's fur, focusing on areas prone to pests.

4. Use daily or as needed.

3) Castor Oil, Neem Oil, and Lemon Eucalyptus Blend

- **Ingredients:**
    - 1 tablespoon castor oil
    - 5 drops neem oil
    - 5 drops lemon eucalyptus essential oil

- **Instructions:**

1. Combine all oils in a small bowl.

2. Mix thoroughly and apply a small amount to your hands.

3. Gently rub the blend onto your pet's fur, especially around the neck, ears, and tail.

4. Repeat weekly for prevention.

4) Castor Oil and Peppermint Oil Mixture

- **Ingredients:**
    - 2 tablespoons castor oil
    - 10 drops peppermint essential oil
    - 1/2 cup apple cider vinegar

- **Instructions:**

1. Mix castor oil and peppermint oil in a bowl.

2. Add apple cider vinegar and blend thoroughly.

3. Apply the mixture to a cloth and wipe it over your pet's fur, focusing on legs and belly.

4. Use caution near sensitive areas and avoid direct contact with eyes.

5) Castor Oil, Geranium Oil, and Cedarwood Oil Spray

- **Ingredients:**
    - 2 tablespoons castor oil
    - 5 drops geranium essential oil
    - 5 drops cedarwood essential oil
    - 1 cup distilled water

- **Instructions:**

1. Combine castor oil and essential oils in a spray bottle.

2. Add distilled water and shake well before use.

3. Spray lightly on your pet's fur, rubbing in with your hands.

4. Use daily during peak pest seasons.

Chapter 9: Enhancing coat health

9.1 Promoting a shiny and healthy coat

Promoting a shiny and healthy coat in pets is essential for their well-being and appearance. Castor oil can play a significant role in achieving this through its moisturizing and nourishing properties. Here's how castor oil can be beneficial and some practical ways to use it:

9.1.1 Benefits of Castor Oil for Pet's Coat

Moisturizing: Castor oil is rich in fatty acids that deeply penetrate the skin and coat, providing hydration and preventing dryness. This helps in maintaining a smooth and shiny appearance.

Nourishing: The nutrients in castor oil, including vitamin E, proteins, and minerals, nourish the hair follicles and strengthen the hair shafts, promoting healthy growth and reducing breakage.

Anti-inflammatory: Castor oil has anti-inflammatory properties that can help soothe irritated skin and reduce itching, which often leads to a healthier coat.

Antimicrobial: It also possesses antimicrobial properties, which can help combat fungal or bacterial infections that may affect the skin and coat.

9.1.2 Practical Applications of Castor Oil for a Shiny and Healthy Coat

Topical Application

Coat Conditioning: Mix a small amount of castor oil with your pet's shampoo during bath time. Ensure thorough rinsing to avoid any residue.

Leave-in Treatment: Dilute castor oil with a carrier oil like coconut or olive oil and massage it into your pet's coat. Leave it on for several hours or overnight before bathing.

Regular Grooming

*Brushing:*Apply a few drops of castor oil to a brush and gently groom your pet's fur. This helps distribute the oil evenly and stimulates blood circulation to the skin.

Paw and Pad Care: For dogs and cats with dry or cracked paw pads, massage a small amount of castor oil into the pads to soften and protect them.

Health Supplements

*Internal Use:*Consult with a veterinarian before giving castor oil internally to your pet. Small amounts may be added to food as a dietary supplement to support skin health from the inside out.

DIY Castor Oil Blends

Coconut and Castor Oil Blend: Mix equal parts of coconut and castor oil. Apply a small amount to your hands and rub it gently into your pet's fur.

Olive Oil and Castor Oil Mixture: Combine olive oil and castor oil in equal proportions. Massage into the coat, paying attention to dry or rough areas.

Precautions

Always perform a patch test on a small area of your pet's skin before complete application to ensure they do not have any adverse reactions.

Avoid applying castor oil near your pet's eyes, mouth, or sensitive areas unless directed by a veterinarian.

If your pet shows signs of discomfort or irritation after using castor oil, discontinue use and consult with a veterinarian.

By incorporating castor oil into your pet's grooming routine, you can enhance the health and appearance of their coat. Consistency is key, so use these methods regularly to maintain a shiny, healthy coat and keep your pet feeling their best.

9.2 Prevention and treatment of dandruff

Preventing and treating dandruff in pets is crucial for maintaining their skin health and comfort. Dandruff, characterized by dry, flaky skin and often accompanied by itching, can be caused by various factors such as allergies, skin infections, diet deficiencies, or environmental factors. Castor oil, known for its moisturizing and nourishing properties, can effectively help prevent and manage dandruff in pets.

Causes of Dandruff in Pets

Dry Skin: Insufficient moisture in the skin can lead to flakiness and dandruff formation.

Allergies: Allergic reactions to food, environmental allergens, or certain grooming products can contribute to skin irritation and dandruff.

Parasites: Fleas, mites, or other parasites can irritate the skin, leading to dandruff as a secondary symptom.

Infections: Bacterial or fungal infections can disrupt the skin's natural balance, causing dandruff and discomfort.

Benefits of Castor Oil for Treating Dandruff

Moisturizing: Castor oil is rich in fatty acids that deeply penetrate the skin, providing hydration and preventing dryness, which helps alleviate dandruff.

Anti-inflammatory: It has natural anti-inflammatory properties that can help soothe irritated skin and reduce itching, common symptoms associated with dandruff.

Antimicrobial: Castor oil's antimicrobial properties can help combat fungal or bacterial infections on the skin, addressing underlying causes of dandruff.

Nourishing: The nutrients in castor oil, including vitamin E and proteins, nourish the skin and coat, promoting overall skin health and reducing flakiness.

Practical Applications of Castor Oil for Dandruff Treatment

1. Topical Application:

   o *Direct Application:* Apply a small amount of castor oil directly onto your pet's dry or flaky skin patches. Gently massage it into the skin to ensure absorption.

   o *Oil Blend:* Mix castor oil with a carrier oil like coconut or olive oil in equal parts. Apply this blend to your pet's coat and skin, focusing on areas prone to dandruff.

2. Bath Time Solutions:

   o *Shampoo Additive:* Add a few drops of castor oil to your pet's regular shampoo during bath time. Ensure thorough rinsing to remove any residue.

   o *Leave-in Conditioner:* Dilute castor oil with water and spray it onto your pet's coat as a leave-in conditioner after bathing.

3. Regular Grooming:

   o *Brushing:* Use a brush or comb to distribute a small amount of castor oil throughout your pet's fur. This helps moisturize the skin and reduce flakiness.

4. Health Supplements:

   o *Internal Use:* Consult with a veterinarian before administering castor oil internally to your pet. Small amounts may be added to food as a dietary supplement to support skin health from the inside out.

5. Preventative Measures:

   o Ensure your pet's diet includes essential fatty acids and nutrients that promote skin health.

   o Regular grooming and hygiene practices can help prevent dandruff and maintain a healthy coat.

Precautions

- Always perform a patch test on a small area of your pet's skin before full application to check for any adverse reactions.

- Avoid applying castor oil near your pet's eyes, mouth, or sensitive areas unless directed by a veterinarian.

- If dandruff persists or worsens despite using castor oil, consult with a veterinarian to rule out underlying health conditions.

By incorporating castor oil into your pet's grooming routine and overall care, you can effectively prevent and manage dandruff, promoting a healthier skin and coat. Consistency in application and addressing potential underlying causes are key to achieving long-term relief from dandruff in pets.

9.3 DIY conditioning treatments

Creating DIY conditioning treatments for pets using castor oil can be a beneficial way to promote a healthy coat and skin. These treatments utilize castor oil's moisturizing and nourishing properties to address dryness, flakiness, and overall coat health. Here are several effective DIY conditioning treatments that you can prepare for your pet:

Castor Oil and Coconut Oil Blend:

- Combine equal parts of castor oil and coconut oil in a bowl.
- Mix thoroughly until well blended.
- Apply the mixture to your pet's clean, dry coat, focusing on areas prone to dryness or flakiness.
- Gently massage the oil into the skin and coat to ensure even distribution.
- Allow the mixture to sit for at least 20-30 minutes before rinsing thoroughly with lukewarm water.
- This blend helps moisturize the skin, reduce flakiness, and promote a shiny coat.

Castor Oil and Olive Oil Mask:

- Mix 1 tablespoon of castor oil with 2 tablespoons of olive oil in a small bowl.
- Stir well until the oils are thoroughly combined.
- Apply the mixture to your pet's coat and gently massage it into the skin.
- Cover your pet with a towel or cloth to prevent them from licking the oil.
- Leave the mask on for about 30 minutes to an hour to allow the oils to penetrate the skin and coat.
- Rinse off with lukewarm water and shampoo if necessary.
- This mask helps hydrate the skin, improve coat texture, and reduce dandruff.

Castor Oil and Aloe Vera Gel Treatment:

- Mix 1 tablespoon of castor oil with 1 tablespoon of pure aloe vera gel in a bowl.
- Blend the ingredients until they form a smooth paste.
- Apply the mixture to your pet's coat, focusing on areas that need extra conditioning.
- Massage gently to ensure the mixture reaches the skin.

- Leave it on for 20-30 minutes before rinsing thoroughly with lukewarm water.

- Aloe vera gel soothes irritated skin, while castor oil provides deep moisturization and nourishment.

Castor Oil and Honey Conditioning Mask:

- Combine 1 tablespoon of castor oil with 1 tablespoon of raw honey in a bowl.

- Mix well until the ingredients are thoroughly combined.

- Apply the mixture to your pet's clean coat, focusing on dry or flaky areas.

- Massage gently to promote absorption and circulation.

- Allow the mask to sit for 20-30 minutes before rinsing off with lukewarm water.

- Honey is a natural humectant that attracts moisture to the skin, complementing the moisturizing properties of castor oil.

Castor Oil and Yogurt Treatment:

- Mix 1 tablespoon of castor oil with 2 tablespoons of plain yogurt in a bowl.

- Stir until the ingredients are well blended.

- Apply the mixture to your pet's coat and gently massage it into the skin.

- Leave it on for 20-30 minutes before rinsing thoroughly with lukewarm water.

- Yogurt contains probiotics and enzymes that can help nourish the skin and promote a healthy coat, while castor oil provides essential fatty acids for moisturization.

Application Tips

- Before applying any DIY conditioning treatment, ensure your pet's coat is clean and free from dirt or debris.

- Use lukewarm water for rinsing as it helps to effectively remove the oil without leaving a residue.

- Monitor your pet during the treatment to prevent them from licking or ingesting the oils, especially if they have sensitive skin or allergies.

DIY conditioning treatments using castor oil offer a natural and effective way to enhance your pet's coat health, address dryness and flakiness, and promote overall skin wellness. These treatments can be tailored to your pet's specific needs and provide a soothing and nourishing experience for their skin and coat. Regular use of these treatments can help maintain a healthy and shiny coat, ensuring your pet looks and feels their best.

9.4 Routine care and maintenance

Routine care and maintenance for pets is crucial to ensure their overall health and well-being. Incorporating castor oil into their care regimen can offer various benefits, from maintaining skin hydration to promoting coat shine and addressing minor skin issues. Here are some essential tips and practices for routine care and maintenance using castor oil.

1) Regular Brushing and Grooming

Brushing your pet's coat regularly helps distribute natural oils and prevents matting. Before brushing, apply a small amount of castor oil to a brush to help detangle and add shine to their fur.

This routine promotes a healthy coat and stimulates blood circulation, enhancing overall skin health.

2) Moisturizing and Hydration

Dry skin can lead to itchiness and discomfort for pets.

Apply a small amount of castor oil directly onto dry patches or areas prone to dryness, such as elbows, paws, or noses. Massage the oil gently into the skin to promote absorption and provide long-lasting hydration.

3) Ear Care

Keep your pet's ears clean and free from excessive wax buildup by using a damp cotton ball or pad.

Add a drop of castor oil to the cotton ball before wiping the outer ear area to help remove dirt and debris gently. Avoid inserting anything into the ear canal to prevent injury.

4) Paw Pad Protection

Paw pads can become dry and cracked, especially in harsh weather conditions. Apply a thin layer of castor oil to your pet's paw pads to help moisturize and protect them from drying out.

This practice is particularly beneficial during winter or in hot, dry climates.

5) Skin Irritation and Minor Wounds

For minor cuts, scrapes, or skin irritations, clean the affected area with a mild antiseptic solution.

Apply castor oil to the affected area to soothe and moisturize the skin, promoting faster healing.

Ensure your pet does not lick the area immediately after application to prevent ingestion.

6) Preventive Care

Incorporate castor oil into your pet's bath routine by adding a few drops to their shampoo or bath water.

This helps maintain a healthy coat and skin, reducing the risk of dryness and flakiness.

7) Supplemental Nutrition

Discuss with your veterinarian the option of adding castor oil to your pet's diet as a supplement.

Castor oil contains essential fatty acids that can support skin health and coat shine from within. Ensure proper dosage and consult with a professional before introducing any new supplements.

8) Monitoring and Observation

Regularly monitor your pet's skin and coat for any changes, such as dryness, redness, or hair loss. Promptly address any concerns by consulting with your veterinarian to determine the appropriate course of action.

Incorporating castor oil into your pet's routine care and maintenance can provide numerous benefits for their skin and coat health. From moisturizing dry patches to promoting overall hydration and addressing minor skin issues, castor oil offers a natural and effective solution. By following these tips and practices, you can help keep your pet's skin and coat in optimal condition, ensuring they look and feel their best every day. Always prioritize your pet's safety and well-being by consulting with a veterinarian for personalized care advice and recommendations.

Chapter 10: Oral Health

10.1 Using castor oil for gum and tooth care

Using castor oil for gum and dental care can offer natural benefits that promote oral health and hygiene. Here's how castor oil can be effectively utilized in maintaining healthy gums and teeth:

<u>**Antibacterial and Antimicrobial Properties**</u>: Castor oil possesses antibacterial and antimicrobial properties that can help combat harmful bacteria in the mouth. These properties are beneficial for reducing plaque formation, which is a primary cause of gum disease and tooth decay.

<u>**Reduction of Inflammation**</u>: The anti-inflammatory properties of castor oil can help reduce swelling and inflammation in the gums. This is particularly useful for individuals suffering from gingivitis or periodontal disease, where inflamed gums can lead to discomfort and potential oral health complications.

1. Oil Pulling Technique: Oil pulling is a traditional practice that involves swishing oil around the mouth to draw out toxins and bacteria. Using castor oil for oil pulling can help remove bacteria and debris from the teeth and gums, promoting a cleaner mouth and fresher breath.

Instructions for Oil Pulling:

- Take a tablespoon of castor oil and swish it around in your mouth for 15-20 minutes.

- Spit out the oil into a trash can (to avoid clogging drains) and rinse your mouth thoroughly with warm water.

- Practice oil pulling regularly, preferably in the morning before brushing your teeth.

2. **Promotion of Oral Hydration**: Castor oil can help moisturize and hydrate the gums, which is essential for maintaining their health and preventing dryness. Dry gums can lead to discomfort and increased susceptibility to oral infections.

3. **Application on Gums**: Apply a small amount of castor oil directly to the gums using a clean finger or cotton swab. Gently massage the oil into the gums for a few minutes.

   o Leave the oil on for 5-10 minutes before rinsing your mouth with water.

   o Repeat this process daily to help reduce inflammation and promote gum health.

4. **DIY Toothpaste or Mouthwash**: You can create a natural toothpaste or mouthwash using castor oil along with other beneficial ingredients like baking soda, coconut oil, and essential oils.

   o **DIY Toothpaste Recipe:**

- Mix equal parts of castor oil and baking soda to form a paste.

- Add a few drops of peppermint or tea tree essential oil for flavor and additional antibacterial properties.

- Use this paste to brush your teeth as you would with regular toothpaste.

  o **DIY Mouthwash Recipe:**

- Combine one tablespoon of castor oil with one cup of warm water.

- Add a few drops of tea tree or peppermint essential oil for flavor and antibacterial benefits.

- Use this solution as a mouthwash after brushing your teeth to help kill bacteria and freshen breath.

5. **Natural Cavity Prevention**: The antibacterial properties of castor oil can contribute to preventing cavities by reducing the growth of bacteria that cause tooth decay. Regular use of castor oil in oral care routines can complement brushing and flossing efforts in maintaining oral hygiene.

6. **Consultation with veterinarian**: While castor oil offers natural benefits for oral health, it's essential to consult with a dentist before incorporating it into your dental care regimen, especially if you have existing oral health conditions or allergies.

Castor oil can be a valuable addition to your oral care routine due to its antibacterial, anti-inflammatory, and moisturizing properties. Whether used for oil pulling, applied directly to gums, or incorporated into DIY toothpaste and mouthwash recipes, castor oil offers natural support for gum and dental health. By integrating castor oil into your daily oral hygiene practices, you can help promote healthier gums, fresher breath, and overall improved oral well-being.

10.2 Treating oral infections naturally

Treating oral infections naturally can be effectively supported by the antimicrobial and anti-inflammatory properties of castor oil. Here's how castor oil can be utilized as a natural remedy for various oral infections:

1. Antimicrobial Benefits: Castor oil contains ricinoleic acid, which exhibits strong antimicrobial properties. These properties help in combating bacteria, viruses, and fungi that can cause oral infections such as gingivitis, periodontitis, and oral thrush.

2. Application for Gingivitis and Periodontitis: Gingivitis, characterized by inflammation of the gums, and periodontitis, involving deeper infection and potential damage to the tooth-supporting structures, can benefit from castor oil's anti-inflammatory effects. Massaging the affected gums with castor oil can help reduce swelling and pain.

   o Procedure:

- Apply a small amount of castor oil directly to the inflamed gums.

- Gently massage the oil into the gums using clean fingers or a cotton swab.

- Leave the oil on for 10-15 minutes before rinsing thoroughly with warm water.

- Repeat this process 2-3 times daily until symptoms improve.

3. Oral Thrush Treatment: Oral thrush, caused by the Candida fungus, manifests as white patches on the tongue, inner cheeks, or roof of the mouth. Castor oil's antifungal properties can help eliminate Candida and relieve discomfort associated with oral thrush.

   o Usage:

      ▪ Apply a small amount of castor oil directly to the affected areas using a clean cotton swab.

      ▪ Leave it on for 15-20 minutes before rinsing your mouth with warm water.

      ▪ Repeat this application 2-3 times daily until the symptoms of oral thrush resolve.

4. Oil Pulling Technique: Oil pulling with castor oil is an effective method to draw out toxins and bacteria from the mouth, thereby supporting the treatment of oral infections. The practice helps maintain oral hygiene by reducing plaque buildup and promoting healthy gums.

   o Steps for Oil Pulling:

      ▪ Take a tablespoon of castor oil and swish it around in your mouth for 15-20 minutes.

      ▪ Spit out the oil into a trash can (to avoid clogging drains) and rinse your mouth thoroughly with warm water.

      ▪ Practice oil pulling daily, preferably in the morning before brushing your teeth, to enhance oral health and alleviate oral infections.

5. DIY Mouthwash for Oral Infections: Creating a homemade mouthwash using castor oil and essential oils can provide additional antimicrobial benefits to combat oral infections effectively.

   o Recipe:

      ▪ Mix one tablespoon of castor oil with one cup of warm water.

      ▪ Add 3-5 drops of tea tree oil or peppermint oil for their antimicrobial properties and flavor.

      ▪ Use this solution as a mouthwash after brushing your teeth to help kill oral bacteria and promote healing of oral infections.

6. Consultation with a veterinarian: While castor oil offers natural benefits for treating oral infections, it's essential to consult with a dentist, especially for persistent or severe conditions. They can provide appropriate guidance and ensure the infection is properly diagnosed and treated.

10.3 Recipes for homemade toothpaste

Creating homemade toothpaste for pets can be a beneficial way to maintain their dental health using safe and natural ingredients. Here are some effective recipes using castor oil:

1) Basic Castor Oil Toothpaste

   o **Ingredients:**

      ▪ 2 tablespoons baking soda

- 1 tablespoon coconut oil
- 1 tablespoon castor oil
- A few drops of peppermint oil (optional, for flavor)

  o **Instructions:**

1. Mix all ingredients in a bowl until they form a smooth paste.
2. Store the toothpaste in a small, airtight container.
3. Use a soft-bristled toothbrush or finger brush to apply a small amount to your pet's teeth and gums.
4. Gently brush in circular motions for about 2 minutes.
5. Rinse your pet's mouth thoroughly with water.

2) Herbal Castor Oil Toothpaste

  o **Ingredients:**

- 2 tablespoons baking soda
- 1 tablespoon coconut oil
- 1 tablespoon castor oil
- 1 teaspoon dried parsley (for fresh breath)
- 1 teaspoon dried mint (optional, for additional freshness)

  o **Instructions:**

1. Mix baking soda, coconut oil, and castor oil in a bowl until well combined.
2. Add dried parsley and mint (if using) and mix thoroughly.
3. Store the toothpaste in a sealed container.
4. Use a toothbrush or finger brush to apply a small amount to your pet's teeth.
5. Brush gently for 2-3 minutes, focusing on the gum line and hard-to-reach areas.
6. Rinse your pet's mouth with water to remove any residue.

3) Vegetable Glycerin Castor Oil Toothpaste

  o **Ingredients:**

- 2 tablespoons baking soda
- 1 tablespoon castor oil

- 1 tablespoon vegetable glycerin

- 1/4 teaspoon fine sea salt (optional, for extra cleansing)

- 3-5 drops of essential oil (such as peppermint or tea tree, for flavor and antibacterial properties)

- o **Instructions:**

1. In a bowl, combine baking soda, castor oil, vegetable glycerin, and sea salt (if using).

2. Add a few drops of essential oil for flavor and additional benefits.

3. Mix well until all ingredients are thoroughly incorporated.

4. Transfer the toothpaste to a clean, airtight container for storage.

5. Apply a small amount to your pet's toothbrush or finger brush and brush gently.

6. Rinse your pet's mouth with water afterward.

4) Coconut Oil and Castor Oil Toothpaste

- o **Ingredients:**

- 2 tablespoons baking soda

- 1 tablespoon coconut oil

- 1 tablespoon castor oil

- 1 teaspoon cinnamon powder (optional, for a pleasant taste and antibacterial properties)

- o **Instructions:**

1. Mix baking soda, coconut oil, castor oil, and cinnamon powder (if using) in a bowl until smooth.

2. Store the toothpaste in a container with a lid.

3. Apply a small amount to your pet's toothbrush or finger brush.

4. Gently brush your pet's teeth and gums for about 2 minutes.

5. Rinse thoroughly with water to remove any remaining toothpaste.

These homemade toothpaste recipes are formulated with castor oil to help maintain your pet's dental health naturally. Regular brushing with these toothpastes can help prevent plaque buildup, freshen breath, and promote healthy gums.

10.4 Maintenance of general oral hygiene

Maintaining overall oral hygiene for pets is essential for their health and well-being. Regular dental care can prevent dental diseases such as periodontal disease, gingivitis, and tooth decay, leading to more severe health issues if left untreated. Here are some essential practices and tips for maintaining your pet's oral hygiene:

1) Regular Brushing

Regular brushing is one of the most effective ways to prevent dental problems in pets. Use a toothbrush specifically designed for pets, a finger brush, and pet-safe toothpaste. Brushing should ideally be done daily or at least several times a week to remove plaque and food particles that can lead to tartar buildup.

2) Choosing the Right Toothbrush and Toothpaste

Use a toothbrush with soft bristles that are gentle on your pet's gums and teeth. Pet-specific toothpaste is crucial as human toothpaste can be harmful if ingested by pets. Toothpaste flavors like poultry, beef, or seafood are often more appealing to pets, making the brushing experience more pleasant.

3) Regular Dental Check-ups

Regular dental check-ups are a crucial part of maintaining your pet's oral health. These appointments with your veterinarian provide a comprehensive dental exam, professional cleanings, and early detection of any emerging dental issues. They also offer personalized guidance on proper dental care techniques for your pet's breed and age, giving you peace of mind about your pet's oral health.

4) Monitor Dental Health Signs

Be vigilant for signs of dental problems such as persistent bad breath, swollen or bleeding gums, yellow or brown tartar buildup on teeth, difficulty chewing, pawing at the mouth, or reluctance to eat. If you notice any of these signs, it's important to seek veterinary intervention promptly to prevent the progression of dental disease.

5) Provide Dental Chews and Toys

Introducing dental chews and toys that promote dental health is a proactive step in reducing plaque and tartar buildup. These products, when approved by veterinary dental associations, can help mechanically scrub teeth as pets chew. By supervising your pet's use of these items, you're taking a responsible approach to your pet's dental health.

6) Diet and Nutrition

A balanced diet that supports dental health is crucial. Some specially formulated pet foods include ingredients that promote dental health by reducing plaque and tartar. Discuss with your veterinarian to choose the best diet for your pet's oral health needs.

7) Avoid Harmful Habits

Discouraging habits that can contribute to dental issues, such as chewing on hard objects or consuming sugary treats, is a powerful way to protect your pet's oral health. By being mindful of these factors, you're taking control and actively preventing potential dental problems.

8) Professional Dental Cleanings

In addition to regular home care, consider professional dental cleanings your veterinarian performs as recommended. These cleanings involve scaling and polishing to remove stubborn tartar and plaque that cannot be effectively removed at home.

9) Special Considerations for Pets

Different pets may require different approaches to dental care based on their age, breed, and overall health. For example, smaller and certain breeds like brachycephalic (short-nosed) dogs may be more prone to dental issues and require more frequent dental care.

10) Environmental Enrichment

Providing pets environmental enrichment and mental stimulation can indirectly support their dental health. Engaging pets in interactive play and activities can help reduce stress and prevent behaviors like excessive chewing, which can impact oral health.

By implementing these practices, you can help ensure your pet maintains good oral hygiene. Regular attention to your pet's dental health prevents dental diseases and contributes to their overall health and longevity. Always consult your veterinarian for personalized advice and recommendations regarding your pet's dental care routine.

Chapter 11: Castor oil supplementation in daily pet care

11.1 Developing a routine with castor oil

Developing a routine with castor oil can benefit various health and wellness aspects. Integrating castor oil into your routine can provide numerous benefits, whether used topically or internally. Here's how you can establish a routine with castor oil:

Understanding Castor Oil Benefits

Castor oil, with its versatile properties, has been traditionally used for its anti-inflammatory, antimicrobial, and moisturizing benefits. Rich in ricinoleic acid, it can promote skin health, hair growth, and wound healing when applied topically. When taken internally, it can support digestive health and relieve constipation. This versatility empowers you to address various health concerns with a single natural remedy.

Choosing High-Quality Castor Oil

Ensuring the effectiveness and safety of your castor oil is paramount. Opt for organic, cold-pressed, and hexane-free castor oil to guarantee purity and retain its beneficial compounds. This emphasis on quality provides a sense of security in your health and wellness journey.

Skin and Hair Care Routine

Incorporate castor oil into your skincare regimen as a moisturizer or facial cleanser. For added benefits, you can mix it with other oils like coconut or almond oil. Apply castor oil to the scalp for hair care to promote hair growth and nourish hair follicles. Leave it on for a few hours or overnight before washing it with shampoo.

Castor Oil Packs

Castor oil packs are a popular method for providing localized benefits. To create a castor oil pack, saturate a piece of cloth with castor oil and apply it to the desired area, such as the abdomen for digestive health or joints for pain relief. Cover with plastic wrap and a heating pad to enhance absorption and relax muscles.

Internal Use for Digestive Health

Castor oil can be taken internally to help relieve constipation and promote regular bowel movements. It acts as a natural laxative by stimulating intestinal contractions. However, use caution with internal use and consult with a healthcare provider for proper dosage and guidance.

Incorporating into Daily Routine

Establish a consistent schedule for using castor oil to maximize its benefits. For example, castor oil packs can be applied twice to thrice a week for targeted relief or as a nightly moisturizer for skin and hair. Consistency is critical to achieving desired results.

Safety Considerations

While castor oil is generally safe for topical use, it can cause skin irritation or allergic reactions in some individuals. Perform a patch test before using it on larger areas of the skin. When using internally, follow recommended dosages to avoid potential side effects such as nausea or diarrhea.

Monitoring Results

Keep track of how your body responds to castor oil over time. Notice any improvements in skin texture, hair growth, digestive regularity, or pain relief. Adjust your routine as needed based on your personal experience and health goals.

Consulting Healthcare Professionals

If you have specific health concerns or medical conditions, consult a healthcare professional before incorporating castor oil into your routine, especially for internal use. They can provide personalized recommendations and monitor your progress.

Long-Term Benefits

Over time, integrating castor oil into your routine can lead to long-term benefits for your overall health and well-being. It supports natural healing processes, improves skin and hair health, and contributes to digestive regularity, promoting a holistic approach to wellness.

By developing a consistent and thoughtful routine with castor oil, you can harness its therapeutic properties effectively for various health benefits. Whether used topically or internally, incorporating castor oil into your daily regimen can support your journey toward better health and vitality.

11.2 Combining castor oil with other natural remedies

Combining castor oil with other natural remedies can enhance its therapeutic effects and provide comprehensive health benefits. Here are several effective combinations that leverage the synergistic properties of castor oil with other natural remedies:

Castor Oil and Essential Oils: essential oils are concentrated plant extracts known for their medicinal properties. When combined with castor oil, it can enhance its benefits. For example, adding a few drops of lavender essential oil to castor oil can promote relaxation and soothe skin irritation. Peppermint oil combined with castor oil can help alleviate headaches and provide a cooling sensation when applied topically.

Turmeric and Castor Oil Paste: Turmeric is renowned for its anti-inflammatory and antioxidant properties. Mixing turmeric powder with castor oil creates a paste that can be applied to joints affected by arthritis or muscle soreness. When massaged into the affected area, this blend can help reduce inflammation and alleviate pain.

Ginger and Castor Oil Compress: ginger is another potent anti-inflammatory herb that complements castor oil's therapeutic benefits. Making ginger tea and using it to soak a cloth for a warm compress can provide relief for menstrual cramps or abdominal pain. Adding a few drops of castor oil to the compress can further enhance its effectiveness in reducing discomfort.

Castor Oil and Aloe Vera Gel: Aloe vera gel is well-known for its soothing and healing properties for the skin. Mixing aloe vera gel with castor oil creates a moisturizing blend that can be applied to sunburns, cuts, or minor wounds. This combination helps hydrate the skin, reduce inflammation, and promote faster healing.

Castor Oil and Coconut Oil: coconut oil is deeply moisturizing and has antimicrobial properties. Mixing castor oil with coconut oil creates a nourishing blend that can be used as a hair conditioner or scalp treatment. This combination helps strengthen hair, reduce dandruff, and improve overall scalp health.

Castor Oil and Epsom Salt Bath: Epsom salt baths are famous for relaxing muscles and promoting detoxification. Adding a few tablespoons of castor oil to an Epsom salt bath can enhance its muscle-relaxing benefits. This combination is beneficial for soothing sore muscles, reducing stress, and promoting overall relaxation.

Honey and Castor Oil Mask: Honey is naturally antibacterial and moisturizing, making it an excellent addition to facial masks. Mixing honey with castor oil creates a hydrating and cleansing mask that can help unclog pores, reduce acne, and improve skin texture. This blend is gentle yet effective for promoting clear and radiant skin.

Castor Oil and Chamomile Tea Infusion: chamomile tea is known for its calming and anti-inflammatory properties. Using chamomile tea with castor oil creates a soothing eye compress that reduces puffiness and dark circles. This combination is gentle on the delicate skin around the eyes and helps promote relaxation.

Castor Oil and Shea Butter Salve: Shea butter is deeply moisturizing and rich in vitamins and antioxidants. Combining shea butter with castor oil creates a healing salve that can be used to treat dry, cracked skin, eczema, or psoriasis. This blend provides intense hydration and helps repair the damaged skin barrier.

Castor Oil and Apple Cider Vinegar Rinse: apple cider vinegar is known for its pH-balancing and antibacterial properties. Diluting apple cider vinegar with water and adding a few drops of castor oil creates a scalp rinse that can help clarify the scalp, balance pH levels, and promote healthy hair growth.

Combining castor oil with other natural remedies allows you to customize treatments based on your specific health needs and preferences. Whether used topically or internally, these combinations can amplify the therapeutic benefits of castor oil and support overall health and well-being.

11.3 Monitoring and adjustment of treatment plans

Monitoring and adjusting treatment plans using natural remedies like castor oil is crucial to ensuring effectiveness and safety. Here are several key considerations and practices for monitoring and adjusting treatment plans:

Observation and Symptom Tracking

Begin by closely observing the pet's response to the treatment. Keep track of any changes in symptoms, such as improvements or worsening conditions. This can include noting changes in energy levels, appetite, skin condition, and overall behavior.

Consultation with a Veterinarian

Regular consultation with a veterinarian is essential, especially when using natural remedies. A veterinarian can guide dosage, application frequency, and potential interactions with other medications or treatments. They can also help monitor progress and adjust the treatment plan as needed.

Start with Small Dosages

Start with small dosages or concentrations when introducing a new treatment or remedy. This approach allows you to assess the pet's tolerance and observe any adverse reactions. Gradually increase the dosage, if necessary, under the guidance of a veterinarian.

Regular Health Assessments

Proactively schedule regular health assessments with a veterinarian to evaluate the pet's overall health and monitor any changes in conditions. This proactive approach helps detect issues early and ensures the treatment plan aligns with the pet's evolving health needs, making you a responsible and caring pet owner.

Reviewing Effectiveness

Continuously evaluate the effectiveness of the treatment plan. Discuss alternative options with the veterinarian if the desired results are not achieved within a reasonable timeframe. They may recommend adjustments to the dosage, frequency, or combination of natural remedies.

Adapting to Individual Responses

Pets may respond differently to natural remedies based on age, breed, underlying health conditions, and individual tolerance. Adjust the treatment plan based on these factors to optimize effectiveness and minimize risks.

Monitoring for Side Effects

Monitor the pet for any potential side effects or adverse reactions to the treatment. Common signs may include gastrointestinal upset, allergic reactions, or changes in behavior. Discontinue use immediately and consult a veterinarian if any adverse reactions occur.

Educational Resources and Support

Stay informed about the latest research and educational resources on natural remedies and pet care. This knowledge empowers pet owners to make informed decisions and collaborate effectively with veterinarians in managing their pet's health, instilling a sense of confidence and knowledge.

Environmental and Lifestyle Factors

Consider environmental factors that may impact the pet's health and treatment outcomes. This includes diet, exercise, stress levels, and exposure to allergens or toxins. Appropriate adjustments in these areas can support the effectiveness of natural remedies like castor oil.

Documenting Progress

Maintain detailed records of the treatment plan, including dosage, application methods, and observations. Documenting progress lets you track improvements or setbacks and provides valuable information for future adjustments, giving you a sense of control and organization in managing your pet's health.

These practices allow pet owners to effectively monitor and adjust treatment plans using natural remedies such as castor oil. Collaborating with a veterinarian ensures that the treatment approach is safe, tailored to the pet's needs, and supports their overall health and well-being.

Chapter 12: Frequently Asked Questions (FAQs)

1) Is castor oil safe for pets?

Castor oil can be safe for pets when used appropriately and under veterinary guidance. However, it's essential to consult with a veterinarian before using castor oil, especially for internal or topical applications. Pets may have different sensitivities and health conditions that can influence the safety and effectiveness of castor oil.

2) What are the benefits of using castor oil for pets?

Castor oil is known for its anti-inflammatory, antimicrobial, and moisturizing properties. It can help promote healthy skin and coat, alleviate pain and inflammation in joints, and support digestive health. Additionally, some pet owners use castor oil to manage conditions like dry skin, allergies, and minor wounds.

3) How can castor oil be used for pets?

Castor oil can be used topically by applying it to the pet's skin or coat to promote healing and moisture retention. It can also be used as a massage oil for joint pain relief or as a natural remedy for minor skin irritations. For internal use, such as for digestive issues, it's essential to follow veterinary recommendations for dosage and administration.

4) Can castor oil be used to treat fleas and ticks on pets?

Castor oil is sometimes used in natural flea and tick prevention methods. It's believed to create an unfavorable environment for pests due to its odor and texture. However, its effectiveness may vary, and it's important to use it in combination with other preventive measures and under veterinary guidance.

5) Is castor oil ingestion safe for pets?

While castor oil is generally considered safe for external use on pets, ingestion of castor oil can be toxic. Castor oil contains ricin, a toxic compound that can cause gastrointestinal upset, dehydration, and other serious health issues if ingested in large quantities. Always keep castor oil and any other potentially harmful substances out of reach of pets.

6) How do I apply castor oil to my pet?

When applying castor oil topically, start with a small amount and gently massage it into your pet's skin or coat. Use circular motions to ensure even distribution. Avoid applying near the eyes, mouth, or genital areas unless specifically directed by a veterinarian. For internal use, follow veterinary instructions carefully.

7) Are there any side effects of using castor oil on pets?

Some pets may experience mild skin irritation or allergic reactions when using castor oil topically. Signs of sensitivity include redness, itching, or swelling at the application site. Discontinue use and consult a veterinarian if any adverse reactions occur. Internal use should only be done under veterinary supervision to minimize potential risks.

8) Can castor oil be used on all types of pets?

Castor oil is commonly used on dogs and cats, but its suitability for other pets may vary. Always consult with a veterinarian before using castor oil on exotic pets, birds, or small mammals. Different species may have different reactions to castor oil, so veterinary guidance is essential.

9) Is organic castor oil better for pets?

Organic castor oil is generally preferred as it reduces the risk of exposure to pesticides and other harmful chemicals. Look for cold-pressed, organic castor oil to ensure purity and quality. However, regardless of the type of castor oil used, it's important to prioritize veterinary guidance and safety considerations.

10) How do I choose the right castor oil product for my pet?

Choose a high-quality, pure castor oil product that is free from additives, fragrances, and preservatives. Look for cold-pressed, organic options whenever possible. Consider consulting with a veterinarian to ensure the chosen product is safe and appropriate for your pet's specific needs.

BOOK 9: Castor Oil in Aromatherapy

Castor Oil in Aromatherapy

Enhancing Well-Being with Nature's Essence

By

Vincent Vega

Disclaimer notice

Please be aware that the information provided in this document is intended solely for educational and entertainment purposes. Every effort has been made to ensure the content is accurate, reliable, current, and complete.

However, no guarantees, either explicit or implicit, are made. Readers acknowledge that the author is not providing legal, financial, medical, or professional advice.

The content has been sourced from various references. It is strongly recommended that you consult a licensed professional before attempting any of the of the methods described in this document.

By reading this document, you agree that the author is not liable for any direct or indirect losses resulting from the use of the information within, including but not limited to errors, omissions, or inaccuracies.

Chapter 1: Introduction to castor oil and aromatherapy

1.1 Historical background

Castor oil dates back to ancient civilizations, where it was revered for its versatile therapeutic and medicinal properties. The castor bean plant, scientifically known as Ricinus communis, has been cultivated for thousands of years. Evidence of its use has been found in ancient Egypt, where it was employed in various applications, including as a fuel for lamps, a laxative, and a balm for skin ailments. The ancient Egyptians, renowned for their advancements in medicine and cosmetics, utilized castor oil extensively daily. The Ebers Papyrus, one of the oldest medical texts dating back to 1550 BCE, mentions the use of castor oil for medicinal purposes, highlighting its importance in ancient Egyptian healthcare.

In ancient India, castor oil was a staple in Ayurvedic medicine, the traditional system of medicine that dates back over 3,000 years. Ayurvedic practitioners valued castor oil for its purgative properties and ability to balance the doshas, or the fundamental energies that govern physiological and psychological processes. It was commonly used to treat digestive issues and skin disorders and to promote overall health and well-being. Castor oil's significance in Ayurvedic medicine continues to this day, where it remains a popular remedy for a wide range of ailments.

The use of castor oil also extended to ancient Greece and Rome. The Greek physician Dioscorides, in his seminal work "De Materia Medica," written in the first century CE, documented the medicinal properties of castor oil, referring to it as "kiki." He noted its efficacy as a laxative and its utility in treating various skin conditions. The Romans, who were heavily influenced by Greek medical practices, adopted castor oil and incorporated it into their medical treatments.

Castor oil's reputation as a potent natural remedy has spread across continents throughout the centuries. In Africa, it was used in traditional medicine to treat various ailments, from skin infections to digestive issues. Indigenous communities in the Americas also recognized the value of castor oil, using it for its healing properties and as a remedy for various health conditions.

1.2 Botanical source and extraction process

Castor oil is derived from the seeds of the castor bean plant, Ricinus communis, a hardy perennial shrub that belongs to the Euphorbiaceae family. The plant is characterized by its large, glossy leaves and clusters of spiny, seed-bearing capsules. It thrives in tropical and subtropical regions, with India, Brazil, and China being the leading producers of castor oil today. The plant's adaptability to diverse climatic conditions and its resilience to pests and diseases make it an ideal crop for cultivation worldwide.

The extraction process of castor oil begins with the harvesting of ripe castor seeds, which are typically done by hand to ensure the integrity of the seeds. Once harvested, the seeds undergo a drying process to reduce moisture content, which is essential for effective oil extraction. The dried seeds are then subjected to mechanical and chemical processes to extract the oil.

The first step in the oil extraction process is cleaning and dehulling the seeds. This involves removing the outer husk to expose the inner kernel containing the oil. The cleaned seeds are then crushed to break them into smaller pieces, facilitating the release of oil. The ground seeds are heated to enhance the oil extraction process, as heat helps to soften the seeds and increase oil yield.

The castor oil can be extracted using various methods, the two most common being cold pressing and solvent extraction. Cold pressing is a mechanical process that involves pressing the crushed seeds at low temperatures to extract the oil. This method is favored for producing high-quality, unrefined castor oil, as it preserves the oil's natural nutrients and beneficial compounds. Solvent extraction, on the other hand, involves using chemical solvents to dissolve the oil from the seed material. While this method can produce a higher yield of oil, it may also result in the loss of some beneficial properties due to the use of chemicals and higher temperatures.

Once the oil is extracted, it is purified to remove impurities and enhance its quality. The purified oil is then packaged and distributed for various uses, including medicinal, industrial, and cosmetic applications. Castor oil's versatility and beneficial properties make it a valuable resource in aromatherapy.

1.3 Chemical composition and properties

Castor oil is renowned for its unique chemical composition, which is primarily characterized by a high concentration of ricinoleic acid, a monounsaturated fatty acid that constitutes about 90% of its fatty acid content. This high ricinoleic acid content sets castor oil apart from other vegetable oils, endowing it with a range of potent therapeutic properties.

Ricinoleic acid, the key component of castor oil, is a powerhouse of health benefits. Its anti-inflammatory, antimicrobial, and analgesic effects make castor oil a reliable remedy for a variety of health conditions, from reducing pain and inflammation to promoting wound healing and inhibiting harmful bacteria growth. Its ability to stimulate the lymphatic system further underscores its role in detoxification and immune system maintenance.

Besides ricinoleic acid, castor oil contains other beneficial fatty acids, including oleic acid, linoleic acid, and stearic acid. Oleic acid, a monounsaturated fatty acid, contributes to the oil's moisturizing properties, making it an excellent emollient for skin care. Linoleic acid, a polyunsaturated fatty acid, is essential for maintaining skin barrier function and reducing inflammation. Stearic acid, a saturated fatty acid, provides cleansing properties and helps in protecting the skin's surface.

The presence of triglycerides in castor oil, esters derived from glycerol and three fatty acids, contributes to its thick and dense consistency. This unique texture makes castor oil popular in the cosmetic and pharmaceutical industries for formulating creams, lotions, and ointments.

Castor oil also contains small amounts of other compounds, such as tocopherols (vitamin E) and phytosterols, which provide antioxidant benefits. These compounds help protect the skin from oxidative stress, which can lead to premature aging and other skin issues. Combining these components gives castor oil its multifaceted therapeutic properties, making it a valuable ingredient in aromatherapy and other natural health practices.

1.4 Fundamentals of aromatherapy

Aromatherapy is a holistic healing practice that uses natural plant extracts, primarily essential oils, to promote health and well-being. This ancient practice dates back thousands of years and has been used by various cultures, including the Egyptians, Greeks, Romans, and Chinese, to treat various physical and psychological ailments.

The fundamental principle of aromatherapy is the therapeutic application of essential oils, which are concentrated extracts obtained from plants' leaves, flowers, stems, bark, and roots. These oils contain volatile compounds responsible for the plant's aroma and therapeutic properties. When inhaled or applied to the skin, these volatile compounds interact with the body's chemistry, producing various physiological and psychological effects.

Aromatherapy offers several methods of application, each with its specific benefits. These methods include inhalation, topical application, massage, bathing, and compresses, each providing unique ways to experience the therapeutic effects of essential oils.

Inhalation is one of the most common methods of using essential oils. It involves breathing in the aromatic molecules through the nose, interacting with the olfactory system. The olfactory receptors send signals to the brain, particularly the limbic system, which is involved in regulating emotions, memory, and mood. This makes inhalation an effective way to address emotional and mental health issues such as stress, anxiety, and depression.

Topical Application: essential oils can be applied directly to the skin, often diluted in a carrier oil like castor oil to prevent irritation and enhance absorption. The skin absorbs the oils, allowing their active compounds to enter the bloodstream and exert their therapeutic effects. Topical application is commonly used for treating localized conditions such as muscle pain, skin infections, and inflammatory conditions.

Massage: combining essential oils with massage therapy enhances the therapeutic effects of both practices. Physically manipulating tissues during a massage improves circulation, relieves muscle tension, and promotes relaxation, while the essential oils provide additional benefits such as pain relief, anti-inflammatory effects, and emotional calming.

Bathing: adding essential oils to bathwater allows for both inhalation and skin absorption. This method is particularly useful for full-body relaxation and can help with conditions such as insomnia, muscle aches, and stress.

Compresses: soaking a cloth in water mixed with essential oils and applying it to the skin can provide targeted relief for specific areas of pain or inflammation. Compresses can be used hot or cold depending on the condition being treated.

The effectiveness of aromatherapy depends on the quality of the essential oils used, the method of application, and the individual's unique response to the oils. Essential oils are potent substances, and their use requires knowledge and caution to avoid adverse reactions.

While not an essential oil itself, castor oil plays a crucial role as a carrier oil in aromatherapy. Its thick consistency and high content of ricinoleic acid make it particularly effective in enhancing the absorption of essential oils through the skin, thereby amplifying their therapeutic effects. By combining castor oil with essential oils, practitioners can create customized blends tailored to individual needs, addressing a wide range of physical and emotional health issues.

1.5 Definition and principles of aromatherapy

Aromatherapy is a holistic healing practice that utilizes natural plant extracts, particularly essential oils, to promote physical, emotional, and psychological well-being. The term "aromatherapy" was coined by French chemist René-

Maurice Gattefossé in the early 20th century, following his discovery of the healing properties of lavender oil for treating burns. Aromatherapy operates on the premise that aromatic compounds in essential oils interact with the body's systems to stimulate healing processes, enhance mood, and improve overall health.

The principles of aromatherapy are grounded in the therapeutic application of essential oils. Essential oils are volatile, aromatic compounds extracted from various parts of plants, including leaves, flowers, stems, bark, and roots. These oils contain the essence of the plant's fragrance and therapeutic properties, harnessed for healing. The fundamental principles of aromatherapy include:

Holistic Approach

Aromatherapy emphasizes treating the whole person rather than just addressing specific symptoms. It considers an individual's physical, emotional, mental, and spiritual aspects, aiming to restore balance and harmony.

Natural Healing

Aromatherapy relies on essential oils' natural properties to support the body's innate ability to heal itself. It avoids synthetic substances, focusing instead on pure, natural plant extracts.

Individualized Treatment

Each person is unique, and their response to essential oils can vary. Aromatherapy practitioners tailor treatments to the individual's specific needs, preferences, and health conditions, ensuring a personalized approach to healing.

Integration with Other Therapies

Aromatherapy can be used alongside other complementary and conventional therapies to enhance effectiveness. It is often integrated with practices such as massage, reflexology, and herbal medicine to provide a comprehensive healing experience.

Preventative Care

Aromatherapy is used to treat existing conditions, prevent illness, and maintain overall health. Regularly using essential oils can help strengthen the immune system, reduce stress, and promote well-being.

1.6 Overview of essential oils and their therapeutic uses

Essential oils are the cornerstone of aromatherapy, each with unique properties and therapeutic benefits. Here is an overview of some commonly used essential oils and their uses in aromatherapy:

Lavender (Lavandula angustifolia): known for its calming and relaxing properties, lavender oil is widely used to reduce stress, anxiety, and insomnia. It also has antiseptic and anti-inflammatory properties, making it useful for treating minor burns, cuts, and skin irritations.

Peppermint (Mentha piperita): peppermint oil is invigorating and refreshing, often used to enhance mental clarity and focus. It is also effective in relieving headaches, muscle pain, and digestive issues due to its analgesic and anti-spasmodic properties.

Eucalyptus (Eucalyptus globulus): eucalyptus oil is renowned for its respiratory benefits. It helps clear nasal congestion, ease coughs, and improve breathing. Its antimicrobial properties also make it worthwhile for disinfecting wounds and treating infections.

Tea Tree (Melaleuca alternifolia): with potent antibacterial, antiviral, and antifungal properties, tea tree oil is a powerful remedy for various skin conditions, including acne, fungal infections, and cuts. It is also used in household cleaning products for its disinfectant qualities.

Chamomile (Matricaria recutita / Chamaemelum nobile): chamomile oil is known for its soothing and anti-inflammatory effects. It is often used to calm irritated skin, reduce inflammation, and promote relaxation and sleep.

Rose (Rosa damascena): Rose oil is prized for its emotional and skin-care benefits. It helps alleviate anxiety, depression, and stress while rejuvenating and moisturizing the skin. Its antiseptic properties make it beneficial for treating skin wounds and infections.

Lemon (Citrus limon): lemon oil is uplifting and energizing, often used to improve mood and concentration. It also has detoxifying and immune-boosting properties, making it useful for cleansing the body and supporting overall health.

Frankincense (Boswellia carterii): Frankincense oil is known for its spiritual and meditative benefits. It enhances meditation, reduces stress, and promotes a sense of inner peace. Its anti-inflammatory properties also make it beneficial for joint pain and skin care.

Geranium (Pelargonium graveolens): geranium oil balances hormones and emotions, effectively relieving symptoms of PMS and menopause. It also has astringent and antiseptic properties, beneficial for skin care and wound healing.

Ylang-ylang (Cananga odorata): Ylang-ylang oil is renowned for its aphrodisiac and mood-enhancing effects. It helps reduce stress, anxiety, and depression while also promoting relaxation and emotional balance.

The therapeutic uses of essential oils in aromatherapy are vast and varied. They can be used for physical ailments, such as pain, inflammation, and infections, as well as for emotional and mental health issues like stress, anxiety, and depression. The versatility of essential oils allows them to be incorporated into various applications, including inhalation, topical application, massage, and baths, providing a comprehensive approach to holistic healing.

Aromatherapy, with its rich history and foundational principles, utilizes the powerful properties of essential oils to promote health and well-being. By understanding the unique benefits of each essential oil and how they can be applied, individuals can harness aromatherapy's therapeutic potential for a wide range of physical, emotional, and psychological needs.

1.7 Importance of castor oil in aromatherapy

Castor oil plays a significant role in aromatherapy due to its unique properties and versatility as a carrier oil. While essential oils are the primary therapeutic agents in aromatherapy, carrier oils like castor oil are crucial for diluting these potent substances, ensuring safe application, and enhancing the overall efficacy of treatments. Castor oil's distinctive characteristics make it an invaluable addition to aromatherapy.

One of the primary reasons for castor oil's importance in aromatherapy is its exceptional ability to penetrate deep into the skin and tissues. This property allows it to effectively carry essential oils into the body, maximizing their therapeutic effects. Like many other carrier oils, castor oil does not merely sit on the skin's surface; instead, it facilitates deeper absorption, ensuring that the active compounds in essential oils reach their intended targets within the body.

Castor oil's rich, thick consistency makes it an ideal medium for prolonged massage sessions and topical applications. Its viscosity provides a smooth glide during massage, enhancing the practitioner's ability to work on more profound muscle layers and connective tissues. This is particularly beneficial in treatments to relieve muscle tension, reduce pain, and promote relaxation. The oil's lubricating properties also help to prevent friction and irritation during massage, ensuring a comfortable and therapeutic experience for the recipient.

In addition to its mechanical benefits, castor oil boasts a range of therapeutic properties that complement the effects of essential oils. Its anti-inflammatory, antimicrobial, and analgesic properties make it a powerful agent for addressing various skin conditions, infections, and inflammatory issues. When combined with essential oils known for their healing effects, such as tea tree or lavender oil, castor oil enhances the overall potency of the blend, providing more effective relief and faster healing.

Moreover, castor oil's unique fatty acid composition, particularly its high ricinoleic acid content, contributes to its effectiveness in aromatherapy. Ricinoleic acid is known for reducing pain and inflammation, making castor oil an excellent choice for treating joint pain, arthritis, and muscle soreness. Its ability to boost lymphatic circulation further supports detoxification processes and immune system function, aligning with the holistic goals of aromatherapy to promote overall well-being.

1.8 Unique properties of castor oil that enhance aromatherapy

Castor oil possesses several unique properties that enhance its effectiveness in aromatherapy, setting it apart from other carrier oils. These properties include its deep-penetrating ability, anti-inflammatory and antimicrobial effects, high ricinoleic acid content, and suitability for various therapeutic applications.

Deep Penetration

Castor oil is renowned for penetrating deeply into the skin and underlying tissues. This property is particularly advantageous in aromatherapy, as it allows essential oils to be absorbed more effectively and reach their target areas within the body. This deep penetration enhances vital oils' therapeutic effects, whether intended to relieve muscle pain, reduce inflammation, or promote skin healing.

Anti-inflammatory and Antimicrobial Properties

Castor oil's anti-inflammatory and antimicrobial effects make it a valuable addition to aromatherapy blends. These properties help to soothe and heal irritated or infected skin, making castor oil an ideal carrier for essential oils with similar therapeutic effects. For example, when combined with lavender or tea tree oil, castor oil can enhance the blend's ability to treat skin infections, reduce redness, and alleviate discomfort.

High Ricinoleic Acid Content

The presence of ricinoleic acid, a monounsaturated fatty acid, is a defining feature of castor oil. Ricinoleic acid is known for its potent anti-inflammatory and analgesic properties, making castor oil particularly effective in treating conditions such as arthritis, muscle pain, and inflammatory skin disorders. This fatty acid also promotes the health of the lymphatic system, aiding in detoxification and immune system support, which are essential components of holistic health practices like aromatherapy.

Versatility in Applications

Castor oil's thick, dense nature makes it suitable for various therapeutic applications in aromatherapy. It can be used in massage therapy to provide a smooth glide and enhance deep tissue work, in topical treatments to deliver essential oils effectively, and in compresses to target specific areas of pain or inflammation. Its versatility ensures that it can be adapted to meet the diverse needs of aromatherapy clients.

Moisturizing and Healing

Castor oil's emollient properties make it an excellent moisturizer, capable of softening and hydrating the skin. This is particularly beneficial in aromatherapy treatments focused on skin health and beauty. By combining castor oil with essential oils known for their skin-healing properties, practitioners can create powerful blends that nourish the skin, promote healing, and address issues such as dryness, eczema, and psoriasis.

Castor oil's unique properties significantly enhance the practice of aromatherapy. Its deep-penetrating ability, anti-inflammatory and antimicrobial effects, high ricinoleic acid content, versatility, and moisturizing capabilities make it an indispensable carrier oil in creating effective and holistic aromatherapy treatments.

1.9 Synergistic effects with essential oils

Castor oil's unique properties make it an exceptional carrier oil in aromatherapy, enhancing the synergistic effects when combined with essential oils. Synergy in aromatherapy refers to the phenomenon where the combined effects of two or more substances produce a greater therapeutic outcome than the sum of their effects. This synergistic interaction between castor oil and essential oils can significantly amplify the overall benefits of aromatherapy treatments.

One of the key aspects of this synergy is castor oil's exceptional ability to penetrate deeply into the skin and underlying tissues. This deep penetration ensures that the therapeutic compounds in essential oils are efficiently delivered to their target areas within the body. For example, when essential oils known for their analgesic properties, such as peppermint or eucalyptus, are blended with castor oil, they can provide more effective pain relief and muscle relaxation. The castor oil not only carries the essential oils deeper into the tissues but also enhances their absorption and efficacy.

Moreover, castor oil's high content of ricinoleic acid, a potent anti-inflammatory and analgesic agent, complements the therapeutic properties of many essential oils. When combined with anti-inflammatory essential oils like lavender, chamomile, or frankincense, the result is a powerful blend that can significantly reduce inflammation, soothe irritated skin, and alleviate pain. The anti-inflammatory properties of castor oil and essential oils work together to provide more comprehensive relief for conditions such as arthritis, muscle soreness, and inflammatory skin disorders.

Castor oil's antimicrobial properties further enhance the effects of antimicrobial essential oils such as tea tree, thyme, and oregano. This combination can be particularly effective in treating skin infections, wounds, and fungal conditions. Castor oil helps to deliver the essential oils deeply into the affected areas while also contributing its own antimicrobial action, resulting in a more potent and effective treatment.

In addition to its therapeutic benefits, castor oil's moisturizing and emollient properties make it an ideal base for essential oils used in skin care. Essential oils such as rose, geranium, and sandalwood, known for their skin-nourishing and rejuvenating effects, can be blended with castor oil to create luxurious and effective skin treatments. Castor oil provides deep hydration and helps lock in moisture, while essential oils deliver therapeutic benefits, improving skin texture, elasticity, and overall health.

Another aspect of the synergistic effects of castor oil with essential oils is the enhancement of emotional and mental well-being. Essential oils such as ylang-ylang, bergamot, and clary sage, known for their mood-enhancing and stress-relieving properties, can be combined with castor oil to create soothing massage oils or bath blends. The castor oil's ability to prolong the duration of massage sessions and its gentle, calming effects on the skin help to amplify the emotional and psychological benefits of the essential oils.

The synergistic effects of castor oil with essential oils in aromatherapy result in enhanced therapeutic outcomes. When combined with the potent effects of essential oils, the deep penetration, anti-inflammatory, antimicrobial, and moisturizing properties of castor oil create powerful and effective treatments for a wide range of physical, emotional, and skin-related conditions. This synergy not only maximizes the benefits of aromatherapy but also ensures a holistic and comprehensive approach to health and well-being.

Chapter 2: Application methods in aromatherapy

2.1 Techniques for applying castor oil to the skin

Several effective techniques can be used to apply castor oil to the skin, each suited to different therapeutic goals and skin conditions. Castor oil's thick, viscous nature makes it ideal for treatments that require prolonged contact with the skin, ensuring deep penetration and sustained effects.

Direct Application

Direct application involves applying castor oil straight onto the skin without dilution. This method is beneficial for treating localized areas of concern, such as dry patches, scars, or minor skin irritations. To apply castor oil directly:

Cleanse the skin thoroughly to remove any dirt and impurities.

Warm a small amount of castor oil slightly by rubbing it between your palms.

Massage the oil gently into the skin using circular motions, allowing it to absorb fully.

Leave the oil on the skin for at least 20-30 minutes before wiping off any excess with a soft cloth. You can leave it on overnight and wash it off in the morning for the best results.

Compress

Castor oil in a compress is highly effective for deeper penetration and targeting specific areas of pain or inflammation. Here's how to make and use a castor oil compress:

Fold a flannel or cotton cloth into several layers and soak it in castor oil.

Apply the oil-soaked cloth to the affected area.

Cover the compress with a plastic wrap to prevent oil from leaking.

Place a heating pad or hot water bottle over the compress to enhance absorption.

Leave the compress on for 30-60 minutes, allowing the heat to help the oil penetrate deeper into the tissues.

After removing the compress, clean the area with a mild soap and water to remove any residual oil.

Massage

Incorporating castor oil into massage therapy can enhance the therapeutic effects of the treatment. Its lubricating properties allow for smooth gliding over the skin while providing deep moisturization. For a castor oil massage:

Warm a small amount of castor oil to body temperature.

Apply the oil to the skin in the area to be massaged.

Use gentle, rhythmic motions to massage the oil into the skin, focusing on areas of tension or pain.

Continue massaging for 15-30 minutes, adding more oil as needed to maintain lubrication.

After the massage, allow the oil to remain on the skin for additional hydration or wash off the excess if desired.

Facial Treatment

Castor oil can be used as a facial treatment to cleanse and nourish the skin. It is particularly beneficial for dry, acne-prone, or mature skin. For a facial treatment:

To reduce the viscosity of castor oil, mix a small amount with a lighter carrier oil, such as jojoba or almond oil.

Apply the oil blend to the face, massaging it gently into the skin.

Leave the oil on for 10-15 minutes to allow deep penetration.

Use a warm, damp washcloth to gently wipe away the oil, removing impurities and leaving the skin feeling soft and hydrated.

2.2 Combining castor oil with essential oils for greater Benefits

Combining castor oil with essential oils can significantly enhance the therapeutic benefits, creating powerful blends tailored to specific health and wellness needs. The carrier properties of castor oil make it an excellent medium for diluting and delivering essential oils to the skin effectively.

For Pain Relief

To create a blend for alleviating muscle pain, joint discomfort, or inflammation.

Mix 2 tablespoons of castor oil with 10 drops of peppermint oil (known for its analgesic properties) and 5 drops of lavender oil (known for its anti-inflammatory and calming effects).

Massage the blend into the affected areas, using circular motions to ensure deep penetration.

Apply a warm compress or heating pad to enhance absorption and provide additional relief.

For Skin Healing and Moisturization

To formulate a blend that promotes skin healing, reduces scarring, and provides deep hydration.

Combine 2 tablespoons of castor oil with 5 drops of tea tree oil (known for its antimicrobial properties) and 10 drops of rosehip oil (known for its skin regenerative properties).

Apply the blend to clean skin, focusing on areas with scars, blemishes, or dry patches.

Leave the oil blend on the skin for at least 20-30 minutes or overnight for intensive treatment.

<u>For Stress Relief and Relaxation</u>

To create a soothing blend for reducing stress and promoting relaxation.

Mix 2 tablespoons of castor oil with 8 chamomile oil (known for its calming properties) and 5 drops of ylang-ylang oil (known for its mood-enhancing effects).

Use the blend for a full-body massage or add it to a warm bath.

Inhale deeply during the massage or bath to benefit from the aromatic properties of the essential oils.

<u>For Respiratory Support</u>

To support respiratory health and relieve congestion

Combine 2 tablespoons of castor oil with 10 drops of eucalyptus oil (known for its decongestant properties) and 5 drops of rosemary oil (known for its respiratory support).

Massage the blend onto the chest and back, focusing on areas around the lungs and throat.

Use a warm compress to enhance the blend's effectiveness and promote deeper inhalation of the essential oils.

By blending castor oil with essential oils, practitioners can create customized treatments that address various physical and emotional health issues. Castor oil's deep-penetrating and moisturizing properties complement the therapeutic effects of essential oils, resulting in more effective and comprehensive aromatherapy applications.

2.3 Massage therapy

Massage therapy, a widely practiced therapeutic technique, has deep roots in ancient civilizations such as those in China, Egypt, Greece, and India. This rich history lends a sense of tradition and trust to the practice, which involves manipulating muscles, connective tissues, tendons, and ligaments to enhance physical and emotional well-being. It is one of the oldest healing arts, with evidence of its use dating back to ancient times. Massage therapy encompasses various styles and techniques designed to address specific health concerns and promote overall wellness.

The primary benefits of massage therapy include relaxation, stress reduction, pain relief, improved circulation, and enhanced lymphatic drainage. Massage therapists can help alleviate muscle tension, reduce inflammation, and improve mobility by applying pressure and manipulating soft tissues. This practice also stimulates the release of endorphins, the body's natural painkillers, contributing to an enhanced sense of well-being.

Massage therapy can be categorized into several types, each with unique techniques and benefits.

<u>Swedish Massage</u>

This is the most common type of massage, known for its gentle and relaxing techniques. It involves long, flowing strokes, kneading, and circular movements on the superficial layers of muscles. Swedish massage is excellent for overall relaxation and improving circulation.

Deep Tissue Massage

This technique targets the deeper layers of muscles and connective tissues. It is particularly effective for treating chronic pain, muscle knots, and tension. Deep tissue massage uses slower, more forceful strokes to reach deep muscles and fascia.

Sports Massage

Designed specifically for athletes, sports massage focuses on preventing and treating injuries, improving performance, and enhancing flexibility. It combines techniques from Swedish and deep tissue massage, stretching, and other therapeutic modalities.

Trigger Point Therapy

This technique targets specific areas of muscle tension known as trigger points. Therapists can relieve pain and dysfunction in other body parts by applying focused pressure to these points.

Aromatherapy Massage

This type of massage incorporates essential oils to enhance the therapeutic effects. The aromatic compounds in the oils help promote relaxation, reduce stress, and address various physical and emotional issues.

Hot Stone Massage

In this technique, smooth, heated stones are placed on specific body points to warm and loosen tight muscles. The stones can also be used to extend the therapist's hands to provide deeper pressure.

2.4 Role of castor oil in massage practices

Castor oil is significant in massage therapy due to its unique properties and benefits. Known for its thick, dense consistency and rich nutrient profile, castor oil is an excellent carrier oil for massage, enhancing the therapeutic effects of various massage techniques.

Lubrication and Glide

Castor oil's thick, oily texture provides excellent lubrication, allowing massage therapists to glide smoothly over the skin without causing friction. This is particularly beneficial in techniques requiring prolonged skin contact, such as deep tissue and Swedish massages. The oil's viscosity ensures that a small amount goes a long way, making it a cost-effective and efficient choice for long massage sessions. This practicality and resourcefulness make castor oil a valuable addition to any massage practice.

Deep Penetration and Moisturization

One of the standout features of castor oil is its ability to penetrate deeply into the skin and underlying tissues. This deep penetration allows for more effective delivery of therapeutic compounds, making it ideal for addressing muscle tension, pain, and inflammation. Additionally, castor oil is highly moisturizing, making it beneficial for dry or irritated skin. It helps to lock in moisture, leaving the skin feeling soft and hydrated after the massage.

Anti-inflammatory and Pain-relieving Properties

Castor oil contains ricinoleic acid, a fatty acid with potent anti-inflammatory and analgesic properties. When used in massage therapy, castor oil can help reduce inflammation and relieve pain in conditions such as arthritis, muscle soreness, and joint pain. Its natural anti-inflammatory effects make it a valuable addition to therapeutic massages to manage chronic pain and inflammatory conditions.

Enhancing Aromatherapy

Castor oil is an excellent carrier oil for essential oils in aromatherapy massage. Its ability to blend well with essential oils ensures that the oils' therapeutic properties are effectively delivered to the body. For instance, combining castor oil with lavender or peppermint oil can enhance the calming and pain-relieving effects of the massage, providing a more holistic and integrated approach to healing. The unique properties of castor oil, such as its deep penetration and moisturizing effects, can amplify the benefits of aromatherapy, making it an invaluable addition to massage practices.

Improved Circulation and Detoxification

Castor oil in massage can help stimulate blood flow and lymphatic circulation. Improved circulation ensures that oxygen and nutrients are efficiently delivered to tissues, promoting healing and recovery. Additionally, the oil's ability to boost lymphatic drainage aids in detoxification, helping to remove toxins and reduce swelling and edema.

Castor oil's unique properties make it a highly effective and versatile choice in massage therapy. Its lubrication, deep penetration, anti-inflammatory effects, and ability to enhance aromatherapy make it an invaluable tool for massage therapists. Whether it's used for deep tissue massage to address chronic pain, or in aromatherapy massage to enhance relaxation, castor oil can provide more effective and holistic treatments, addressing various physical and emotional health concerns.

2.5 Compresses and packs

Compresses and packs are traditional therapeutic applications used to deliver heat, moisture, and medicinal substances to specific areas of the body. In aromatherapy and holistic medicine, compresses and packs are often used to address a variety of conditions such as pain, inflammation, and detoxification. Castor oil packs, in particular, have gained popularity for their deep penetrating properties and multiple health benefits.

Castor oil compresses and packs are made by soaking a piece of cloth in castor oil and applying it to the skin. This technique is effective for localized treatment, allowing the therapeutic properties of castor oil to penetrate deeply into the tissues. The heat applied to the compress or pack enhances the absorption and effectiveness of the oil.

2.6 Instructions for the preparation and use of castor oil compresses

2.6.1 Materials Needed

- Cold-pressed castor oil

- A piece of flannel or cotton cloth (preferably unbleached)

- Plastic wrap

- Heating pad or hot water bottle

- Towel

- Old clothing or sheets (to protect from oil stains)

2.6.2 Step-by-Step Instructions

<u>Prepare the Area</u>

Choose a comfortable, quiet place where you can relax while using the castor oil pack. Spread an old towel or sheet to protect the area from oil stains, as castor oil can be quite messy.

<u>Soak the Cloth</u>

Cut the flannel or cotton cloth into a size that will adequately cover the area you want to treat. Typically, a piece about 12 inches by 18 inches works well for most applications.

Fold the cloth into three or four layers to increase its absorbency.

Pour enough castor oil over the cloth to saturate it, but not so much that it's dripping. You can do this by placing the cloth in a glass dish or plastic bag and pouring the oil over it until it is fully soaked.

<u>Apply the Pack</u>

Place the oil-saturated cloth directly onto the area of concern. Common areas for castor oil packs include the abdomen (for digestive and reproductive issues), joints (for arthritis and inflammation), and the lower back (for pain and detoxification).

Cover the pack with a piece of plastic wrap to prevent the oil from leaking out and staining your clothes or bedding.

<u>Apply Heat</u>

Place a heating pad or hot water bottle over the plastic-covered pack. The heat will help to increase circulation, enhance the absorption of the castor oil, and improve the effectiveness of the treatment.

Adjust the heat to a comfortable level. It should be warm but not so hot that it causes discomfort or burns your skin.

2.6.3 Relax and Allow Absorption

Relax in a comfortable position and allow the castor oil pack to work for 45-60 minutes. During this time, you can read, meditate, listen to music, or simply rest.

To maximize the therapeutic benefits, some people prefer to use the castor oil pack overnight. If you choose to do this, be sure to secure the pack well and protect your bedding with additional layers of towels or old sheets.

2.6.4 Clean Up

After the treatment, carefully remove the pack and wipe the area with a clean towel or cloth to remove any residual oil. You can also use a mixture of baking soda and water to help remove the oil from your skin.

Store the oil-soaked cloth in a plastic bag or glass container for future use. The same cloth can be reused several times, typically for a few weeks, before needing to be replaced. Simply add a little more castor oil to the cloth as needed.

2.6.5 Frequency of Use

For best results, use the castor oil pack three to four times per week. Consistent use over several weeks is often necessary to see significant benefits.

2.6.6 Benefits of Castor Oil Packs

Castor oil packs are renowned for their numerous health benefits. Some of the primary benefits include.

Pain Relief

Castor oil packs can help alleviate pain and discomfort from conditions such as arthritis, muscle soreness, and joint pain. The anti-inflammatory properties of castor oil, combined with the soothing heat from the pack, provide effective pain relief.

Detoxification

Castor oil packs stimulate the lymphatic system and enhance liver function, promoting the elimination of toxins from the body. This detoxifying effect can improve overall health and boost the immune system.

Digestive Health

Applying castor oil packs to the abdomen can help improve digestion, reduce bloating, and alleviate constipation. The packs can also support reproductive health by reducing menstrual cramps and improving circulation to the pelvic region.

Skin Health

Castor oil's moisturizing and healing properties make it beneficial for various skin conditions. Using castor oil packs can help soothe dry, irritated skin, reduce inflammation, and promote healing of wounds and scars.

Castor oil packs are a simple yet powerful tool in holistic health practices. Their ability to penetrate deeply into the tissues, combined with their anti-inflammatory and detoxifying properties, makes them effective for a wide range of health issues. Regular use of castor oil packs can lead to improved physical well-being and enhanced overall health.

2.7 Therapeutic indications and benefits

Castor oil has numerous therapeutic indications and benefits, making it versatile and valuable in holistic health practices. From traditional medicinal uses to modern aromatherapy and natural health care applications, castor oil offers a range of benefits for physical, emotional, and even spiritual well-being.

2.7.1 Anti-inflammatory Properties

One of the primary therapeutic benefits of castor oil is its potent anti-inflammatory properties. This is mainly due to its high ricinoleic acid content, a monounsaturated fatty acid known for its anti-inflammatory effects. When applied topically or used in packs, castor oil can help reduce inflammation and alleviate pain associated with arthritis, muscle strains, and joint pain. Its ability to penetrate deeply into tissues enhances its effectiveness in targeting inflammation at the source.

2.7.2 Pain Relief

Castor oil is also valued for its analgesic properties, contributing to its pain relief effectiveness. Castor oil helps to soothe pain and discomfort, whether applied directly to sore muscles or in massage therapy. This makes it beneficial for individuals seeking natural alternatives to conventional pain medications.

2.7.3 Skin Care

Castor oil is widely used in skin care due to its moisturizing, nourishing, and healing properties. It helps to hydrate the skin, improve elasticity, and reduce the appearance of wrinkles and fine lines. Castor oil also treats various skin conditions such as acne, dermatitis, eczema, and psoriasis. Its antimicrobial properties further support skin health by preventing bacterial overgrowth and infections.

2.7.4 Digestive Health

Castor oil has traditionally been used internally to promote digestive health and relieve constipation. It acts as a mild laxative, stimulating bowel movements and aiding in the elimination of toxins from the body. However, due to its potent effects, internal use of castor oil should be done cautiously and under the guidance of a healthcare professional.

2.7.5 Hair and Scalp Care

Castor oil is a popular remedy for promoting hair growth and maintaining scalp health. It nourishes the hair follicles, strengthens the hair shaft, and prevents split ends and breakage. Massaging castor oil into the scalp improves circulation and stimulates hair growth. Regular use of castor oil can lead to thicker, healthier hair and a revitalized scalp.

2.7.6 Immune System Support

Castor oil's antimicrobial and antifungal properties contribute to its ability to support the immune system. Castor oil helps the body maintain optimal immune function by reducing microbial growth and fighting infections. This is particularly beneficial during cold and flu season or when dealing with minor infections.

2.7.7 Detoxification

Castor oil packs are often used as a detoxification tool to support liver function and enhance lymphatic drainage. The packs help remove toxins from the body, improving overall detoxification pathways. Regular castor oil packs can aid in cleansing the body and promoting systemic health.

2.8 Inhalation and diffusion

Essential oil inhalation and diffusion are integral practices in aromatherapy, harnessing the therapeutic benefits of aromatic compounds for physical, emotional, and mental well-being. Essential oils are highly concentrated plant extracts that capture the essence and fragrance of plants. When inhaled or diffused, these aromatic molecules interact with the olfactory system and can have profound effects on the body and mind.

Direct Inhalation

Direct inhalation involves breathing in essential oils directly from the bottle or a few drops on a tissue. This method allows quick absorption of the aromatic compounds into the bloodstream through the lungs. Direct inhalation benefits respiratory conditions, emotional support, and enhancing mental clarity and focus.

Diffusion

Diffusion disperses essential oils into the air using devices such as diffusers, nebulizers, or humidifiers. These devices break down essential oils into microscopic particles suspended in the air, creating a therapeutic atmosphere throughout a room or space. Diffusion is a popular method for continuously enjoying critical oils' aromatic and therapeutic benefits.

Respiratory Health

Many essential oils, such as eucalyptus, peppermint, and tea tree, have decongestant, expectorant, and antimicrobial properties that support respiratory health. Inhalation of these oils can help clear nasal passages, reduce congestion, and relieve symptoms of colds, flu, sinusitis, and allergies. Diffusing essential oils in the home or workplace can create a supportive environment for respiratory wellness.

Emotional and Mental Well-being

Aromatherapy is widely used to promote emotional balance, reduce stress, and uplift mood. Essential oils like lavender, bergamot, and frankincense are renowned for their calming and anxiety-relieving effects. Inhalation of these oils triggers the limbic system in the brain, which regulates emotions and memories, promoting relaxation and emotional well-being.

Cognitive Function

Certain essential oils, such as rosemary, lemon, and peppermint, are known for their stimulating and cognitive-enhancing effects. Inhalation of these oils can improve concentration, memory retention, and mental clarity. Diffusing these oils in study or workspaces can enhance focus and productivity.

Antimicrobial and Air Purification

Essential oils with antimicrobial properties, such as tea tree, cinnamon, and thyme, can purify the air and reduce airborne pathogens. Diffusing these oils can help create a cleaner and healthier indoor environment, particularly during increased illness or high-traffic areas.

Inhalation and diffusion of essential oils offer versatile and effective ways to experience their therapeutic benefits. Integrating aromatherapy into daily routines can promote overall wellness and enhance quality of life, whether for respiratory health, emotional well-being, cognitive function, or air purification. Combining the therapeutic indications of castor oil with the aromatic benefits of essential oils provides a holistic approach to health and healing, supporting the body, mind, and spirit.

2.9 Use of castor oil in aromatherapy diffusers

Aromatherapy diffusers are popular devices that disperse essential oils into the air, creating a therapeutic atmosphere that can benefit physical, emotional, and mental well-being. While castor oil itself is not typically used in diffusers due to its thick consistency, it can serve as a valuable carrier oil for blending with essential oils to enhance their aromatic and therapeutic effects.

Blending with Essential Oils

Castor oil's role in aromatherapy diffusers primarily involves serving as a carrier for essential oils. Due to its viscosity and texture, castor oil is ideal for diluting and carrying more volatile essential oils, allowing them to be safely dispersed in the air. Castor oil helps slow their evaporation rate and extends their aromatic presence in the air when blended with essential oils.

Enhancing Aromatic Experience

Essential oils are highly concentrated plant extracts that contain aromatic compounds known as volatile organic compounds (VOCs). These compounds evaporate quickly when air exposure, releasing their characteristic scents and therapeutic properties. By blending essential oils with castor oil, individuals can create unique aromatic blends that offer prolonged diffusion in the room. This enhances the overall aromatic experience and allows for sustained exposure to the therapeutic benefits of the essential oils.

Aromatic Profiles

Castor oil has a slightly nutty aroma that blends well with many essential oils. When selecting essential oils to blend with castor oil for diffuser use, consider the aromatic profile and the desired therapeutic properties. For example:

Relaxation and Sleep

Lavender, chamomile, and sandalwood essential oils are renowned for their calming and soothing effects. Blending these oils with castor oil in a diffuser creates a relaxing ambiance that promotes relaxation and supports restful sleep.

Mental Clarity and Focus

Essential oils such as peppermint, rosemary, and lemon are known for their stimulating and cognitive-enhancing properties. When diffused with castor oil, these oils can help improve concentration, mental clarity, and productivity.

Respiratory Support

Eucalyptus, tea tree, and pine essential oils have decongestant, expectorant, and antimicrobial properties that support respiratory health. Diffusing these oils with castor oil can help clear nasal passages, reduce congestion, and ease symptoms of respiratory conditions like colds and allergies.

Choose Your Essential Oils

Select two or three essential oils that complement each other regarding aroma and therapeutic benefits.

Prepare the Blend

Mix 10-15 drops of essential oils in a small glass bottle or container with 1-2 tablespoons of castor oil. Adjust the ratio based on the desired strength of the aroma.

Blend Thoroughly

Stir or shake the mixture well to ensure the essential oils are evenly distributed in the castor oil.

Use in the Diffuser

Add 5-10 drops of the blended oil mixture into your aromatherapy diffuser, following the manufacturer's water levels and settings instructions.

Enjoy

Turn on the diffuser and allow the aromatic blend to disperse into the air. Enjoy the therapeutic benefits of the essential oils and the extended diffusion provided by the castor oil.

2.10 Mixing essential oils for respiratory and emotional benefits

Blending castor oil with essential oils for respiratory and emotional benefits can create potent synergies that support overall well-being. Whether used in massage oils, bath blends, or aromatherapy diffusers, these blends harness castor oil's and essential oils' therapeutic properties to address a wide range of specific health concerns, reassuring individuals about the effectiveness of these holistic healing solutions.

Respiratory Benefits. Respiratory issues such as congestion, sinusitis, and seasonal allergies can be effectively managed with the right blend of essential oils and castor oil. Essential oils like eucalyptus, peppermint, and tea tree have decongestant, expectorant, and antimicrobial properties that help clear airways, reduce inflammation, and fight respiratory infections. When blended with castor oil for topical application or diffusion, these oils provide targeted relief and support respiratory health.

Emotional Benefits. Essential oils play a crucial role in aromatherapy for emotional well-being, offering natural remedies for stress, anxiety, depression, and mood swings. When inhaled or applied topically, oils such as lavender, bergamot, and frankincense have calming, uplifting, and mood-stabilizing effects. By blending these oils with castor oil, individuals can create their own personalized blends, empowering them to take control of their emotional balance, reduce tension, and enhance overall mental health.

Balancing Blends. When blending essential oils with castor oil for respiratory and emotional benefits, consider the following combinations:

Calming Blend. Combine lavender, chamomile, and ylang-ylang essential oils with castor oil to create a soothing blend that promotes relaxation and reduces stress.

Energizing Blend. Blend peppermint, rosemary, and lemon essential oils with castor oil to create a refreshing blend that boosts energy levels, improves focus, and enhances mental clarity.

Respiratory Support Blend. Mix eucalyptus, tea tree, and pine essential oils with castor oil for a respiratory support blend that clears congestion, strengthens the immune system, and promotes easier breathing.

2.10.1 Application Methods

Topical Application

Dilute the essential oil blend with castor oil and apply it directly to the chest, back, or throat area for respiratory support. Massage gently into the skin to enhance absorption and effectiveness.

Aromatherapy Diffusion

Add the blended oil mixture into an aromatherapy diffuser and diffuse it throughout the room to enjoy respiratory benefits and emotional support. This method allows for continuous inhalation of the aromatic compounds.

Bath Blend

Add a few drops of the blended oil mixture to a warm bath and Epsom salts or bath gel for a relaxing and therapeutic soak. The bath steam helps release the essential oil vapors, promoting respiratory health and emotional relaxation.

Blending essential oils with castor oil enhances their therapeutic benefits and extends their aromatic presence when used in aromatherapy diffusers. Whether for respiratory support, emotional balance, or overall well-being, these blends offer natural and effective solutions, instilling confidence in individuals about their choice of holistic healing. By incorporating these blends into daily routines, individuals can harness the power of aromatherapy to support holistic healing and enhance quality of life.

Chapter 3: Supplement castor oil with essential oils

3.1 Principles of mixing castor oil with essential oils

Blending castor oil with essential oils involves art and science, requiring understanding each oil's properties, aromas, and therapeutic benefits. Mastering blending techniques ensures effective synergy and optimal results, whether creating blends for massage oils, bath products, or aromatherapy diffusers.

Essential oils are highly concentrated plant extracts derived from various parts of plants, including flowers, leaves, stems, and roots. Each essential oil possesses unique aromatic profiles and therapeutic properties due to its complex chemical composition. Understanding these properties is crucial when blending with castor oil:

3.1.1 Aromatic Profile

Essential oils vary widely in aroma, ranging from floral and citrusy to earthy and spicy. Some oils are more potent than others, requiring careful consideration of their intensity when blending. For example, lavender and chamomile offer calming scents for relaxation blends, while peppermint and eucalyptus provide invigorating notes for respiratory blends.

3.1.2 Therapeutic Benefits

Each essential oil offers distinct therapeutic benefits, such as anti-inflammatory, antimicrobial, or calming effects. Combining oils with complementary properties enhances their overall efficacy. For instance, blending tea tree oil's antimicrobial properties with lavender's soothing effects can create a potent skin-care blend.

3.1.3 Chemical Composition

Essential oils contain bioactive compounds like terpenes, phenols, and esters, determining their therapeutic actions. When blending, consider how these compounds interact to achieve desired outcomes. Some oils may synergize to amplify their effects, while others may counteract or balance each other.

3.1.4 Carrier Oil Dilution

Castor oil, known for its thick consistency, serves as an ideal carrier oil for diluting essential oils. Typically, essential oils are diluted in castor oil at 1-5% concentration, depending on the application. For example, a 1% dilution equates to 1 drop of essential oil per teaspoon (5 mL) of castor oil, suitable for facial serums or sensitive skin blends. A 5% dilution, on the other hand, allows for more potent formulations for body massage or therapeutic purposes.

3.1.5 Scent Harmony

Balancing aromas ensures a pleasant and harmonious blend that appeals to personal preferences and therapeutic goals. Start by selecting a base note (e.g., cedarwood), middle note (e.g., lavender), and top note (e.g., citrus) to create a well-rounded fragrance profile. Experiment with different combinations to achieve desired aromatic effects.

3.1.6 Targeted Formulations

Tailor blends to address specific concerns, such as skin conditions, respiratory issues, or emotional well-being. For example, a rosemary, peppermint, and castor oil blend supports scalp health and hair growth. In contrast, blending bergamot, ylang-ylang, and castor oil promotes relaxation and stress relief.

3.1.7 Layering Techniques

Layering involves adding essential oils in sequence to achieve depth and complexity in fragrance. Start with a base note, followed by middle and top notes, allowing each oil to harmonize before adding the next. This method creates a balanced blend with a lasting aroma profile.

3.1.8 Practical Application in Aromatherapy

In aromatherapy, blending castor oil with essential oils maximizes therapeutic benefits through various applications.

Massage Oils

Combine castor oil with essential oils like lavender and chamomile for soothing massages that promote relaxation and alleviate muscle tension.

Bath Blends

Add a few drops of blended oils to bath water or bath salts for a luxurious soak that enhances skin hydration and provides aromatherapeutic benefits.

Diffuser Blends

Create personalized diffuser blends by mixing castor oil with essential oils such as lemon, eucalyptus, and tea tree for respiratory support or bergamot, frankincense, and sandalwood for emotional balance.

Mastering blending techniques and principles allows for creative expression in aromatherapy while harnessing castor oil's and essential oils' natural healing properties. Whether crafting blends for personal use or professional practice, understanding these fundamentals ensures safe, effective, and enjoyable aromatherapy experiences.

3.2 Recommended ratios and formulations

Creating effective castor oil blends with essential oils requires careful consideration of ratios and formulations to achieve desired therapeutic outcomes while ensuring safety and efficacy. The following recommendations serve as guidelines for blending castor oil with essential oils for various applications:

3.2.1 Dilution Ratios

For Facial and Sensitive Skin, a gentle formulation is key. A lower dilution of 1% to 2%, which equates to 1-2 drops of essential oil per teaspoon (5 mL) of castor oil, is ideal. This formulation is not only suitable for facial serums and spot treatments but also for individuals with sensitive skin, providing a gentle and effective solution.

For a versatile blend that offers therapeutic benefits, opt for a moderate dilution of 2% to 5%. This equates to 2-5 drops of essential oil per teaspoon (5 mL) of castor oil. This concentration is perfect for muscle relaxation, pain relief, and skin nourishment during massage sessions, showcasing the blend's versatility.

For localized treatments or acute conditions, such as joint pain, inflammation, or skin ailments, increase the dilution to 5% to 10%. To enhance effectiveness without compromising safety, use 5-10 drops of essential oil per teaspoon (5 mL) of castor oil.

3.2.2 Formulations Based on Application: Versatile and Effective

For conditions like acne, eczema, or dry skin, blend castor oil with essential oils like lavender, tea tree, and geranium. These formulations cleanse, moisturize, and rejuvenate the skin while addressing specific concerns.

Hair Care. Combine castor oil with rosemary, peppermint, and jojoba oil for scalp health and hair growth. This blend stimulates circulation, strengthens hair follicles, and promotes thicker, healthier hair growth.

Respiratory Support. Create diffuser blends with castor oil and essential oils such as eucalyptus, peppermint, and lemon to clear nasal passages, reduce congestion, and support respiratory health.

Emotional Well-being. Develop blends with castor oil and calming essential oils like chamomile, bergamot, and frankincense for stress relief, relaxation, and emotional balance. These blends are designed to provide you with a sense of comfort and peace.

3.3 Synergistic Effects

Synergistic effects occur when two or more substances work together to produce a greater combined effect than the sum of their individual effects. When blending castor oil with essential oils, synergies can enhance therapeutic benefits and optimize holistic healing approaches:

1. Enhanced Absorption: Castor oil acts as a carrier oil, enhancing the absorption of essential oils into the skin or respiratory system. This increases the bioavailability of active compounds, facilitating quicker and more effective therapeutic outcomes.

2. Complementary Actions: Essential oils possess diverse therapeutic properties that complement each other when blended with castor oil. For example, pairing anti-inflammatory oils like lavender and chamomile with analgesic oils such as peppermint and ginger creates a synergistic blend for pain relief and muscle relaxation.

3. Balanced Formulations: By blending oils with varying properties, such as antibacterial, antiviral, and immune-stimulating effects, synergies strengthen overall formulations. For instance, combining tea tree oil's antimicrobial properties with citrus oils' immune-boosting effects supports both skin health and immune system function.

4. Holistic Benefits: Synergistic blends of castor oil and essential oils offer holistic benefits that address multiple aspects of health and well-being. Whether promoting physical healing, emotional balance, or mental clarity, these synergies align with the principles of integrative medicine and natural health care.

Understanding recommended ratios and formulations for blending castor oil with essential oils ensures safe and effective use in various applications, from skin and hair care to respiratory support and emotional well-being. Harnessing synergistic effects through thoughtful blending enhances therapeutic outcomes, promoting holistic health and vitality. Whether crafting blends for personal use or professional practice, these principles guide the creation of customized aromatherapy formulations that support overall wellness and enhance quality of life.

3.4 How castor oil enhances the effectiveness of essential oils

Castor oil serves as a valuable carrier oil in aromatherapy, enhancing the effectiveness of essential oils through various mechanisms that optimize their therapeutic benefits. Here's how castor oil contributes to and amplifies the efficacy of essential oils.

Castor oil has a unique molecular structure allows it to penetrate deeply into the skin or mucous membranes. When combined with volatile essential oils, which evaporate quickly, castor oil acts as a carrier that slows down evaporation and facilitates better absorption of essential oil constituents into the body. This ensures a more sustained release of active compounds, prolonging their therapeutic effects.

Essential oils contain bioactive molecules such as terpenes, phenols, and esters, providing therapeutic benefits. Castor oil helps these compounds penetrate the skin's barrier more effectively, increasing their bioavailability and allowing them to exert their effects at a cellular level. This enhances essential oils' overall potency and efficiency in addressing various health concerns.

Castor oil's emollient and moisturizing properties help strengthen the skin's natural barrier function. By creating a protective layer on the skin, castor oil prevents moisture loss and improves the absorption of essential oils without causing irritation or sensitivity. This makes it suitable for individuals with sensitive or dry skin who may benefit from the soothing effects of essential oils.

Essential oils are prized for their aromatic qualities, which can positively impact mood, emotions, and cognitive function. Essential oils remain volatile and fragrant for longer periods when blended with castor oil in diffusers or topical applications. Castor oil's viscosity slows the evaporation rate of essential oils, ensuring a sustained release of fragrant molecules into the air or skin. This allows individuals to enjoy prolonged aromatherapeutic benefits throughout the day or during specific treatments.

Castor oil enhances the synergistic effects of essential oil blends by providing a stable base that harmonizes the aromatic profiles and therapeutic properties of different oils. Whether creating blends for massage oils, bath products, or treatments, castor oil is a unifying element that balances and enhances the overall formulation. This synergy promotes holistic healing and supports comprehensive approaches to health and well-being.

Due to its versatile nature, castor oil can be used in various applications alongside essential oils. From skincare routines and hair treatments to respiratory support and emotional wellness practices, castor oil enriches the efficacy and versatility of essential oil therapies. Its compatibility with different oils and ability to adapt to diverse therapeutic needs make castor oil a valuable asset in holistic health practices.

Castor oil's role as a carrier oil complements the therapeutic properties of essential oils by improving absorption, enhancing bioavailability, prolonging aromatic presence, supporting skin barrier function, and promoting synergistic formulations. Whether used alone or in combination with essential oils, castor oil contributes to the effectiveness of aromatherapy treatments, enriching the overall experience and promoting optimal health outcomes.

3.5 Personalization of aromatherapy treatments

Aromatherapy offers a personalized approach to health and well-being by harnessing the therapeutic properties of essential oils. Customizing aromatherapy treatments involves tailoring blends and applications to address individual needs, preferences, and health goals. Whether used for physical ailments, emotional support, or overall wellness, personalized aromatherapy treatments empower individuals to optimize their healing journey through holistic and natural practices.

Customizing aromatherapy treatments begins with thoroughly assessing the individual's health history, current symptoms, and wellness goals. Aromatherapists or healthcare practitioners conduct consultations to gather information about conditions, allergies, or sensitivities that may impact the choice of essential oils and application methods.

Identifying specific health concerns or objectives guides the selection of essential oils and formulation of treatment plans. Whether addressing chronic pain, stress management, skin conditions, respiratory issues, or emotional well-being, understanding the primary concerns allows for targeted and effective aromatherapy interventions.

Preferences in aroma, texture, and application methods are crucial in customizing aromatherapy treatments. Some individuals may prefer floral scents for relaxation, while others favor citrus or herbal aromas for energy and focus. Preferences also extend to the carrier oils used, such as castor oil for its moisturizing properties or jojoba oil for its similarity to skin sebum.

3.5.1 Tailoring Essential Oil Blends

Based on individual needs and preferences, aromatherapists choose essential oils known for their specific therapeutic properties. For example, lavender and chamomile are favored for their calming effects, while eucalyptus and peppermint are used for respiratory support. Each essential oil is selected not only for its aroma but also for its biochemical composition and targeted benefits.

Blending essential oils requires expertise in balancing aromas and therapeutic effects. Aromatherapists consider factors such as top, middle, and base notes to create well-rounded blends that deliver both immediate and prolonged benefits. Techniques like layering, where oils are added sequentially to build complexity, and dilution ratios ensure safe and effective formulations tailored to individual sensitivities and application methods.

Combining essential oils enhances synergistic effects, where oils work together to amplify therapeutic outcomes. For example, blending lavender with bergamot creates a harmonious blend that promotes relaxation and uplifts mood. Understanding the complementary actions of oils allows for strategic formulations that simultaneously address multiple aspects of well-being.

3.5.2 Application Methods

Customized blends are often applied topically through massage oils, lotions, or compresses. Diluting essential oils in carrier oils like castor oil ensures safe application and enhances absorption into the skin. Aromatherapists adjust concentrations based on skin type, sensitivity, and targeted therapeutic effects, ensuring optimal efficacy without irritation.

Essential oils are inhaled via diffusers, dispersing aromatic molecules into the air and offering respiratory benefits and emotional support. Customized diffuser blends to cater to individual preferences in fragrance and therapeutic goals, creating calming atmospheres for relaxation, stimulating environments for focus, or supportive blends for respiratory health.

Adding essential oil blends to baths or foot soaks enhances relaxation, relieves muscle tension, and supports skin health. Combining oils with bath salts or carrier oils like castor oil facilitates dispersion in water, allowing for full-body absorption of aromatic compounds and therapeutic benefits.

3.5.3 Monitoring and Adjusting

Aromatherapists monitor client responses to treatments, adjusting blends and applications as needed to optimize effectiveness. Regular feedback ensures treatments remain aligned with evolving health goals and preferences, fostering a collaborative approach to holistic healing.

Personalizing aromatherapy treatments involves adhering to safety guidelines and precautions to prevent adverse reactions. Aromatherapists educate clients on proper dilution ratios, potential contraindications, and sensitivity tests to promote essential oils' safe and beneficial use.

Customizing aromatherapy treatments involves a holistic approach, considering individual needs, preferences, and health objectives. By tailoring essential oil blends, selecting appropriate application methods, and monitoring client responses, aromatherapists empower individuals to experience the therapeutic benefits of aromatherapy in a personalized and effective manner. This individualized approach promotes overall well-being, supports natural healing processes, and enhances quality of life through the art and science of aromatherapy.

Chapter 4: Sample recipes for various conditions

1) Sleep Aid Blend

Ingredients:

- 3 drops Lavender (Lavandula angustifolia)
- 2 drops Cedarwood (Juniperus virginiana)
- 1 drop Vetiver (Vetiveria zizanioides)
- 1 tablespoon Castor Oil (Ricinus communis)

Instructions:

1. Mix the essential oils with castor oil in a glass bottle.
2. Apply a small amount of the blend to the wrists, chest, or back of the neck before bedtime.
3. Alternatively, add a few drops to an aromatherapy diffuser to create a calming sleep environment.

Benefits: Lavender induces relaxation, cedarwood promotes tranquility, and vetiver enhances grounding, making this blend effective for promoting restful sleep and reducing insomnia.

2) Digestive Comfort Massage Oil

Ingredients:

- 3 drops Peppermint (Mentha × piperita)
- 2 drops Ginger (Zingiber officinale)
- 1 drop Roman Chamomile (Chamaemelum nobile)
- 1 tablespoon Castor Oil (Ricinus communis)

Instructions:

1. Combine the essential oils with castor oil in a glass bottle.
2. Massage the blend onto the abdomen in a clockwise direction to alleviate digestive discomfort and bloating.

3. Use as needed for digestive support after meals or during periods of discomfort.

Benefits: Peppermint and ginger oils aid digestion and reduce nausea, while roman chamomile soothes digestive spasms, promoting digestive comfort and overall gastrointestinal health.

3) Focus and Concentration Blend

Ingredients:

- 2 drops Rosemary (Rosmarinus officinalis)

- 2 drops Lemon (Citrus limon)

- 1 drop Basil (Ocimum basilicum)

- 1 tablespoon Castor Oil (Ricinus communis)

Instructions:

1. Mix the essential oils with castor oil in a glass bottle.

2. Apply a small amount to the temples, wrists, or chest to enhance mental clarity and concentration.

3. Use during study sessions, work tasks, or whenever improved focus is needed.

Benefits: Rosemary enhances cognitive function, lemon promotes alertness, and basil reduces mental fatigue, making this blend ideal for boosting productivity and mental clarity.

4) Allergy Relief Inhalation Blend

Ingredients:

- 2 drops Lavender (Lavandula angustifolia)

- 2 drops Peppermint (Mentha × piperita)

- 1 drop Eucalyptus (Eucalyptus globulus)

- 1 tablespoon Castor Oil (Ricinus communis)

Instructions:

1. Combine the essential oils with castor oil in a personal inhaler or diffuser.

2. Inhale deeply to alleviate allergy symptoms such as congestion and sinus pressure.

3. Use throughout the day as needed for ongoing relief during allergy season.

Benefits: Lavender and peppermint reduce inflammation, while eucalyptus opens airways and relieves respiratory congestion, providing natural relief from allergy symptoms.

5) Immune Support Roll-On Blend

Ingredients:

- 2 drops Tea Tree (Melaleuca alternifolia)
- 2 drops Lemon (Citrus limon)
- 1 drop Frankincense (Boswellia carterii)
- 1 tablespoon Castor Oil (Ricinus communis)

Instructions:

1. Mix the essential oils with castor oil in a roll-on bottle.
2. Apply to pulse points or lymphatic areas (wrists, neck, behind ears) to support immune function.
3. Use daily as a preventive measure during cold and flu season or when feeling run down.

Benefits: Tea tree and lemon oils boost immune response, while frankincense supports overall health and wellness, fortifying the body's natural defenses against illness.

6) Headache Relief Compress

Ingredients:

- 2 drops Peppermint (Mentha × piperita)
- 2 drops Lavender (Lavandula angustifolia)
- 1 drop Rosemary (Rosmarinus officinalis)
- 1 tablespoon Castor Oil (Ricinus communis)

Instructions:

1. Dilute the essential oils in a bowl of warm water with castor oil.
2. Soak a cloth in the mixture, wring out excess, and apply to the forehead or back of the neck.
3. Relax for 10-15 minutes while inhaling deeply to alleviate tension and headache symptoms.

Benefits: Peppermint relieves headaches and migraines, lavender calms the nervous system, and rosemary reduces tension, providing effective relief from headache discomfort.

7) Anti-inflammatory Joint Support Blend

Ingredients:

- 3 drops Ginger (Zingiber officinale)

- 2 drops Black Pepper (Piper nigrum)

- 1 drop Marjoram (Origanum majorana)

- 1 tablespoon Castor Oil (Ricinus communis)

Instructions:

1. Mix the essential oils with castor oil in a glass bottle.

2. Apply to affected joints and massage gently to reduce inflammation and relieve joint pain.

3. Use regularly for chronic conditions or as needed for acute flare-ups.

Benefits: Ginger and black pepper oils have anti-inflammatory properties, while marjoram soothes muscle tension, making this blend effective for arthritis pain and joint stiffness.

8) Hormonal Balance Roller Blend

Ingredients:

- 2 drops Clary Sage (Salvia sclarea)

- 2 drops Geranium (Pelargonium graveolens)

- 1 drop Ylang Ylang (Cananga odorata)

- 1 tablespoon Castor Oil (Ricinus communis)

Instructions:

1. Blend the essential oils with castor oil in a roller bottle.

2. Apply to the abdomen or lower back area to support hormonal balance and relieve menstrual discomfort.

3. Use daily during hormonal fluctuations or as part of a natural hormone support regimen.

Benefits: Clary sage regulates hormones, geranium balances emotions, and ylang ylang enhances mood, promoting overall hormonal health and well-being.

9) Scar Healing Serum

Ingredients:

- 2 drops Helichrysum (Helichrysum italicum)

- 2 drops Frankincense (Boswellia carterii)

- 1 drop Carrot Seed (Daucus carota)

- 1 tablespoon Castor Oil (Ricinus communis)

- 1 tablespoon Rosehip Seed Oil (Rosa rubiginosa)

Instructions:

1. Combine the essential oils with castor oil and rosehip seed oil in a dark glass bottle.

2. Apply a small amount to scars or stretch marks to promote skin regeneration and reduce discoloration.

3. Use daily as part of a skincare routine to improve the appearance of scars over time.

Benefits: Helichrysum and frankincense oils aid in cell regeneration, carrot seed oil supports skin elasticity, and rosehip seed oil hydrates and nourishes, making this blend effective for scar healing and skin rejuvenation.

10) Anti-Anxiety Room Spray

Ingredients:

- 3 drops Bergamot (Citrus bergamia)

- 2 drops Lavender (Lavandula angustifolia)

- 1 drop Cedarwood (Juniperus virginiana)

- 1 tablespoon Castor Oil (Ricinus communis)

- 2 tablespoons Witch Hazel (Hamamelis virginiana)

- 2 tablespoons Distilled Water

Instructions:

1. Mix the essential oils with castor oil in a spray bottle.

2. Add witch hazel and distilled water to the bottle, shake well to combine.

3. Use as a room spray to promote relaxation, reduce anxiety, and create a calming atmosphere.

Benefits: Bergamot and lavender oils reduce stress and anxiety, while cedarwood promotes emotional stability and relaxation, making this blend ideal for promoting a tranquil environment.

11) Skin Irritation Soothing Balm

Ingredients:

- 2 drops Chamomile (Chamaemelum nobile)

- 2 drops Lavender (Lavandula angustifolia)

- 1 drop Geranium (Pelargonium graveolens)

- 1 tablespoon Castor Oil (Ricinus communis)

- 1 tablespoon Coconut Oil (Cocos nucifera)

Instructions:

1. Blend the essential oils with castor oil and coconut oil in a small container.

2. Apply a small amount to irritated or inflamed skin to soothe irritation and promote healing.

3. Use as needed for eczema, insect bites, rashes, or sunburn relief.

Benefits: Chamomile and lavender oils calm inflammation, geranium balances skin, and coconut oil moisturizes and protects, providing effective relief for various skin irritations.

BOOK 10: Castor Oil in Home Remedies

Castor Oil in Home Remedies

Harnessing Nature's Power for Everyday Healing

By

Vincent Vega

Disclaimer notice

Please be aware that the information provided in this document is intended solely for educational and entertainment purposes. Every effort has been made to ensure the content is accurate, reliable, current, and complete.

However, no guarantees, either explicit or implicit, are made. Readers acknowledge that the author is not providing legal, financial, medical, or professional advice.

The content has been sourced from various references. It is strongly recommended that you consult a licensed professional before attempting any of the of the methods described in this document.

By reading this document, you agree that the author is not liable for any direct or indirect losses resulting from the use of the information within, including but not limited to errors, omissions, or inaccuracies.

Chapter 1: Castor oil in home remedies

1.1 Benefits and versatility of castor oil in home remedies

Castor oil, a time-honored remedy derived from the seeds of the Ricinus communis plant, has been revered for centuries for its therapeutic properties and wide-ranging applications in home remedies. Known for its rich composition of fatty acids, particularly ricinoleic acid, along with antioxidants and anti-inflammatory compounds, castor oil offers numerous benefits for both external and internal use.

1.1.1 Skincare Benefits

One of the most popular uses of castor oil is in skincare. Its emollient properties make it an excellent moisturizer for dry, rough skin. When applied topically, it penetrates deeply into the skin, hydrating and nourishing it without clogging pores. This makes it beneficial for conditions like eczema and psoriasis, relieving itching and inflammation. Castor oil is also effective in healing minor cuts, scrapes, and burns due to its antimicrobial properties, promoting faster wound healing.

1.1.2 Haircare Benefits

Castor oil is widely used to promote hair growth and improve hair health. It contains nutrients like vitamin E, omega-6 fatty acids, and proteins that nourish the hair follicles, stimulating growth and reducing hair loss. Regular application of castor oil to the scalp can also strengthen hair shafts, making them less prone to breakage. It is particularly beneficial for those suffering from dry, damaged hair or scalp conditions like dandruff, as it moisturizes the scalp and helps maintain its pH balance.

1.1.3 Digestive Health

Internally, castor oil is known for its powerful laxative effect, making it a popular remedy for relieving constipation. When ingested, it stimulates the smooth muscles of the intestines, promoting bowel movements. It is important to use castor oil internally cautiously and under medical supervision due to its potency. In addition to its laxative properties, castor oil supports digestive health by reducing inflammation in the gut and promoting regularity.

1.1.4 Pain Relief and Anti-inflammatory Properties

Castor oil is also valued for its analgesic and anti-inflammatory properties. When applied to sore muscles or joints, it can relieve pain and inflammation associated with arthritis or muscle strain. Its ability to penetrate deep into tissues helps relax muscles and reduce stiffness. Castor oil packs, which involve applying a cloth soaked in castor oil to the affected area, are a traditional remedy for pain relief and detoxification.

1.1.5 Immune System Support and Detoxification

Rich in antioxidants, castor oil supports overall immune function by scavenging free radicals and reducing oxidative stress. It is believed to enhance lymphatic circulation, which is crucial to immune system health and detoxification. Castor oil packs applied over the abdomen are thought to stimulate lymphatic drainage, aiding in removing toxins and waste products from the body. This detoxifying effect can contribute to improved overall health and vitality.

1.1.6 Practical Applications in Home Remedies

Beyond its medicinal uses, castor oil finds applications in various home remedies and natural health practices. It is used in oil pulling for oral health, where swishing a small amount of oil in the mouth helps remove bacteria and promote gum health. Due to its moisturizing and conditioning properties, castor oil is also incorporated into homemade beauty products like lip balms, moisturizers, and hair masks.

1.1.7 Environmental and Sustainability Considerations

From an environmental perspective, castor oil is derived from a renewable source—the castor bean plant—which grows in tropical and subtropical regions. It is biodegradable and has minimal environmental impact compared to synthetic chemicals often found in commercial skincare and haircare products. Individuals can reduce their ecological footprint and support sustainable practices by choosing castor oil for home remedies.

Castor oil's versatility and numerous health benefits make it a valuable addition to home remedies. Whether used for skincare, haircare, digestive health, pain relief, immune support, or detoxification, its natural composition and effectiveness have made it a staple in traditional medicine practices worldwide. Integrating castor oil into daily health and wellness routines offers a holistic approach to maintaining overall well-being and supporting natural healing processes, empowering individuals with a comprehensive health solution.

1.2 Importance of using natural remedies and sustainability

Recently, there has been a growing interest and preference for natural remedies like castor oil, driven by concerns over synthetic chemicals, environmental impact, and holistic health benefits. Understanding the importance of natural remedies and their sustainability is crucial in making informed choices for personal health and global well-being.

1.2.1 Holistic Approach to Health

Natural remedies, such as castor oil, offer a holistic approach to health and wellness by harnessing the healing properties of plants and natural substances. Unlike synthetic drugs that often target specific symptoms, natural remedies work synergistically with the body's natural processes, supporting overall health rather than just alleviating symptoms. This holistic approach considers the interconnectedness of physical, mental, and emotional well-being, promoting a balanced and sustainable approach to health maintenance.

1.2.2 Minimizing Exposure to Synthetic Chemicals

One primary reason for choosing natural remedies is to reduce exposure to synthetic chemicals found in many conventional medications and personal care products. Artificial chemicals, such as parabens, phthalates, and sulfates, are used as preservatives, fragrances, and cleansing agents in commercial products. Prolonged exposure to these chemicals has been linked to various health concerns, including hormone disruption, allergies, and environmental pollution. Natural remedies like castor oil offer a safer alternative without compromising efficacy.

1.2.3 Environmental Sustainability

The use of natural remedies contributes to environmental sustainability in several ways. First, plants used in natural remedies are often renewable resources that can be cultivated sustainably without depleting natural ecosystems. Castor oil, for example, is derived from the seeds of the castor bean plant (Ricinus communis), which grows in tropical and subtropical regions and requires minimal water and resources compared to synthetic alternatives.

Secondly, natural remedies tend to have a lower environmental impact throughout their lifecycle. They are biodegradable, meaning they break down naturally without accumulating in the environment or causing long-term harm to ecosystems. In contrast, synthetic chemicals used in pharmaceuticals and personal care products can persist in the environment for years, polluting waterways, soil degradation, and adverse effects on wildlife.

1.2.4 Supporting Local and Global Communities

Choosing natural remedies often supports local and global communities involved in sustainable agriculture and traditional medicine practices. Many natural remedies, including castor oil, are sourced from small-scale farmers and cooperatives in developing countries. By purchasing sustainably sourced castor oil and other natural products, consumers can contribute to fair trade practices, economic empowerment, and improved livelihoods for local communities.

1.2.5 Preserving Traditional Knowledge and Cultural Heritage

Natural remedies are often deeply rooted in traditional knowledge and cultural practices passed down through generations. Indigenous communities and traditional healers have long relied on plants and natural substances for their medicinal properties and therapeutic benefits. By embracing natural remedies like castor oil, individuals can help preserve traditional knowledge systems and cultural heritage, fostering respect for diverse healing traditions and promoting cultural sustainability.

1.2.6 Personal Empowerment and Wellness

Beyond environmental and community benefits, using natural remedies empowers individuals to take charge of their health and well-being. Natural remedies like castor oil are readily accessible and affordable and can be used safely for various health concerns, from skincare and haircare to digestive health and pain relief. They offer a proactive approach to self-care, promoting preventive health measures and reducing reliance on synthetic medications that may have adverse side effects.

The importance of using natural remedies like castor oil extends beyond personal health benefits to encompass environmental sustainability, community support, and cultural preservation. By choosing natural remedies, individuals contribute to a healthier planet and support ethical practices prioritizing human and ecological well-being. Embracing natural remedies is not just a trend but a commitment to a more sustainable and holistic approach to health and wellness for current and future generations.

Chapter 2: Common domestic uses of castor oil

2.1 Skin care remedies

Castor oil is renowned for its exceptional moisturizing, healing, and anti-inflammatory properties, making it a versatile and powerful ingredient in skincare routines. From hydrating dry skin to healing wounds, castor oil offers numerous benefits that promote healthy and radiant skin. Understanding its versatility empowers you to make informed choices for your skincare routine.

<u>Moisturizing and Nourishing Dry Skin</u>

One of the primary benefits of castor oil in skincare is its ability to deeply moisturize and nourish dry skin. Rich in fatty acids, particularly ricinoleic acid, castor oil penetrates the skin's layers, restoring moisture and preventing water loss. This makes it an excellent choice for individuals with dry or rough skin, providing long-lasting hydration without leaving a greasy residue. Regular application of castor oil can soften the skin, smooth rough patches, and improve overall skin texture.

<u>Healing Minor Cuts, Scrapes, and Burns</u>

Castor oil's antimicrobial and anti-inflammatory properties effectively treat minor cuts, scrapes, and burns in a natural and gentle way. When applied topically, it forms a protective barrier over the wound, shielding it from bacteria and environmental irritants while promoting healing. Its gentle nature makes it suitable for sensitive skin and minor injuries to children, offering a safe and secure natural alternative to conventional antiseptic creams.

<u>Treating Acne and Skin Inflammation</u>

Despite being an oil, castor oil can be beneficial for acne-prone skin. Its antibacterial and anti-inflammatory properties help reduce acne-causing bacteria and inflammation associated with breakouts. Castor oil's ability to regulate sebum production can also prevent clogged pores and reduce the formation of blackheads and whiteheads. Castor oil can promote clearer, healthier-looking skin without exacerbating acne when used as a cleanser or incorporated into skincare products like facial masks or spot treatments.

<u>Anti-aging Benefits and Wrinkle Reduction</u>

Castor oil is increasingly recognized for its anti-aging properties and ability to reduce the appearance of wrinkles and fine lines. Its rich composition of antioxidants, including vitamin E, helps neutralize free radicals that contribute to premature aging and skin damage. Regular application of castor oil stimulates collagen production, enhancing skin elasticity and firmness. This can diminish the visibility of wrinkles, crow's feet, and sagging skin, resulting in a more youthful and radiant complexion.

2.1.1 Using Castor Oil in Skincare

<u>Daily Moisturizer</u>

Apply a few drops of castor oil to cleansed skin as a moisturizer. Massage gently until absorbed, focusing on areas prone to dryness or fine lines.

<u>Healing Wounds</u>

For minor cuts or burns, cleanse the affected area, apply a thin layer of castor oil, and cover with a sterile bandage. Reapply as needed until the wound heals.

<u>Acne Treatment</u>

Mix castor oil with a carrier oil like jojoba or grapeseed oil for a lighter consistency. Apply to clean skin as a spot treatment or overnight mask to reduce inflammation and promote healing.

<u>Anti-aging Serum</u>

Create a homemade anti-aging serum by combining castor oil with rosehip seed oil and a few drops of essential oils like frankincense or rosemary. Apply nightly to clean skin to reduce wrinkles and improve skin elasticity.

While castor oil is generally safe for topical use, it may cause skin irritation or allergic reactions in some individuals, especially those with sensitive skin. It's advisable to perform a patch test extensively before using castor oil and discontinue use if irritation occurs. Avoid contact with eyes and mucous membranes. Pregnant women should consult with a healthcare provider before using castor oil topically.

Castor oil is a valuable natural remedy for achieving healthy, radiant skin. Whether used for moisturizing dry skin, healing wounds, treating acne, or reducing signs of aging, its versatile benefits make it a staple in skincare routines. By incorporating castor oil into daily skincare practices, individuals can nurture their skin's health naturally and effectively.

2.2 Hair care remedies

Castor oil has long been celebrated for its remarkable benefits in hair care, from promoting hair growth to nourishing the scalp and improving overall health. Derived from the seeds of the Ricinus communis plant, castor oil is rich in essential nutrients such as ricinoleic acid, omega-6 fatty acids, and vitamin E, all of which contribute to its effectiveness in enhancing hair quality.

Promoting Hair Growth and Thickness

One of the most well-known benefits of castor oil is its ability to promote hair growth and increase hair thickness. Ricinoleic acid, the primary fatty acid in castor oil, stimulates blood circulation to the scalp when applied topically. This increased blood flow delivers essential nutrients and oxygen to hair follicles, promoting hair growth and strengthening the roots. Regular massaging castor oil into the scalp can rejuvenate dormant hair follicles, encouraging the development of new hair strands and reducing hair thinning over time.

Conditioning Hair and Scalp

Castor oil is a potent natural conditioner that helps moisturize and hydrate hair strands and the scalp. Its thick consistency allows it to coat the hair shaft, sealing in moisture and preventing dryness and frizz. This moisturizing effect makes castor oil particularly beneficial for individuals with dry, damaged, or brittle hair. It softens the hair texture, making it more manageable and less prone to breakage.

Treating Dandruff and Scalp Conditions

Castor oil's antifungal and antibacterial properties make it effective in treating various scalp conditions, including dandruff and scalp infections. A dry, flaky scalp or fungal overgrowth often causes dandruff. Applying castor oil to the scalp can help balance scalp pH, reduce inflammation, and moisturize dry patches, alleviating dandruff symptoms. Its antimicrobial properties also help combat scalp infections, promoting a healthier scalp environment for optimal hair growth.

Enhancing Hair Health and Shine

Regular use of castor oil can significantly improve hair health and impart a natural shine. Vitamin E and omega-6 fatty acids in castor oil nourish the hair follicles and strengthen the hair shaft, reducing split ends and breakage. This results in smoother, silkier hair that reflects light more effectively, enhancing its overall appearance and vitality.

Using Castor Oil in Hair Care

1) Scalp Massage

Warm castor oil slightly and massage it into the scalp using circular motions. Leave it on for at least 30 minutes or overnight for deep penetration before shampooing. This stimulates blood circulation and promotes hair growth.

2) Hair Mask

Mix castor oil with coconut or olive oil to create a nourishing hair mask. Apply the mixture to damp hair, focusing on the ends. Cover with a shower cap and leave it on for 1-2 hours before shampooing. This intensive treatment helps condition and strengthen hair strands.

3) Leave-in Conditioner

For daily use, dilute castor oil with a lighter carrier oil like jojoba or argan oil. Apply a small amount to damp or dry hair, focusing on the ends to tame frizz and add shine without weighing down the hair.

4) Eyelash and Eyebrow Growth

Use a clean mascara wand or cotton swab to apply a small amount of castor oil to eyelashes and eyebrows. Leave it overnight to promote thicker, longer lashes and fuller eyebrows.

While castor oil is generally safe for hair and scalp use, individuals with sensitive skin may experience mild irritation or allergic reactions. It's advisable to perform a patch test before extensively applying castor oil and discontinue use if irritation occurs. Avoid contact with eyes and mucous membranes. Pregnant women should consult with a healthcare provider before using castor oil topically.

Castor oil is a versatile and effective natural remedy for maintaining healthy hair and scalp. Whether used to promote hair growth, condition strands, treat scalp conditions, or enhance hair shine, its nutrient-rich composition offers numerous benefits for all hair types. By incorporating castor oil into regular hair care routines, individuals can naturally achieve stronger, more vibrant hair and scalp health.

2.3 Digestive health remedies

Castor oil has been traditionally used as a natural remedy to support digestive health and relieve constipation. Derived from the seeds of the Ricinus communis plant, castor oil contains ricinoleic acid, a fatty acid known for its potent laxative effects. Castor oil can help alleviate constipation and promote overall digestive wellness when used appropriately and in moderation.

2.3.1 Relieving Constipation

One of the primary benefits of castor oil in digestive health is its ability to relieve constipation effectively. Castor oil works as a stimulant laxative, meaning it stimulates the muscles of the intestines to contract and move stool through the bowels. This action helps soften and lubricate the stool, making it easier to pass. It is particularly beneficial for occasional constipation or when other remedies are ineffective.

Castor oil is typically taken orally in small doses for constipation relief. The dosage varies depending on age and individual tolerance, but starting with a small amount (e.g., 1-2 teaspoons for adults) is generally recommended and increasing gradually if needed. It is crucial to follow dosage guidelines and consult with a healthcare provider, especially for children, pregnant women, or individuals with underlying health conditions.

2.3.2 Supporting Digestive Function

Beyond relieving constipation, castor oil supports overall digestive function by promoting regular bowel movements and intestinal motility. Regular use of castor oil can help maintain bowel regularity and prevent constipation from becoming a chronic issue. Its lubricating properties also contribute to smoother digestion and reduce discomfort associated with bowel movements.

2.3.3 Liver Detoxification and Gallbladder Health

Castor oil is believed to have detoxifying properties that support liver function and gallbladder health. The liver plays a crucial role in detoxification by filtering toxins and waste products from the bloodstream. Castor oil packs applied over the abdomen stimulate lymphatic circulation and enhance liver detoxification processes. This detoxifying effect may help improve overall digestive health and promote well-being.

2.3.4 Internal Anti-inflammatory Benefits

In addition to its digestive benefits, castor oil may have internal anti-inflammatory effects when taken orally. Ricinoleic acid, the active compound in castor oil, has been studied for its potential to reduce inflammation in the gastrointestinal tract. This can benefit individuals with inflammatory bowel conditions like Crohn's disease or ulcerative colitis, although further research is needed to validate these claims.

2.3.5 Using Castor Oil for Digestive Health

To relieve constipation, adults can take 1-2 teaspoons of castor oil orally on an empty stomach. Mixing it with a small amount of juice is advisable to mask the taste. It is best taken in the morning to allow time for bowel movements throughout the day. Ensure to follow dosage instructions carefully and avoid prolonged use to prevent dependency.

Castor oil packs can be applied externally over the abdomen for liver detoxification and digestive support. Soak a flannel cloth in castor oil, place it on the abdomen, and cover it with plastic wrap or a towel. Apply heat using a heating pad for 30-60 minutes. This method stimulates circulation, enhances detoxification, and supports digestive health.

While castor oil is generally considered safe for occasional use as a laxative, it should be used cautiously and under medical supervision, especially for prolonged or frequent use. Overuse of castor oil as a laxative can lead to dehydration, electrolyte imbalance, and dependency on laxatives. Pregnant women, breastfeeding mothers, and individuals with gastrointestinal disorders should consult with a healthcare provider before using castor oil internally.

Castor oil offers effective and natural remedies for promoting digestive health, relieving constipation, and supporting overall well-being. When used responsibly and in moderation, castor oil can be a valuable addition to digestive care routines, providing relief from discomfort and promoting digestive regularity naturally.

Chapter 3: Therapeutic uses of castor oil

3.1 Remedies for pain

Castor oil has been valued for its therapeutic properties in alleviating various types of pain, ranging from joint and muscle discomfort to menstrual cramps and inflammatory conditions. Derived from the seeds of the Ricinus communis plant, castor oil contains ricinoleic acid, a compound known for its anti-inflammatory and analgesic effects. These properties make castor oil a natural choice for pain relief and management.

3.1.1 Alleviating Joint and Muscle Pain

One of the primary uses of castor oil in pain relief is for alleviating joint and muscle pain. When massaged onto affected areas, castor oil penetrates deep into the tissues, reducing inflammation and promoting circulation. This can help relieve pain associated with arthritis, rheumatism, gout, and general muscle soreness. Regular application of castor oil may also improve joint flexibility and mobility over time.

To use castor oil for joint and muscle pain relief, warm the oil slightly and massage it into the affected area using gentle, circular motions. Cover the area with a warm cloth or apply heat using a heating pad to enhance the oil's absorption and therapeutic effects.

3.1.2 Easing Menstrual Cramps and PMS Symptoms

Castor oil is also effective in easing menstrual cramps and symptoms of premenstrual syndrome (PMS). Its anti-inflammatory properties help relax uterine muscles and reduce the intensity of menstrual cramps. Massaging the lower abdomen with castor oil during menstruation can relieve cramping and discomfort. Additionally, castor oil packs applied over the lower abdomen can help alleviate bloating and tension associated with PMS.

3.1.3 Soothing Arthritis and Rheumatic Conditions

Castor oil can relieve individuals suffering from arthritis and rheumatic conditions. Its anti-inflammatory properties help reduce joint swelling and stiffness, improving mobility and easing pain. Regular application of castor oil can complement other arthritis treatments, such as medications and physical therapy, by providing natural pain relief and promoting joint health.

3.1.4 Muscle Relaxation and Tension Relief

Castor oil's ability to penetrate deep into muscles effectively relieves tension and promotes muscle relaxation. Massaging castor oil into the affected areas can help relax muscles and reduce discomfort, whether for post-exercise soreness, tension headaches, or everyday muscle stiffness. Its calming properties can also promote relaxation and reduce stress, contributing to overall well-being.

3.1.5 Using Castor Oil for Pain Relief

1) Topical Application

Apply castor oil directly to the affected area for localized pain relief and massage gently until absorbed. Cover with a warm cloth or use a heating pad to enhance absorption and therapeutic effects.

2) Castor Oil Packs

Create a castor oil pack by soaking a flannel cloth in castor oil, placing it over the affected area, and covering it with plastic wrap or a towel. Apply heat using a heating pad for 30-60 minutes. This method enhances circulation, reduces inflammation, and provides deep pain relief. It's important to ensure that the cloth is saturated with castor oil but not dripping, and the plastic wrap or towel is used to prevent the oil from staining clothes or bedding.

3) Massage Oil Blend

Combine castor oil with essential oils known for their pain-relieving properties, such as peppermint, lavender, or eucalyptus oil. These essential oils can enhance the analgesic and anti-inflammatory effects of castor oil. Massage the blend onto sore muscles or joints for added therapeutic benefits. The combination of castor oil and these essential oils can provide a more comprehensive pain relief solution.

While castor oil is generally safe for topical use, some individuals may experience skin irritation or allergic reactions. It is advisable to extensively perform a patch test before using castor oil and discontinue use if irritation occurs. Avoid contact with eyes and mucous membranes. Pregnant women, breastfeeding mothers, and individuals with sensitive skin should consult with a healthcare provider before using castor oil for pain relief. Additionally, excessive use of castor oil can lead to diarrhea or other digestive issues, so it's important to use it in moderation.

Castor oil offers effective natural remedies for alleviating various types of pain, including joint and muscle discomfort, menstrual cramps, and inflammatory conditions. By harnessing its anti-inflammatory, analgesic, and muscle-relaxing properties, individuals can find relief from pain naturally and improve their overall quality of life. Incorporating castor oil into pain management routines provides a gentle yet effective alternative to conventional pain relief methods.

3.2 Detoxification remedies

Castor oil has been used for centuries as a natural remedy to support detoxification and cleanse the body from toxins. Derived from the seeds of the Ricinus communis plant, castor oil contains ricinoleic acid, a potent compound known for its detoxifying and anti-inflammatory properties. Castor oil can help stimulate detoxification pathways, support organ function, and promote overall health and well-being when used internally or externally.

3.2.1 Supporting Liver Detoxification

The liver is crucial in detoxifying the body by filtering toxins and waste products from the bloodstream. Castor oil is believed to support liver function and enhance detoxification processes. When applied externally as castor oil packs over the abdomen, it stimulates lymphatic circulation and improves blood flow to the liver. This can help increase the liver's efficiency in breaking down toxins and promoting their elimination from the body.

To create a castor oil pack for liver detoxification, soak a flannel cloth in castor oil, place it over the right side of the abdomen (where the liver is located), and cover it with plastic wrap or a towel. Apply gentle heat using a heating pad for 30-60 minutes. This method encourages the absorption of castor oil into the skin and underlying tissues, supporting liver health and detoxification.

3.2.2 Improving Digestive Function

Detoxification involves the liver and the digestive system, including the intestines and colon. Castor oil acts as a natural laxative when taken orally, stimulating bowel movements and promoting the elimination of waste and toxins from the colon. This cleansing effect helps relieve constipation and supports regular bowel movements, essential for overall detoxification and digestive health.

Adults can take 1-2 teaspoons of castor oil orally on an empty stomach to use castor oil for digestive detoxification. Mixing it with a small amount of juice is recommended to mask the taste. Ensure to follow dosage instructions carefully and avoid prolonged use to prevent dependency. Castor oil should be taken in the morning to allow time for bowel movements throughout the day.

3.2.3 Lymphatic System Support

The lymphatic system plays a crucial role in detoxification by transporting toxins and waste products away from tissues and toward lymph nodes for elimination. Castor oil packs applied over lymphatic drainage areas, such as the abdomen, can help stimulate lymphatic circulation and enhance detoxification. This method encourages the movement of lymphatic fluid, promoting the removal of toxins and metabolic waste from the body.

3.2.4 Anti-inflammatory Benefits

In addition to its detoxification properties, castor oil offers anti-inflammatory benefits that support overall health and well-being. Chronic inflammation is linked to various health conditions, including autoimmune disorders, cardiovascular disease, and digestive disorders. Castor oil reduces inflammation, supports the body's natural detoxification processes, and helps maintain a balanced inflammatory response.

3.2.5 Using Castor Oil for Detoxification

1) External Application

Create a castor oil pack by soaking a flannel cloth in castor oil, placing it over the abdomen or liver area, and covering it with plastic wrap or a towel. Apply gentle heat using a heating pad for 30-60 minutes. This method can be performed several times weekly to support detoxification and liver health.

2) Internal Consumption

Adults can take 1-2 teaspoons of castor oil orally on an empty stomach for digestive detoxification. To improve palatability, it is advisable to mix it with a small amount of juice. To prevent dependency, follow dosage instructions carefully and avoid prolonged use.

While castor oil is generally safe for short-term use as a laxative and external application, prolonged or excessive use may lead to dehydration, electrolyte imbalance, or dependency on laxatives. Castor oil detoxification under medical supervision is recommended, especially for pregnant women, breastfeeding mothers, and individuals with gastrointestinal disorders. Perform a patch test before extensively using castor oil on the skin to check for allergic reactions or sensitivities.

Chapter 4: Practical applications and recipes for home remedies

Castor oil is a versatile natural remedy that can be used in various ways to address common health concerns and promote well-being. From skincare and hair care to digestive health and pain relief, here are some practical applications and recipes for incorporating castor oil into your home remedies:

4.1 Skincare Applications

1) Moisturizing Face Serum

- Mix 1 tablespoon of castor oil with 1 tablespoon of argan oil and 5-10 drops of lavender essential oil.

- Apply a few drops to clean, damp skin every night before bed.

- This serum helps hydrate the skin, reduce fine lines, and improve overall skin texture.

2) Healing Balm for Dry Patches

- Combine equal parts of castor oil and shea butter.

- Add a few drops of tea tree essential oil for its antibacterial properties.

- Apply to dry patches or irritated skin as needed for soothing relief and hydration.

3) Anti-aging Eye Cream

- Mix 1 teaspoon of castor oil with 1 teaspoon of coconut oil and 1 teaspoon of vitamin E oil.

- Gently dab around the eyes to reduce puffiness, dark circles, and fine lines.

- Use nightly as part of your skincare routine.

4.2 Hair Care Recipes

1) Deep Conditioning Hair Mask

- Blend 2 tablespoons of castor oil with 1 tablespoon of coconut oil and 1 tablespoon of honey.

- Apply the mixture to damp hair, focusing on the ends.

- Cover with a shower cap and leave for 1-2 hours before shampooing.

- This mask helps nourish hair, reduce frizz, and promote healthy hair growth.

2) Scalp Treatment for Dandruff

- Mix equal parts of castor oil and jojoba oil.

- Add a few drops of tea tree essential oil for its anti-fungal properties.

- Massage into the scalp and leave on for 30 minutes to 1 hour before washing hair.

- Use weekly to help eliminate dandruff and soothe scalp irritation.

4.3 Digestive Health Remedies

1) Gentle Laxative Te

- Add 1 teaspoon of castor oil to a cup of herbal tea, such as chamomile or peppermint.

- Drink the tea on an empty stomach in the morning to promote bowel movements.

- Use occasionally for gentle relief from constipation.

2) Liver Detoxifying Castor Oil Pack:

- Soak a piece of flannel cloth in castor oil and place it over the right side of the abdomen (where the liver is located).

- Cover with plastic wrap or a towel and apply gentle heat using a heating pad for 30-60 minutes.

- Perform this detoxifying pack 2-3 times a week to support liver function and overall detoxification.

4.4 Pain Relief Applications

1) Muscle and Joint Pain Relief Salve

- Melt 2 tablespoons of beeswax in a double boiler.

- Stir in 1/2 cup of castor oil and 1/4 cup of coconut oil until well combined.

- Add 20 drops of peppermint essential oil and 10 drops of eucalyptus essential oil.

- Pour into a glass jar and allow to cool and solidify.

- Massage onto sore muscles and joints as needed for pain relief and relaxation.

2) Menstrual Cramp Relief Massage Oil

- Combine 2 tablespoons of castor oil with 1 tablespoon of almond oil.

- Add 5 drops of clary sage essential oil and 3 drops of lavender essential oil.

- Massage gently onto the lower abdomen during menstruation to help ease cramps and discomfort.

4.5 General Applications

1) Immune-Boosting Chest Rub

- Mix 1/4 cup of castor oil with 10 drops of eucalyptus essential oil and 5 drops of tea tree essential oil.

- Rub onto the chest and upper back to relieve congestion and support respiratory health during colds or flu.

2) Stress-Relieving Body Massage Oil

- Combine 1/2 cup of castor oil with 1/4 cup of sweet almond oil.

- Add 10 drops of lavender essential oil and 5 drops of chamomile essential oil.

- Use for a relaxing full-body massage to reduce stress, tension, and promote relaxation.

Perform a patch test before using any new recipe extensively, especially if you have sensitive skin or allergies.

Use castor oil in moderation and follow recommended dosages for internal use to avoid potential side effects such as digestive discomfort.

Consult with a healthcare professional, especially if pregnant, breastfeeding, or have pre-existing medical conditions before using castor oil internally or externally.

These practical applications and recipes demonstrate the versatility and effectiveness of castor oil in home remedies. Whether addressing skincare concerns, promoting hair health, supporting digestive function, relieving pain, or enhancing overall well-being, castor oil offers natural solutions that can be easily incorporated into daily self-care routines. Experiment with these recipes to discover the benefits of castor oil for yourself and enjoy its therapeutic properties.

4.6 Home remedies for children and pets

Castor oil, known for its natural healing properties, can be used safely for various home remedies for both children and pets. Whether addressing minor skin issues, digestive discomfort, or promoting overall wellness, castor oil offers gentle yet effective solutions.

4.6.1 For Children

1) Soothing Diaper Rash Cream

- Mix 1 tablespoon of castor oil with 1 tablespoon of coconut oil and 1 tablespoon of shea butter.

- Add a few drops of lavender essential oil for its calming effects.

- Apply a thin layer to clean, dry skin during diaper changes to soothe and protect against diaper rash.

2) Gentle Constipation Relief

- Mix 1 teaspoon of castor oil into a glass of warm milk or juice (for older children).

- Give once daily as needed to relieve constipation. Start with a lower dosage and adjust as necessary based on the child's age and response.

3) Earache Relief Compress

- Warm a small amount of castor oil and soak a cotton ball or cloth in it.

- Gently place the warm compress over the affected ear for soothing relief from earaches.

- Ensure the oil is comfortably warm and not hot to avoid burns.

4.6.2 For Pets

1) Healing Paw Balm:

- Mix equal parts of castor oil and coconut oil.

- Add a few drops of lavender or chamomile essential oil (ensure pet-safe oils).

- Apply a small amount to dry or cracked paw pads to soothe and moisturize. This is especially beneficial for pets exposed to harsh weather conditions.

2) Fur and Skin Conditioner:

- Add a teaspoon of castor oil to your pet's shampoo or dilute it with water for a final rinse.

- Massage into fur and skin to help alleviate dryness and itchiness. Rinse thoroughly and dry your pet well after bathing.

3) Digestive Support for Pets:

- Mix a small amount of castor oil into your pet's food or water, following veterinary advice for appropriate dosage.

- This can help promote regular bowel movements and support digestive health, particularly for pets experiencing occasional constipation.

Use castor oil externally for children and avoid oral administration without consulting a pediatrician. Perform a patch test before applying to sensitive skin areas.

Use castor oil cautiously for pets, especially cats, as they may be more sensitive to certain oils. Always use pet-safe essential oils and consult a veterinarian before administering internally.

Castor oil provides versatile and gentle home remedies for addressing common issues in both children and pets. By leveraging its natural healing properties, you can safely incorporate castor oil into your family's and pet's wellness routines, promoting comfort, health, and well-being naturally. As with any home remedy, it's essential to start with small amounts and monitor the response to ensure safety and effectiveness for your little ones and furry friends alike.

Conclusion

As we conclude this comprehensive exploration of castor oil, it's crucial to recognize the empowering journey we've shared through these ten volumes. Each book meticulously unveiled castor oil's rich history, versatile applications, and profound benefits, demonstrating its pivotal role in natural and holistic healing. What started as a quest for natural health solutions has evolved into a comprehensive guide, equipping you with knowledge, tools, and practical applications to take charge of your well-being.

Throughout this collection, we've delved deep into the multifaceted uses of castor oil. From skincare and hair care to digestive health and pain relief, castor oil has proven to be a remarkably versatile and effective remedy. We explored its historical significance, uncovering how ancient civilizations revered this oil for its healing properties and how modern science continues to validate these age-old practices. Understanding its chemical composition and therapeutic potential has highlighted how castor oil can seamlessly integrate into contemporary wellness routines.

One of the central themes running through these volumes is the profound importance of natural remedies in our modern lives. In a world increasingly dominated by synthetic products and quick fixes, turning to nature's bounty offers a return to simplicity, safety, and sustainability. Castor oil is a beacon of this philosophy, providing gentle yet powerful solutions for various health concerns. It bridges the gap between ancient wisdom and modern needs, offering a path to holistic well-being that is accessible and effective.

The arguments presented in this collection are not just theoretical; they are rooted in extensive research, practical experience, and time-tested traditions. Each recipe, application, and technique has been carefully selected to ensure it delivers tangible benefits. The strength of these arguments lies in their reliability—whether you seek to enhance your skincare regimen, improve your hair health, support your digestive system, alleviate pain, or explore the wonders of aromatherapy, castor oil emerges as a dependable ally.

This collection touches upon broader themes relevant to our overall approach to health and wellness. It emphasizes the importance of mindful living, the benefits of embracing natural and sustainable practices, and the empowering effect of taking control of our health. By incorporating castor oil into your daily routines, you are not just addressing specific ailments but fostering a holistic lifestyle that values balance, self-care, and connection to nature.

May you feel inspired to experiment, personalize, and fully integrate its benefits into your life. The knowledge contained within these pages is a testament to the enduring relevance of castor oil and the power of natural remedies.

Remember, the journey to wellness is ongoing. As you continue to explore and embrace the possibilities castor oil offers, you join a legacy of individuals who have trusted nature's gifts for their health and happiness. This collection is your gateway to a more natural, empowered, and healthier life. Thank you for embarking on this journey with me—may it enrich your life as profoundly as it has mine.

Made in the USA
Columbia, SC
29 July 2024